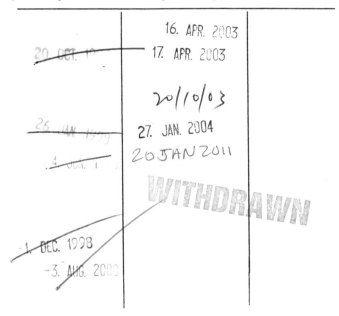
Christensen, A./Uzzell, B. P.

Brain Injury and Neuropsychological
Rehabilitation

**INSTITUTE
for RESEARCH
in BEHAVIORAL NEUROSCIENCE**

Jason W. Brown, Series Editor

BROWN

Agnosia and Apraxia: Selected Papers
of Liepmann, Lange, and Pötzl

BROWN

Neuropsychology of Visual Perception

CHRISTENSEN/UZZELL

Brain Injury and Neuropsychological Rehabilitation:
International Perspectives

GOLDBERG

Contemporary Neuropsychology
and the Legacy of Luria

PERECMAN

The Frontal Lobes Revisited

PERECMAN

Integrating Theory and Practice
in Clinical Neuropsychology

Brain Injury and Neuropsychological Rehabilitation:
International Perspectives

Edited by

ANNE-LISE CHRISTENSEN
Center for Rehabilitation of Brain Injury,
Copenhagen, Denmark

BARBARA P. UZZELL
Del Oro Institute for Rehabilitation,
Houston, Texas

LEA LAWRENCE ERLBAUM ASSOCIATES, PUBLISHERS
1994 Hillsdale, New Jersey   Hove, UK

Cover design by Kate Dusza

Lawrence Erlbaum Associates, Inc., Publishers
365 Broadway
Hillsdale, New Jersey, 07642

Library of Congress Cataloging-in-Publication Data

Brain injury and neuropsychological rehabilitation : International
  perspectives / edited by Anne-Lise Christensen, Barbara P. Uzzell.
      p.   cm.
  Includes bibliographical references and indexes.
  ISBN-0-8058-1447-7 (cloth). — ISBN 0-8058-1448-5 (pbk.)
  1. Brain damage—Patients—Rehabilitation—Congresses.
  2. Clinical neuropsychology—Congresses. I. Christensen, Anne-
Lise. II. Uzzell, Barbara P.
  [DNLM: 1. Brain Injuries—rehabilitation—congresses.
  2. Neuropsychology—congresses. WL 354 B8133 1994]
  RC387.5.B727   1994
  617.4'81044—dc20
  DNLM/DLC
  for Library of Congress   93-21071
                                               CIP

Books published by Lawrence Erlbaum Associates are printed on acid-free
paper, and their bindings are chosen for strength and durability.

Printed in the United States of America
10 9 8 7 6 5 4 3 2 1

Contents

Contributors

Diane Bistany, General Insurance Corporation, Financial Centre, P.O. Box 10350, Stamford, Connecticut 06904-2350

Tom G. Bolwig, Department of Psychiatry, State University Hospital/Rigshospitalet, Blegdamsvej 9, 2100 Copenhagen Ø, Denmark

D. Neil Brooks, The Kemsley Unit, St. Andrew's Hospital, Billing Road, Northampton, NN1 5DG, UK

Anne-Lise Christensen, Center for Rehabilitation of Brain Injury, University of Copenhagen, Njalsgade 88, 2300 Copenhagen S, Denmark

D. Nathan Cope, Paradigm Health Corporation, 1001 Galaxy Way, Suite 410, Concord, California 94520

Leonard Diller, New York University Medical Center, The Howard A. Rusk Institute of Rehabilitation Medicine, 400 East 34th Street, New York, New York 10016

Esben Dragsted, Dragsted Lawyers, Toldbodgade 29, 1253 Copenhagen K, Denmark

David W. Ellis, Mediplex Rehab-Camden, 2 Cooper Plaza, Camden, New Jersey 08103

Marylou M. Glasier, Institute for Animal Behavior, Rutgers University, University Heights, Hill Hall, Newark, New Jersey 07102

Zeev Groswasser, Kupat Cholim, Loewenstein Hospital Rehabilitation Center, Sackler Faculty of Medicine, Tel-Aviv University, 278 Ahuza Street, P.O. Box Ra'anana 43100, Israel

Stuart W. Hoffman, Institute for Animal Behavior, Rutgers University, University Heights, Hill Hall, Newark, New Jersey 07102

Sandra Horn, Department of Psychology, University of Southampton, University Road, Highfield, Southampton SO9 4XY, UK

Lise Randrup Jensen, Center for Rehabilitation of Brain Injury, Njalsgade 88, 2300 Copenhagen S, Denmark

Pierre-Alain Joseph, Neurologie B, C.H.U. 17X, 49033 Angers Cedex, France

Ritva Laaksonen, The KL Institute, Eteläinen Hesperiankatu 16 B 8, 00100 Helsinki, Finland

Anders Larsen, Local Governments' Research Institute (AKF), Nyropsgade 37, 1602 Copenhagen V, Denmark

Lindsay Mclellan, University of Southampton, Rehabilitation Research Unit, Southampton General Hospital, Tremona Road, Southampton SO9 4XY, UK.

Jill Mehlbye, Local Governments' Research Institute (AKF), Nyropsgade 37, 1602 Copenhagen V, Denmark

C. Potagas, M.D., Premetis 3, 16121 Athens, Greece

George P. Prigatano, Neurological Rehabilitation, Barrow Neurological Institute, St. Joseph's Hospital and Medical Center, 350 West Thomas Road, Phoenix, Arizona 85013-4496

Gitte Rasmussen, Center for Rehabilitation of Brain Injury, University of Copenhagen, Njsalsgade 88, 2300 Copenhagen S, Denmark

Jarl Risberg, CBF-Laboratory, Clinical-Neurophysiological Department, Lasarettet, 221, 85 Lund, Sweden

Agnes Shiel, University of Southampton, Rehabilitation Research Unit, Southampton General Hospital, Tremona Road, Southampton SO9 4XY, UK

Franz J. Stachowiak, Rheinische Landesklinik Bonn (ZOK), Julius Vorster Strasse 10, 5300 Bonn 3, Germany

Donald G. Stein, Rutgers University, University Heights, Hill Hall, Newark, New Jersey 07102

Thomas W. Teasdale, Center for Rehabilitation of Brain Injury, University of Copenhagen, Njalsgade 88, 2300 Copenhagen S, Denmark

Lance E. Trexler, CNR Clinics, 8925 North Meridian Street, Suite 100, Indianapolis, Indiana 46260-2384

Jean-Luc Truelle, Centre de Médico-Chirugical Foch, Service de Neurologie, 40, rue Worth BP 36, 92151 Surenes Cedex, France

Barbara P. Uzzell, Del Oro Institute of Rehabilitation, 8081 Greenbriar Drive, Houston, Texas 77054

Martin Watson, Occupational Therapy, Physiotherapy Department, University of East Anglia, Norwich NR4 7T, UK

Patrick M. Webb, Center for Neuropsychological Rehabilitation, Inc., 8925 North Meridian Street, Suite 100, Indianapolis, Indiana 46260-2384

Barbara Wilson, MRC Applied Psychology Unit, 15 Chaucer Road, Cambridge CB2 2EF, UK

Giuseppe Zappala, Center for Neuropsychological Rehabilitation, Inc., 8925 North Meridian Street, Suite 100, Indianapolis, Indiana 46260-2384

George A. Zitnay, National Head Injury Foundation, Inc., 1140 Connecticut Avenue N.W., Suite 812, Washington, D.C. 20036

Preface

Most individuals with brain damage experience a curtailment or loss of lifestyle without rehabilitation. Improved methods and appropriately timed medical interventions now make it possible for more individuals to survive brain insults, and to be assisted by rehabilitation neuropsychologists in achieving renewed commitment to life. Damage to the brain, the organ of human emotions and cognition, reduces psychological functioning and realistic adaptation, and the patient and his/her family are often encapsulated in the time prior to injury. To regain part or most of the lifestyle lost, an honest, dedicated, and realistic approach is required.

Neuropsychological rehabilitation can provide tools for this task, provided that the most comprehensive, elaborate, and knowledge-based methods are integrated in the training, and provided that knowledge from many disciplines and from community environments and family is encompassed.

Neuropsychological rehabilitation today has increased throughout the world. In different ways it was initiated in the Soviet Union and in Israel following involvement in wars, and in the United States in the last two decades, due primarily to increasing amount of traumatic motor vehicle accidents. Neuropsychological rehabilitation continues to evolve and undergo change.

Five years ago we recorded in a book a body of knowledge central to neuropsychological rehabilitation from the neurosciences and psychology, which was presented at a conference, "Neuropsychological Rehabilitation—Current Knowledge and Future Directions," in Copenhagen. In the present book, knowledge representing the development of neuropsychological rehabilitation during the past 5 years is collected from a second conference in Copenhagen, Denmark, "Progress in Neuropsychological Rehabilitation." The chapters in this book are written by professionals who were invited to share their experiences from different areas within the field. They were invited to communicate because of their expertise with processes involved in neuropsychological rehabilitation. Some authors have contributed chapters to both books, illustrating the perspective in development. Other authors are contributing for the first time, and as such, are evidence of growth and expansion of rehabilitation in content and geographical distribution. There is a stronger representation from Europe because of expansion of neuropsychological rehabilitation throughout the continent.

The conference was planned with the purpose of stressing the different areas of importance in rehabilitation. After a historical review, the chapters follow a visible sequence with content of biology, neuropsychology, and neuropharmacology. Experts discuss the most advanced medical knowledge of the effect of injury on states of the organism. In the next chapters, the concern is directed toward the stages of development after brain injury and the various methods adapted by the professionals from neuropsychology, psychotherapy, physical training, and psychosocial functioning.

The second part of the book is dedicated to outcome and the economics of rehabilitation, followed by chapters concerning the future. Plans and visions are described from various parts of the world and within different areas regarding neuropsychological rehabilitation. A panel discussion ensues addressing the overall question: Is rehabilitation worthwhile and ethical? The reactions of the participants shed light on the essence and practice of today's neurorehabilitation and, at the same time, the influence of cross-cultural exchange of knowledge is made evident.

Our experiences with this conference makes us continue to be exuberant about the ever-increasing fund of knowledge and its application, as well as concerned for quality assurance in the health-care field. After another 5 years have passed, we wish to meet again to witness the evolutionary status of the field.

We wish to express appreciation to the generosity of the Egmont Foundation in making the conference possible. We want to offer much-deserved thanks to contributing authors and conference participants who provided thought-provoking material, ideas, and perspectives within the field of neuropsychological rehabilitation. We would like to acknowledge Dr. Sheldon Berrol's contributions to the field of rehabilitation, and we miss his thoughts in this book due to his untimely death. Special appreciation goes to the editorial assistance of Lise Bjerregaard Lambek and Anne Marie Petersen, and to our colleague Tom W. Teasdale. Without them, this book would not have been possible.

—Anne-Lise Christensen
—Barbara P. Uzzell

Foreword

Esben Dragsted
*Chairman of the Board of Trustees of the
Egmont Foundation, Copenhagen, Denmark*

For historical and personal reasons it is a particular satisfaction for me to write a few opening words to this book, emanating as it does from the work of the Center for Brain Injury at the University of Copenhagen and its many collaborators. In 1985, a grant from the Danish Egmont Foundation made possible the establishment of the Center under the direction of Professor Anne-Lise Christensen. As chairman of the Board of Trustees of the Foundation, it has therefore been very gratifying for me to see the Center grow into a healthy and productive independence. The Center has been successful, not only in helping unfortunate victims of brain injury toward a better and more fulfilling life, but also in awakening public concern to their situation, and in pursuing research aimed at improving methods of assisting them. Brain injury is, however, an international issue, and since its inception, the Center has developed an ever-growing contact and collaboration with other specialists and experts, particularly in Europe and North America.

In recognition of the status of the Center, the Foundation was happy to sponsor the truly international conference in Copenhagen, the papers from which form the basis of the chapters of the present volume. These chapters, meticulously edited and integrated by Anne-Lise Christensen and Barbara Uzzell, thus contain an imposingly wide-ranging distillation of the most recent knowledge and experience, drawn from so many countries, all focused on the vital central concern of improving the lot of the brain-injured person. I am confident that the book will contribute to furthering that improvement.

CHAPTER ONE

Finding the Right Treatment Combinations: Changes in Rehabilitation Over the Past Five Years

Leonard Diller

ABSTRACT

Progress toward finding the right treatment combinations has advanced along a number of fronts in the past 5 years. These include developments in identifying behavioral characteristics at both ends of severity in the recovery from traumatic brain injury. At the most severe end is the application of newer assessment devices, and at the opposite end is the clarification of the definition of *minor traumatic brain injury*. In the middle range there have been two major developments. First, there has been a proliferation of therapeutic modalities to establish competence in functional settings. Among them are the increase of group methods, the applications of the family coach model as a tool, the use of supported employment, and the introduction of computers for orthotic devices or cognitive aids. Second, there has been a large number of reports on varieties of cognitive remediation. These reports are reviewed with regard to the nature of outcomes that are achieved and their experimental designs. Along with the increase and diversity of procedures, there is a reemphasis on psychological constructs related to ego psychology such as awareness and self-efficacy as relevant modulating variables in facilitating response to treatment.

The ideal situation is one in which a patient with a known condition is treated with a known intervention toward a known outcome. In practice, we treat patients with partial knowledge of their conditions, with partial knowledge of the effects of interventions, and with

1

imperfect knowledge of outcomes. We are still far from the ideal situation. Progress over the past 5 years has been slow for those who are impatient, but significant because there now exist more publications and conferences that are peer reviewed to address more precise questions and evaluate procedures more specifically and critically. There have been several major trends including (a) defining patient characteristics in a more salient way, (b) identifying newer treatment modalities, and (c) critical discussing the efficacy of cognitive remediation and clarifying factors, which may modulate responsiveness to treatment. Finding the right treatment combination is more difficult in the face of much diversity, but also more challenging in the light of opportunities offered by newer initiatives. In effect, interventions in psychological modalities must resonate with advances in neurophysiological developments to define biological parameters of the conditions being treated and with developments in service delivery in order to make interventions worthwhile. It also builds on procedures that are being developed with clinical experience.

DEFINING POPULATIONS MORE PRECISELY

In the field of traumatic brain injury (TBI), one major bottleneck in undertaking major clinical trials to assess treatments in fields as diverse as carotid artery surgery or management of depression on an outpatient basis has been a lack of agreement on a proper typology. Severity of TBI as a critical typology was supported by the emergence of the Glasgow Coma Scale (GCS). If there is a continuum for severity of TBI, progress has been made at opposite ends of the spectrum: The most severe patients are defined as minimally responsive, and the least severe persons are said to have so-called minor TBI. Definitions help specify problems that are being treated before interventions can be assessed.

Minimally Responsive Patient

The treatment of the minimally responsive patient via neurostimulation, sensory stimulation, or psychopharmacological means has been marked thus far by an absence of controlled studies. The recovery from coma is important for its own sake as well as its prognostic significance. A confounding problem is that diagnostic heterogeneity does not conform with behavioral homogeneity. Clinical syndromes (coma, vegetative state, persistent vegetative state, akinetic mutism, locked-in syndrome) and neuropathologic syndromes have to be reconciled with behavioral measures. To this end, a number of measures have been developed in the past 5 years: the Coma-Near Coma Scale, Coma Recovery Scale, Sensory Stimulation Assessment Measure, and the Western Neuro-Sensory Stimulation Profile (Giacino, 1992). These scales are more focused than previous measures; they are sensitive to more subtle changes and predict outcome. Whyte (1992) noted that variability is a common characteristic that may not be assessed in conventional rehabilitation instruments. Unlike other areas of rehabilitation, assessment is more transdisciplinary, based on ratings of targeted behavior.

Minor Traumatic Brain Injury

At the opposite end of the spectrum of severity, people with minor TBI have also become the subject of more intensive investigation. Zasler (1992) distinguished between separate effects due to whiplash, cranial trauma, and brain trauma, as well as posttraumatic stress disorder. Among the complaints with high incidence are vestibular disturbances, headaches, myofascial pain, dysfunction, depression, and anxiety. Although it has been suggested that people with minor brain injury who show symptoms immediately after the trauma tend to recover by 3 months, later study suggested that minor brain injury accompanied by radiographic evidence of lesion compromises recovery (Williams, Levin, & Eisenberg, 1990). Kay, Newman, Cavallo, and Resnick (1992) found that in 808 cases of minor TBI, 84% returned to work at 3 months, 7% during the first year, and 9% did not return to work. Complaints diminished, although at 1 year headaches still occurred in 23%, dizziness in 11%, and memory problems in 13% of the cases. Mateer (1992) and her colleagues identified deficit in attention as the primary problem in minor TBI. In a study of attentional disturbances in minor TBI, functional and dysfunctional people were distinguished by slowing of information processing and heightened susceptibility to interference. Problems of recall in memory were secondary to these disturbances. These factors distinguished people with subjective complaints from those without complaints (Newman, 1992). Progress in definitions depends on examining relationships between neuroimaging, clinical, and behavioral measures relative to each other.

With significant advances in measurement at opposite ends of the severity scales, the coming decade is positioned to examine interventions for these populations more precisely.

ADVANCES IN TREATMENT MODALITIES

In the 1,500 TBI treatment programs listed in the directory of the National Directory of Head Injury Services (1992), the vast majority deals with patients in the middle of the extremes. Because the variety of interventions is too great to review in a brief space, I divide them into two types: those emphasizing contextual approaches and those featuring cognitive remediation. The latter are grouped separately because the sheer number of empirical studies ($N = 50$) indicates an accumulating knowledge base and a heavy investment of resources.

Contextually Driven Interventions

With the recognition that rehabilitation should focus on facilitating behaviors that are expressed in nontreatment or naturalistic settings, a variety of treatment modalities that differ considerably from each other have become prominent. Among them are (a) advances in group methods, (b) the use of coaches, (c) newer methods in vocational rehabilitation, and (d) applications of computers as assistive technologies. One could argue that the common element of all of these approaches is to make interventions contextually relevant (i.e., targets of interventions are focused to improve functioning within nonlaboratory settings).

Group approaches have tended to play a more important role in TBI than in other rehabilitation populations. Groups present in vivo opportunities in interpersonal contexts to overcome deficient social skills (Butler & Namerow, 1988) and to elicit behaviors that are not apparent in one-to-one sessions. Groups offer a modality for managing psychosocial as well as cognitive problems. The economy in delivering group approaches also enhances their desirability. Groups have proliferated for a range of purposes from orientation training (Corrigan, Arnett, Hovek, & Jackson, 1985) to training for community reentry (Ylvasker, Szekeres, Henry, Sullivan, & Wheeler, 1987). Groups are evolving for targeted deficits for different levels of patients. They range from building basic skills, such as help in organizing schedules or tracking proceedings in the group discussions, to stress relief or self-regulation (i.e., control of affective flooding and executive dysfunctions; Sherr & Langenbahn, 1992). Although there may be a hierarchy in terms of level of competence and patient needs in assigning membership to a particular group, there is little evidence as to how to proceed (Deaton, 1991). In effect, just as school systems learned that classes were a viable way to educate children, rehabilitation programs are using groups to help individuals learn to adapt to residual problems in living with TBI.

A more recent innovation to deal with community adaptation has been the use of the coach. In the United States, the vocational placement counselor, serving as a coach to facilitate obtaining and holding a job, has received the attention of the rehabilitation community. The use of a personal coach to assist patients and families with cognitive and personal problems in the home has received far less attention. In an early study, it was shown that it is possible to teach spouses of aphasics to serve as coaches for their aphasic partners (Goodkin, Diller, & Shah, 1975). The concept has been extended to show that graduate students could be trained to (a) teach patients and families to compensate for perceptual and cognitive deficits, (b) problem solve with regard to community reentry and family adjustment issues, and (c) teach family members to distinguish deficits from behaviors that may ordinarily be viewed as noncooperation, stubborn, anger, or emotional disturbance (Diller, 1992).

Contextual approaches in vocational rehabilitation have been given added impetus in the rapid growth of supported employment. First developed for use with developmentally disabled, this approach seeks to bypass traditional counseling, vocational aptitude testing, and even work sample approaches. It seeks to have the individual go directly to an employment situation, in which a job coach works with the employer and the patient (Wehman & Kreutzer, 1990) for as long a period of time as necessary. Supported employment has met with some success for people entering jobs with low-level skill demands, performing routine tasks. However, TBI requires more extended support than does placement for other disability groups, therefore its cost-effectiveness may not be as great. A method for assessing "job survival" following placement should provide useful information for assessing effectiveness of vocational programs (Fabian, 1992).

Computers for remedial exercises have been a major growth industry in TBI rehabilitation. Indeed, the proliferation of software for cognitive remediation has been so great that the commercial test corporations (e.g., The Psychological Corporation) offered competitions for development of software, much as the government offers research grants. However, computer applications as cognitive assists extend beyond providing material for remedial exercises. Computers may be used in a more direct, ecologically valid way. Computers can be used to address the multitasking demands of any activity that can be varied in terms of complexity. There is a rapidly growing literature on the use of computers (Levin, 1991; Parenté & DiCesare, 1991) as devices to (a) assist in scheduling activities, (b) cue people who are subject to breakdowns in performing sequential tasks, and (c) coordinate streams of activities. Computers as orthotic aids may receive their greatest boost from their use with normal people. For example, when a simple device is triggered it will emit a signal from a parked car to indicate where it may be located in a shopping mall. The study of forgetting in everyday life, which developed as an emerging field in cognitive psychology, is already beginning to pay dividends in terms of commercial uses that lap over to fit individuals with special needs (Hermann & Petro, 1991). Special accommodations may be needed to fit the needs of people with motor impairments (O'Leary, 1991).

Prediction Studies

On the face of it, prediction studies, which capitalize on individual differences at entry to a program, would appear to be a useful way to find the right patient–treatment combinations. Prediction studies are attractive because they involve collecting data at different points in time and simply correlating them. Earlier reviews for stroke and TBI patients in rehabilitation settings found that predictions were positive, but correlations were not powerful enough for individual use (Acker, 1986; Meier, Strauman, & Thompson, 1987). The criteria and populations varied widely. More recently, Neimann, Ruff, and Baser (1990) found that more severe patients did not do as well as less severe patients in cognitive retraining. Lam, Priddy, and Johnson (1991) found that in a TBI population more intact people did better vocationally than less intact people.

In general, prediction studies attempt to forecast outcome with little regard for the content of specific programs. Hence, the same variables are used to predict success in a vocational program as in a rehabilitation medicine program. Models that work best clinically in rehabilitation settings expose a candidate to a sample of tasks to be mastered and rules to be followed as screening and prediction tools. This holds true for activities of daily living sampled in physical and occupational therapy, learning samples in a school setting, and work samples in an employment situation. The sampling approach is more useful on a clinical level, in contrast to the traditional prediction models, which might be useful in terms of categories of programs or populations. For example, the diagnosis of mental retardation might be useful for eligibility for a given program, but in a population of retarded people within a program it may not be specific enough to provide a good person–program match. In a recent study of a TBI program, where acceptance of disability was both part of the treatment as well as a therapeutic goal, staff ratings of trainee acceptance during the program were the best predictors of vocational outcome (Ezrachi, Ben Yishay, Kay, Diller, & Rattok, 1991).

OUTCOME STUDIES IN COGNITIVE RETRAINING

There are now approximately 50 outcome studies on cognitive remediation in TBI, whereas there were less than 10 a decade ago (Diller
& Gordon, 1981). The studies can be examined in several ways. One
is whether the goals are to improve impairments (structural deficits),
functional limitations (difficulties in performing activities of daily living
without assistance), or handicaps (difficulties in performing normative
roles). Another is the content of the problem or deficit that is being
treated. A third is the nature of the evidence (i.e., case reports,
single-case designs, or control groups). By far the greatest number
of studies have been devoted to improving impairments (i.e., improving
an underlying deficit, such as attention or memory). For the most
part, there has been little attempt to examine the effects of the
interventions in terms of functional limitations or handicaps.

If one examines change in terms of improvement on the task used
in training or in another psychometric task, or in a practical activity
that is useful as an end in itself, studies of attention and memory
for the most part use tests that vary widely in the degree to which
the criteria resemble the training tasks. Many studies use tests as
criteria that differ from training tasks to obviate the argument that
improvement is only task specific. But they must still bridge the gap
between impairment and functional limitations or handicaps. A number of approaches have attempted to address this problem. First,
training an impairment is a way to engage the individual who is otherwise difficult. Some have used impairment training as a precursor
for training in functional situations (Sohlberg & Mateer, 1989).
Elements of the training are then incorporated into functionally
directed activities. Others have used strategies in overcoming
impairments (e.g., self-rehearsal) as a way to deal with a functional
limitation (e.g., reading comprehension and recall; Glasgow, Zeiss,
Barrera, & Lewinsohn, 1977). Second, some use task-specific training,
where the trained task can be used to reduce a functional limitation.
Thus, mnemonic devices have been used to remember telephone
numbers, rather than strings of digits (Parenté, Stapleton, & Wheatley,
1992). Activities of daily living involving the motoric components of
independence, which are part of the normal inpatient retraining
procedures, have been supplemented by task analysis (Mayer, Keating,
& Rapp, 1986). Schachter and Glisky (1986) shaped a patient with
severe cognitive problems to master a computer that could be used
for work. Although these approaches are attractive in terms of program
goals, they have not been examined in terms of cost-effectiveness or
long-term maintenance.

If one examines training in terms of the content or domain, it is apparent that most effort has been put into improving attention and memory. This may be because they are impairments that are easily detected in test procedures, as well as because historically they have lent themselves to laboratory study where conditions can be controlled. Like traditional experimental laboratory studies, they face difficulty in translation into practical activities. Studies of self-regulation and executive dysfunction have emerged as areas of clinical concern that can be treated. Because these areas are closer to presenting symptomatology, they have also built in training procedures that include relief of symptoms and functional limitations. Typically the individual is taught methods of self-regulation in a contrived situation. When the methods are mastered, the individual is guided through his or her expression in naturalistic settings. These studies have met with success (Cicerone & Wood, 1987). Finally, there are holistic programs that integrate cognitive retraining with therapies that are more directed toward psychosocial and vocational goals. These programs seek outcomes that address functional limitations as well as handicaps.

Another way of looking at treatment studies is in terms of whether they are case reports, single-case designs, or control-group studies. Examination in these terms suggests that attention and memory retraining, which have yielded the largest number of studies, also have the most case reports. As a rule, there appear to be more positive findings for case studies than for single-case designs or control-group studies. This suggests that case studies be used as building blocks toward more rigorous studies, rather than as final pieces of evidence. Conversely, single-case designs and control-group designs may profit from prior experience with case studies. The high incidence of negative findings in control-group studies of attention may be a factor of not having worked through the many clinical details in management that cannot be expressed in compressed reports. The absence of replication gives strong testimony to this possibility. Indeed, the one replication study found negative results (Ponsford & Kinsella, 1988), but the patients may not have been treated for a sufficient length of time. In my own experience, many pilot studies must be conducted to answer simple and obvious questions such as (a) style, manner, and presentation of stimuli; (b) criteria for starting and stopping treatment; (c) methods for engaging patients and dealing with patient resistance; and (d) normally reported events including descriptions of patients, assessments, and interventions.

Holistic approaches using multimodalities are the most common clinically. Their efficacy is difficult to document, in the sense of teasing out the contributions of the different therapies to a desired outcome. Although several groups have provided data testifying as to the positive benefits of such programs (Christensen, Pinner, Møller Pedersen, Teasdale, & Trexler, 1992; Prigatano et al., 1984), there is now evidence that different intensities of treatment have different effects with regard to cognitive as opposed to interpersonal outcomes. In a recent study (Rattok et al., 1992), three different groups of TBI patients were equated in terms of neurologic and demographic factors and treated by the same team for the same number of hours. Groups differed in the number of hours spent in cognitive retraining (attention, spatial ability, psychomotor skills, logical reasoning) versus interpersonal training (social skill groups, vocational planning groups). The three groups achieved the same success rate in terms of employment at the completion of the program, as well as at 6-month follow-up. They differed in that the groups with cognitive training improved more on tasks requiring cognitive demands. The interpersonal skill groups improved more on tasks involving interpersonal skills. The group that received training in both improved in both. Hence, one can conclude that there are differential effects for cognitive and interpersonal interventions at the completion of the program.

ADVANCES IN PSYCHOLOGICAL CONSTRUCTS

As treatment has expanded, many concepts that were noted in both cognitive remediation and psychosocial programs have come into greater prominence. Among them are awareness, self-efficacy, and metacognition as critical modulating variables in treatment. They resemble aspects of ego function in the language of an earlier generation of psychologists. The recognition of ego functions in learning is tied to a broader development in general psychology—the return of motivation as an explanatory construct. Thus, in reviewing the changing emphasis in motivation in the *Encyclopedia of Educational Psychology*, Weiner (1990) noted that 40 years ago chapters on motivation were largely about need reduction and drive theory, with key referent studies from the animal literature. Today there is much greater specificity about learning and motivation derived from experimental and normative study in classroom settings. Self-efficacy and "intrinsic motivation" have replaced stimulus–response reenforcement as dominating concern for students of human learning (Schaefele, 1991).

Awareness/unawareness of impairment or disability has received a great deal of discussion from three sources: (a) unawareness as neuropsychological event (Prigatano & Schachter, 1991), (b) denial as psychologic defense or adaptive mechanism to catastrophic loss, and (c) acceptance as a key to program engagement or therapeutic alliance in the rehabilitation process. Because the primary concern is the right patient–treatment combination, a discussion of the rich literature in this area is beyond the scope of this chapter. Several important recent studies have occurred. First, scales have been developed to measure awareness more precisely. This permits the quantification of degree of unawareness so that one can identify a clinically important patient characteristic for determining responsiveness to treatment. Two types of scales have been applied to stroke and TBI populations. The first type consists of examining discrepancies between a patient's account and by outside measures via objective tests (Anderson & Tranel, 1989; Hibbord, Gordon, Stern, Grober, & Sliwinski, 1992). These studies indicate that (a) the greatest discrepancies occur for cognitive impairments, which are invisible, as opposed to physical impairments, which are visible; and (b) for stroke patients, unawareness is related to cognitive competence. The second type of discrepancy measure involves a comparison of ratings of patients, families, and/or staff (Prigatano, Altman, & O'Brien, 1990). Patients who deviate may show different patterns of adjustment to a program. They may also show different patterns of brain damage (Prigatano & Altman, 1990).

Cognitive competence may impact awareness as well as self-report of affective disturbance. This chain of linkage fits Levine's (1990) theory. Awareness of loss following brain damage is a process that is not intuitively obvious, but must be inferred from feedback by others or in response to mishaps in one's own behavior. People with less cognitive competence might be expected to be less likely to make such inferences, particularly if the impairments are invisible. It could also explain a process approach to awareness, which argues that awareness may be considered in terms of intellectual, emergent, and anticipatory qualities, which require somewhat different strategies in assessment and management in TBI (Barco, Crosson, Bolesta, Werts, & Stout, 1991). These different types of awareness may be related to cognitive competence.

An equally important development with regard to unawareness is the demonstration that acceptance of the rehabilitation thesis is the most powerful predictor of vocational placement, offering greater variance than demographic, neurologic, or psychometric factors for predicting outcome (Ezrachi et al., 1991). The thesis involves a series of steps including acknowledgment of TBI, the presence of impairment, the need for a program, acknowledgment that the future may be different, and acknowledgment that the recommendations of the team are reasonable. The therapeutic alliance has been one of the main conditions for success in psychotherapy, and is intuitively appreciated on a clinical level. Empirical demonstration is an important finding for the field of rehabilitation. A refinement of this approach in psychotherapy is a suggestion that a patient and therapist share the responsibility for sessions by dictating summaries of treatment sessions in each other's presence (Albeck & Goldman, 1991). Perhaps we can look forward to a therapeutic goal wherein some individuals with brain damage are able to write their own psychological reports.

Acceptance implies engagement and commitment of the self. Relations between impairments in cognition and self-concept are important, but have not been articulated. Aside from the fact that the cognitive apparatus is diminished, a person may have to recognize that in many ways he or she is different with respect to premorbid capabilities and roles so that an integration of premorbid and postmorbid self must take place. In addition, the role of the disabled has always been denigrated so that the prospect of assuming such a role in the context of bearing the loss of a premorbid sense of self is difficult. Finally, the shaken sense of self that is characteristic of minor TBI (Kay et al., 1992), and the low self-esteem associated with TBI, must contribute to the high incidence of depression. The self-concept has been approached in rehabilitation as a static variable, or as one with only incidental or vague implication for rehabilitation. Although the *self* is a rather difficult concept to define, one aspect is particularly pertinent for rehabilitation—self-efficacy. Self-efficacy suggests that effort makes a difference, and that the performer is responsible for the difference. Passing a test that is too easy or performing poorly on a task that is unimportant does not impact self-efficacy. Self-efficacy is related to perceived competence in a specific situation. It is related to hope, interest, and perception of ability to cope. People with high self-efficacy believe that their efforts make a difference. Studies of limitations of generalization of training in people with brain damage have not separated lack of motivation from lack of mastery. People may see themselves as competent in only one delimited task but fail to see themselves as competent in a similar task (Dittman-Koli, Lachman, Kliegl, & Baltes, 1991). Failure to apply a strategy may therefore not be a cognitive lack, but a motivational one.

These trends fit those emerging in parallel developments with other populations of cognitively impaired. Three decades ago, students of mental retardation introduced metacognition as a moderating influence in enhancing cognitive deficit (Borkowski, Peck, Reid, & Kurtz, 1983). They found that metacognition was closely tied to self-efficacy

(Cavanaugh & Green, 1990). Current students of theories of intellect argue that cognitive processes can be divided into two systems. One is biological and provides the basic architecture system for cognition, such as memory span, speed of encoding, and decoding information. The second is learned and provides the executive system that guides problem solving and metacognition (Campione & Brown, 1978). Although neuropsychologists would reframe the distinction between biological and environmental, the notion of two systems operating in cognition may be a useful guide to students of cognitive remediation.

CONCLUSIONS

The right treatment for the right patient? Important steps have been taken to develop more precise replies to this question. First there is a more careful sorting out of patients at both ends of the spectrum of severity: the most severe and the least severe. These steps involve neurological and behavioral measures. Second, there have been advances in various therapeutic modalities, including innovative therapies delivered in groups, family coaches, supportive employment, and assistive technology. These modalities point toward helping people function at an optimal level in specific contexts. Third, there has been an outpouring of studies on cognitive remediation, but the field does not rest on a firm footing because most studies have dealt with impairments so that gains are difficult to translate into practical benefits. In addition, there is a lack of replicated experimental studies. However, there is also a sense of using cognitive remediation as a step linked to functional outcomes by tying the remediation to functional activities. Fourth, there has been interest in psychological constructs, which serve as moderator variables. Constructs such as awareness and self-efficacy also reflect larger trends in general psychology.

Finding the right treatment for the right patient at this time involves guesswork. With the rapid growth in documenting treatments and descriptions of TBI, we are narrowing the guesses.

ACKNOWLEDGMENTS

This chapter was supported in part by the U.S. Department of Education, National Institute on Disability and Rehabilitation Research, Research and Training Center on Head Trauma and Stroke, Grant No. H133B80028.

REFERENCES

Acker, M. (1986). Relationships between test scores and everyday life in neuropsychological intervention. In B. R. Uzzel & Y. Gross (Eds.), *Clinical neuropsychology of intervention* (pp. 85–118). Boston: Martinus Nijhoff.

Albeck, J. H., & Goldman, C. (1991). Patient–therapist codocumentation implications of jointly authored progress notes for psychotherapy practice, research, training, supervision, and management. *American Journal of Psychotherapy, 45,* 317–332.

Anderson, S. W., & Tranel, D. (1989). Awareness of disease states following cerebral infarct, dementia and head injury. *The Clinical Neuropsychologist, 3,* 327–329.

Barco, P. B., Crosson, B., Bolesta, M. M., Werts, D., & Stout, R. (1991). Training awareness and compensation in post-acute head injury rehabilitation. In J. S. Kreutzer & P. H. Wehman (Eds.), *Cognitive rehabilitation for persons with traumatic brain injury* (pp. 129–146). Baltimore: Paul H. Brookes.

Borkowski, J. H., Peck, I. A., Reid, M. K., & Kurtz, B. E. (1983). Impulsivity and strategy transfer: Metamemory as mediator. *Child Development, 54,* 459–473.

Butler, R. H., & Namerow, N. S. (1988). Cognitive retraining in brain injury rehabilitation. A critical review. *Journal of Neurologic Rehabilitation, 2,* 46–54.

Campione, J. C., & Brown, A. L. (1978). Toward a theory of intelligence. Contributions from research with retarded children. *Intelligence, 2,* 279–304.

Cavanaugh, J. C., & Green, E. Z. (1990). I believe, therefore, I can. Self efficacy beliefs in memory aging. In E. Lovelace (Ed.), *Aging and cognition: Mental processes, self awareness and interventions* (pp. 208–232). Holland: Elsevier Science Publishing.

Christensen, A.-L., Pinner, E. M., Møller Pedersen, P., Teasdale, T. W., & Trexler, L. E. (1992). Psychosocial outcome following individualized neuropsychological rehabilitation of brain damage. *Acta Neurologica Scandinavica, 85,* 32–38.

Cicerone, K. D., & Wood, J. C. (1987). Planning disorder after closed head-injury: A case study. *Archives of Physical and Medical Rehabilitation, 68,* 111–115.

Corrigan, J. D., Arnett, J. A., Hovek, L., & Jackson, R. D. (1985). Reality orientation for brain injured patients: Group treatment and monitoring of recovery. *Archives of Physical Medicine and Rehabilitation, 66,* 626–630.

Deaton, A. (1991). Group interventions for cognitive rehabilitation increasing the challenges. In J. S. Kreutzer & P. H. Wehman (Eds.), *Cognitive rehabilitation for persons with traumatic brain injury* (pp. 201–214). Baltimore: Paul H. Brookes.

Diller, L. (1992). *Psychological and social adjustment after stroke.* Final report to NIDRR (Grant No. H 133A B0057-88).

Diller, L., & Gordon, W. A. (1991). Rehabilitation and clinical neuropsychology. In S. Filskov, & T. Boll (Eds.), *Handbook of clinical neuropsychology* (pp. 702–733). New York: Wiley.

Dittman-Koli, F., Lachman, M. E., Kliegl, R., & Baltes, P. B. (1991). Effects of cognitive training and testing on intellectual efficacy beliefs in elderly adults. *Journal of Gerontology, 46,* 162–164.

Ezrachi, O., Ben Yishay, Y., Kay, T., Diller, L., & Rattok, J. (1991). Predicting employment in traumatic brain injury following neuropsychological rehabilitation. *Journal of Head Trauma Rehabilitation, 6*(3), 71–84.

Fabian, E. S. (1992). Longitudinal outcomes in supported employment. *Rehabilitation Psychology, 37,* 23–37.

Giacino, J. T. (1992, June). *Clinical and neuropathologic syndrome associated with states of minimal responsiveness.* Paper presented at the fourth annual conference on Rebuilding Shattered Lives, Edison, NJ.

Glasgow, R. E., Zeiss, R. A., Barrera, M., & Lewinsohn, P. (1977). Case studies on remediating memory deficits in brain damaged individuals. *Journal of Clinical Psychology, 33,* 1049–1054.

Goodkin, R., Diller, L., & Shah, N. (1975). Training spouses to improve the functional speech of aphasic patients. In B. Lahey (Ed.), *Modification of verbal behavior.* Springfield, IL: Charles C. Thomas.

Hermann, D. J., & Petro, S. (1991). Commercial memory aids. *Applied Cognitive Psychology, 13,* 29–37.

Hibbord, M. R., Gordon, W. A., Stein, P., Grober, S., & Sliwinski, M. J. (1992). Awareness of disability in patients following stroke. *Rehabilitation Psychology. 37,* 103–120.

Kay, T., Newman, B., Cavallo, M., & Resnick, M. (1992). Neuropsychological diagnoses, disentangling multiple determinants of functional disability after mild traumatic brain injury. *Physical Medicine and Rehabilitation: State of the Art Review, 6,* 109–125.

Lam, C. S., Priddy, D. A., & Johnson, P. (1991). Neuropsychological indicators of employability following traumatic brain injury. *Rehabilitation Psychological Bulletin, 35,* 69–75.

Levin, W. (1991). Computer applications in cognitive rehabilitation for persons with traumatic brain injury: A functional approach. In J. S. Kreutzer & P. H. Wehman (Eds.), *Community integration following traumatic brain injury* (pp. 163–180). Baltimore: Paul H. Brookes.

Levine, D. (1990). Unawareness of visual and sensorimotor defects: A hypotheses. *Brain and Cognition, 13,* 233–281.

Mateer, C. (1992). Systems of care for postconcussive syndrome. In L. J. Horn & N. O. Zasler (Eds.), *Physical Medicine and Rehabilitation: State of the Art Review. 6,* 143–160.

Mayer, N. H., Keating, D. J., & Rapp, D. (1986). Skills, routines, and activity patterns of daily living—A functional nested approach. In B. P. Uzzell & Y. Gross (Eds.), *Clinical neuropsychology of intervention* (pp. 205–233). Boston: Dordrecht, & Lanchaster, Martinus Nijhoff.

Meier, M. J., Strauman, S., & Thompson, W. G. (1987). Individual differences in psychological recovery: An overview. In M. J. Meier, A. L. Benton, & L. Diller (Eds.), *Neuropsychological rehabilitation* (pp. 71–110). New York: Guilford.

National Directory of Head Injury Services (1992). Southbridge, MA: National Head Injury Foundation.

Neimann, H., Ruff, R. M., & Baser, C. A. (1990). Computer assisted retraining in head-injured individuals: A controlled efficacy study of an outpatient program. *Journal of Consulting and Clinical Psychology. 58,* 811–818.

Newman, B. (1992, June). *The evaluation of attentional processes after minor traumatic brain injury.* Paper presented at the fourth annual conference on Rebuilding Shattered Lives, Edison, NJ.

O'Leary, S. (1991). Computer access with considerations for patients with traumatic brain injury. *Journal Head Trauma Rehabilitation, 6,* 89–91.

Parenté, R., & DiCesare, A. (1991). Retraining memory: Theory, evaluation, and applications in cognitive rehabilitation for persons with traumatic brain injury: A functional approach. In J. S. Kreutzer & P. H. Wehman (Eds.), *Community integration following traumatic brain injury* (pp. 147–162). Baltimore: Paul H. Brookes.

Parenté, R., Stapleton, C. M., & Wheatley, C. J. (1991). Practical strategies for vocational reentry after traumatic brain injury. *Journal of Head Trauma Rehabilitation. 6,* 35–45.

Ponsford, J. L., & Kinsella, G. (1988). Evaluation of a remedial programme for attentional deficits following closed head injury. *Journal of Clinical and Experimental Neuropsychology, 10*, 693–708.

Prigatano, G. P., & Altman, I. M. (1990). Impaired awareness of behavioral limitations after traumatic brain injury. *Archives of Physical Medicine and Rehabilitation, 71*, 1058–1064.

Prigatano, G. P., Altman, I. M., & O'Brien, K. P. (1990). Behavioral limitation that traumatic brain impaired patients tend to underestimate. *The Clinical Neuropsychologist, 4*, 163–176.

Prigatano, G. P., Fordyce, D. J., Zeiner, H. K., Roueche, J. R., Pepping, M., & Wood, B. C. (1984). Neuropsychological rehabilitation after closed head injury in young adults. *Journal of Neurology, Neurosurgery, and Psychiatry, 47*, 505–513.

Prigatano, G. P., & Schachter, D. L. (Eds.). (1991). *Awareness of deficit after brain injury: Clinical and theoretical issues.* New York: Oxford University Press.

Rattok, J., Ben Yishay, Y., Ezrachi, O., Lakin, P., Piasetsky, E., Ross, B., Silver, S., Vakil, E., Zide, E., & Diller, L. (1992). Outcome of different treatment mixes in a multidimensional neuropsychological rehabilitation program. *Neuropsychology, 6*, 395–416.

Schachter, D., & Glisky, E. I. (1986). Memory remediation: Restoration, alleviation, and the acquisition of domain specific knowledge. In B. P. Uzzell & Y. Gross (Eds.), *Clinical neuropsychology of intervention* (pp. 257–282). Boston: Martinus Nijhoff.

Schaefele, U. (1991). Interest, learning and motivation. *Educational Psychologist, 26*, 299–323.

Sherr, R. L., & Langenbahn, D. (1992). An approach to large scale outpatient rehabilitation. *Neuropsychology, 6*, 417–426.

Sohlberg, M. M., & Mateer, C. A. (1989). Training use of compensatory memory books: A three stage behavioral approach. *Journal of Clinical and Experimental Neuropsychology, 11*, 871–891.

Wehman, P., & Kreutzer, J. (1990). *Vocational rehabilitation for persons with traumatic brain injury.* Gaithersburg, MD: Aspen.

Weiner, B. (1990). History of motivational research in education. *Journal of Educational Psychology, 82*, 616–627.

Whyte, J. M. (1992, June). *Individualized behavioral assessment of the minimally responsive patients.* Paper presented at the fourth annual conference on Rebuilding Shattered Lives, Edison, NJ.

Williams, D. H., Levin, H. S., & Eisenberg, H. M. (1990). Med. head injury classification. *Neurosurgery, 27*, 422–428.

Ylvasker, M., Szekeres, S. F., Henry, K., Sullivan, D. M., & Wheeler, P. (1987). Topics in cognitive rehabilitation therapy. In M. Ylvasker & E. M. R. Gobble (Eds.), *Community reentry for head injured adults* (pp. 137–220). San Diego: Heil Press.

Zasler, N. D. (1992). Mild traumatic brain injury: Facts, fantasies and fables. In L. Horn & N. D. Zasler (Eds.), *Rehabilitation of post-concussive disorders.* Philadelphia: Hanley & Belfus.

CHAPTER TWO

Pharmacological Treatments for Brain-Injury Repair: Progress and Prognosis

Donald G. Stein, Marylou M. Glasier,
and Stuart W. Hoffman

ABSTRACT

It has been only within the last 10 years that research on treatment for central nervous system (CNS) recovery after injury has become more focused on the complexities involved in promoting recovery from brain injury when the CNS is viewed as an integrated and dynamic system. There have been major advances in research in recovery over the last decade, including new information on the mechanics and genetics of metabolism and chemical activity, including the definition of excitotoxic effects and the discovery that the brain secretes complex proteins, peptides, and hormones that are capable of directly stimulating the repair of damaged neurons or blocking some of the degenerative processes caused by the injury cascade. Many of these agents, plus other nontoxic, naturally occurring substances, are being tested as treatment for brain injury. Further work is needed to determine appropriate combinations of treatments and optimum times of administration with respect to the time course of the CNS disorder. Understanding the mechanisms underlying traumatic brain injury and repair must eventually come from a merging of the findings of neurochemical alterations in the whole brain with data from intensive behavioral testing, which will determine the meaning of these findings. For optimum treatment strategies, we also need testing procedures and definitions used in connection with treatment for brain injury.

When the first meeting on neuropsychological rehabilitation was held in Copenhagen in 1988, one of the authors was asked by Drs.

Christensen and Uzzell to provide an overview of some of the conceptual and theoretical issues extant in preclinical research on recovery from brain damage (Stein, 1988). In that overview, emphasis was given to consideration of the contextual issue (i.e., symptoms and syndromes that occur following brain injury depend very much on the context in which the injury occurred and not just on the site of the injury itself). This issue has gained importance as more refined techniques permit access to increasingly better defined views of the living brain. Tremendous progress has been made in brain-imaging techniques that seem to permit one to "localize the injury" and, by extension, assign the nature of the deficit to the damaged tissue. However, we would reiterate that environmental and organismic variables must be taken into account when deciding on the prognosis for recovery, as well as the course of rehabilitation therapy provided for the patient.

Although this holistic perspective can be seen as a point more appropriate for academic discussion than clinical practice, it is an important theoretical issue not only for academicians but also for those directly involved in treatment of brain-injured patients. The issue of plasticity lies at the heart of thinking about (a) how the nervous system is organized, (b) how "plastic" responses may be engendered after injury, and (c) how appropriate treatment strategies may be developed and employed.

It has been only within the last 10 years that some neurologists and neuropsychologists involved with head injury have become more focused on the complexities involved in promoting recovery from brain injury when the central nervous system (CNS) is viewed as an integrated and dynamic system. Prior to this, the main task in dealing with head trauma was first to stabilize the patient and then to diagnose and, in the process, localize the deficits. In general, follow-up therapy was left to rehabilitation specialists and physiatrists whose basic task was to enable the patient to compensate for and cope with his or her disability rather than to promote functional recovery per se. Thus, although a change in attitude about CNS organization is slowly taking place, much emphasis in neuroscience is still on identifying pathways and chemical assays of specific brain regions and demonstrating and perfecting exquisite techniques. Given this molecular perspective, it is not surprising that a widely read textbook in medical neuroscience (Kandel, Schwartz, & Jessell, 1991) states that: "all behavior, including higher mental functioning (affective as well as cognitive), can be localized to specific regions or constellations of regions within the brain. *Descriptive neuroanatomy provides us with a functional guide to local sites within the brain that correspond to specific behaviors*" (p. 15, italics added).

The focus on molecular techniques and ever smaller units of function and brain cartography, which characterizes current thinking about the brain, overlooks the fact that it is a patient that has brain damage and not just a region of the brain itself. The mechanistic-reductionistic perspective offers small hope to patients and provides little basis for formation and testing of hypotheses about the diverse mechanisms underlying functional recovery and CNS repair. It is interesting to note, for example, that at the 1991 International Neurotrauma Society meetings, where the theme was CNS injury and repair, only 6% of the papers reported any data related to functional behavioral assessments—despite the meeting's focus on "recovery of function." Even in the area of brain tissue transplantation, only about 10% of published reports addressed functional and behavioral recovery: the vast majority of papers emphasized biochemical or anatomical changes following intracerebral grafts under the assumption that growth and/or increase in neurotransmitters are necessarily good.

Conceptual development, requiring detailed behavioral assessment, the hallmark of experimental neuropsychology, has given way to an emphasis on localized molecular structure and function. Indeed, the state-of-the-art in behavioral work associated with treatment for recovery from injury was stated clearly by the authors of a best-selling neuropharmacology textbook. Cooper, Bloom, and Roth (1986) stated that: "at the molecular level, an explanation of the action of a drug is often possible, at the cellular level, an explanation is sometimes possible, but at a behavioral level, our ignorance is abysmal" (p. 4).

Current imaging techniques lend themselves to focusing on the tree instead of the forest, and emphasize localization of various activities in response to injury rather than a more systemic change occurring throughout the brain as it undergoes the process of reorganization and repair. In metabolic studies, investigators often focus only on the most intense alterations observed during a given behavior or after an injury. They may ignore the overall pattern and interplay of less intense changes that occur both in the affected hemisphere and on the side contralateral to the injury. Several recent positron emission tomography (PET) studies of regional cerebral blood flow in patients recovering from stroke (Chollet et al., 1991; Weiller, Chollet, Friston, Wise, & Frackowiak, 1992) demonstrated significantly different patterns of activation from those of normal subjects. Importantly, the patterns are shown to be evoked in numerous brain structures involving the whole brain, not just in a few structures to which the deficit might be thought to be "localized."

The elucidation of the mechanisms underlying traumatic brain injury and repair will come from a merging of the findings of molecular biology and neurochemistry concerning alterations in the whole brain with data from intensive behavioral testing in both human and animal models. To understand the subtleties of CNS mechanism and repair, we will need to look carefully at molecular and "localized" findings in conjunction with concomitant distal alterations. Also, we must evaluate these findings in the light of their observed effects on multiple standardized behavioral tasks.

There have been major advances over the last decade. Although specific pharmacologic treatments for brain injuries are not yet on the market, we now have a much broader understanding of the mechanics and genetics of metabolism and chemical activity in neurons and glial cells. This new information has led to a burst of preclinical research activity to develop new substances designed to treat brain injury. In fact, in the past 5 years, there has been a dramatic increase in the number of new biotechnology companies whose specific purpose is to develop new drugs for treating brain injury (e.g., Cephalon, Interneuron, Cortex, Regeneron, etc.).

Only a short time ago, most research on the pharmacology of CNS plasticity was directed to the study of describing how neurons regulate the release and metabolism of neurotramsmitters, whose loss or return was the *sine qua non* for restitution of function. More recent efforts in this field now stress the discovery and characterization of new agents that modulate both neuronal and glial activity under normal and disrupted conditions. Much more emphasis is being placed on the discovery of receptors on both neurons and glial cells and their interdependence in neurotransmitter and neuropeptide release (Barres, 1991; Teichberg, 1991; Martin, 1992), in responses that can influence how the nervous system adapts to environmental conditions and to trauma.

With respect to the development of a specific pharmacology of recovery from brain damage over the last decade, we believe that there were several fundamentally important areas of research that had impact. First, it was confirmed that amino acids involved in CNS metabolism also might serve as neurotransmitters in their own right. In fact, Cooper et al. (1986) argued that: "from a quantitative standpoint (i.e., amounts present in the brain), the amino acids are probably the major neurotransmitters in the mammalian CNS, while the better-known transmitters (acetylcholine, dopamine, etc.) probably account for transmission at only a small percentage of central synaptic sites" (p. 124).

Investigators soon found that the amino acids are not just important for regulation and control of neurotransmission under normal conditions. It was also determined that traumatic brain injury often results in the excessive release of excitatory amino acids such as glutamate. The term *excessive* is used because in higher amounts the same substances required for neural transmission become "toxic" and cause neural death (Faden, Demediuk, Panter, & Vink, 1989; Olney, 1978). Figure 2.1 is a diagram of some of the many events that take place almost immediately after a traumatic injury to the brain. This composite depicts events that produce much of the secondary destruction of neurons and their connections. The secondary effects of the injury outlined in Fig. 2.1 may actually be more respon-

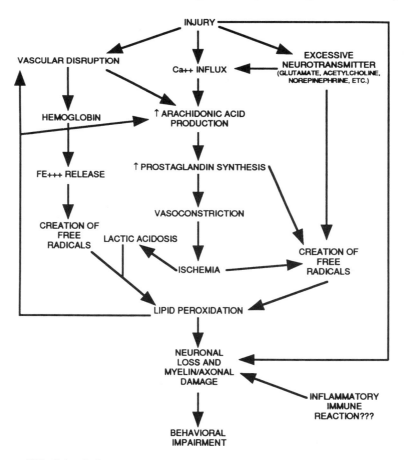

FIG. 2.1. A diagram demonstrating some of the early events that occur following traumatic brain injury. From "Inhibition of Lipid peroxidation in CNS trauma," by E. D. Hall, 1991, *Journal of Neurotrauma* 8, p. 32. Copyright © 1991 by Mary Ann Liebert, Inc. Adapted by permission.

sible for some of the behavioral deficits accompanying the trauma than the initial injury itself. In particular, stroke, ischemia, or direct injury to the brain produces a "glutamate cascade" culminating in an excess of calcium ions entering into vulnerable neurons and destroying them (for details of the process, see the review by Zivin & Choi, 1991).

Once the pathways for the excitotoxic effects had been determined at the beginning of the decade, it then became feasible to develop specific compounds that could be used to antagonize and block the excitotoxic cascade of events leading to cell death, and thus possibly preventing the loss of behavioral functions associated with the damage. For example, there are now agents available that block (antagonize) neuronal glutamate receptors and thus prevent calcium ion toxicity (Boast et al., 1988; McIntosh, Vink, Soares, Hayes, & Simon, 1990; Warner, Neill, Nadler, & Crain, 1991). The effects of these drugs are to reduce cerebral edema and the resultant necrosis of brain tissue, and to attenuate behavioral impairments.

Blocking some of the secondary destructive effects of ions and their toxic by-products, such as free radicals, promises to be a major step in the treatment of brain injury (McCall, Braughler, & Hall, 1987). By quenching the chain reactions initiated by these toxic compounds, CNS protection can be conferred at many different levels. Thus, the hope is to limit the chemical reactions that lead to the spread of secondary injury. The sites of free radical attack occur mainly in the lipid membranes of vascular endothelial cells, glia, and neurons, disrupting their structure and function. In the case of the endothelial cells, their disruption leads to the breakdown of the blood brain barrier (BBB), allowing many other generators of free radicals (such as iron, excitatory amino acids, and clotting factors) to enter the brain, causing edema and further tissue destruction (see Fig. 2.1). The disruption of the BBB can also expose the brain to autoimmune attack by blood macrophages. These inflammatory immune cells possess enzymes in their membranes that produce highly reactive free radicals that can severely damage cell membrane structure. Disruption of neuronal function can be caused by demyelination of axons as well as alterations of membrane fluidity affecting receptors and metabolic enzymes.

To block some of these destructive events, we have studied the effects of alpha tocopherol (vitamin E) on behavioral and anatomical recovery following aspiration injury to the frontal cortex in rats. Our results (Stein, Halks-Miller, & Hoffman, 1991) show that direct application of alpha tocopherol to the wound cavity produces both an increased rate of recovery on a learning task (see Fig. 2.2) and sparing of neuronal tissue (see Fig. 2.3), that is, higher neuronal counts, smaller ventricle size, and reduced gliosis. In another study by Clifton et al. (1989), the systemic administration of an alpha tocopherol derivative had significant protective effects when injected either before or after a fluid percussion injury of the cortex in rats.

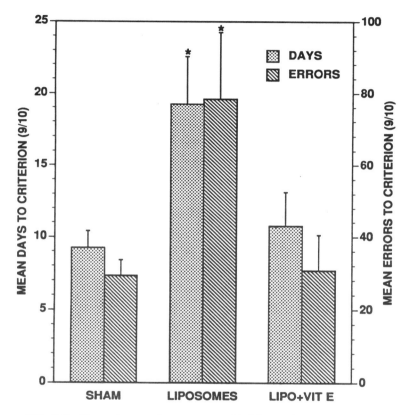

FIG. 2.2. Mean days and errors committed for each group to reach the criterion of 9/10 correct trials in the delayed spatial alternation task. The rats that received the vehicle-only (liposomes) treatments required significantly more days and committed significantly more errors than shams or rats that were treated with vitamin E (Lipo + VIT E) ($p < .05$). *Significantly different from shams and Lipo + VIT E ($p < .05$). From "Intracerebral administration of alpha-topopherol-containing liposomes facilies behavioral recovery in rats with bilateral lesions of the frontal cortex," by D. G. Stein, M. Halks-Miller, and S. W. Hoffman, 1991, *Journal of Neurotrauma, 8,* p. 286. Copyright © 1991 by Mary Ann Liebert, Inc. Adapted by permission.

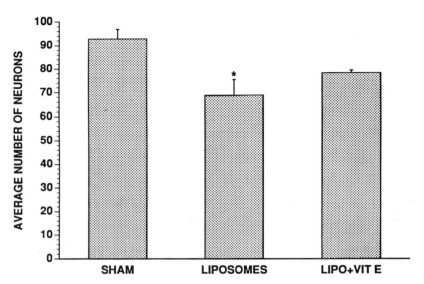

FIG. 2.3. Average number of neurons in the mediodorsal nucleus of the thalamus for each group. The sham controls had significantly more neurons than the rats that received vehicle only ($p < .05$), and the average number of neurons in the vitamin-E treated rats was intermediate to the two groups. *Significantly different from shams ($p < 0.05$). From "Intracerebral administration of alpha-topopherol-containing liposomes facilities behavioral recovery in rats with bilateral lesions of the frontal cortex," by D. G. Stein, M. Halks-Miller, and S. W. Hoffman, 1991, *Journal of Neuroutrauma, 8*, p. 286. Copyright © 1991 by Mary Ann Liebert, Inc. Adapted by permission.

This derivative significantly reduced the mortality rate and increased the rate of motor recovery. These two studies demonstrate the ability of vitamin E (as alpha tocopherol or a derivative) to alleviate deficits following traumatic insult to the brain. The advantages of working with this substance are that it is easily available, inexpensive, and, as far as is known, safe to use.

Another substance that is of plant origin and that has produced beneficial results in both clinical and experimental studies is EGb 761, an extract of the tree *Ginkgo biloba*. This substance consists of many different compounds called ginkgolides that have antioxidant properties and can inhibit the actions of substances that adversely affect the permeability of the blood brain barrier (Braquet et al., 1991; Oberpichler, Sauer, Rolfberg, & Mennel, 1990). In our laboratory, we have found that treatment with EGb 761 in rats given bilateral frontal cortex aspirations produced significant behavioral improvements on a spatial learning task (Attella, Hoffman, Stasio, & Stein, 1989). Rats given EGb 761 made fewer errors and perseverated less frequently to the incorrect side of a T-maze than their lesion-only counterparts, and they also showed more normal exploration behavior in an open-field maze. Anatomical analyses revealed that the treatment with EGb 761 reduced ventricular size, suggesting that EGb 761 prevented the development of cerebral edema. Recently, Brailowsky, Montiel, Hernandez-Echea-garay, Flores-Hernandez, and Hernandez-Pineda (1991) reported similar effects of EGb 761 in ameliorating the effects of cortical hemiplegia in rats with either motor cortex aspiration lesions or cortical depression produced by injection of gamma amino butyric acid (a neurotransmitter) into the brain. In the Brailowsky et al. experiments, both types of "injury" produced short-term deficits in motor behavior. In both injury models, chronic EGb 761 administration reduced the duration of the behavioral deficits, although the effects of the treatments were more clearly seen after the mechanical injury. Although this line of research is still quite new, it demonstrates that recovery from traumatic brain injury can be facilitated by administration of relatively benign, naturally occurring substances that pose little threat to the organism.

The second major step in understanding the mechanisms of recovery came with the discovery that, in response to damage, the brain secretes complex proteins, peptides, and hormones that are capable of directly stimulating the repair of damaged neurons (Barde, 1989; Cotman & Nieto-Sampedro, 1985; Kromer & Cornbrooks, 1987) or blocking some of the degenerative processes caused by the injury cascade. Substances that stimulate new neuronal growth or help to restore damaged membranes are called "neurotrophic factors." When they are extracted from the brain and placed into culture dishes containing neurons, they keep the cells from dying and actually promote growth of new processes called neurites. In vivo, trophic factors serve to guide regenerating or sprouting terminals to their appropriate target areas in the brain (Auburger, Heumann, Hellweg, Korsching, & Thoenen, 1987; Hefti, Hartikka, & Knusel, 1989; Korsching, 1986). Trophic factors appear to have their highest concentrations at or near sites of injury, and they reach their peak after about 1 week postinjury, thereafter declining in concentration and activity (Cotman & Nieto-Sampedro, 1985).

Some researchers have argued that injury-induced activation of specific glial cells is of primary importance in the production of neurotrophic factors after damage to the CNS (Gage, Olejniczak, & Armstrong, 1988). This hypothesis has resulted in consideration of the "beneficial" role of glia in promoting brain-injury repair and functional recovery. Although the eventual formation of a glial scar is thought to be detrimental to recovery, initial effects may be beneficial (Whitaker-Azmitia, Ramirez, Noreika, Gannon, & Azmitia, 1987). One suggested mechanism for a positive effect is through injury-induced activation of astrocytic glia cells, with subsequent expression and production of nerve growth factor (NGF), which promotes cholinergic sprouting responses (Fagan & Gage, 1990; Gage et al., 1988).

The discovery of endogenous, brain-derived, trophic factors, which appear to affect neural growth and viability, has led to the premise that some degenerative disorders such as Alzheimer's disease (AD) might be treatable with specific factors that selectively affect neurons known to figure importantly in systems that become dysfunctional. For example, it has been proposed that treatment with NGF might serve to alleviate a basal forebrain cholinergic deficit which may underlie the loss of cognitive function seen in AD (Hefti et al., 1989; Phelps et al., 1988). The potential for therapeutic use of these proteins has encouraged pharmaceutical and biotechnology companies to find ways to synthesize trophic factors or genetically engineer cells that can be raised and modified in culture and that are capable of producing commercial quantities of substance that might be needed by an injured brain. Altered cells could replace not only trophic factors, but also neurotransmitters or hormones, which could then be provided to patients on a regular basis (Bredesen, Hisanaga, & Sharp, 1990; Chen et al., 1991; Gage, Kawaja, & Fisher, 1991). For example, recent intracerebral application of genetically modified fibroblast cells expressing NGF (Rosenberg et al., 1988) prevented degeneration in 92% of cholinergic neurons subjected to fimbria fornix lesion.

However, we must emphasize that there are grounds for caution, and especially for further research in animals, before treatments can be applied to humans. Pressure from special interest groups and seriously ill patients who (understandably) demand rapid application before all the facts are in has led to clinical trials occurring before the long-term effects of treatments have been determined in the laboratory. An example of this approach is the attempt to provide intracerebral injections of NGF directly to patients with AD. To date, there is no effective way to arrest the cognitive deterioration of these patients. It has been suggested (Butcher & Woolf, 1989) that AD may be initiated by changes in regulatory mechanisms that are responsible for sequential expression of cytoskeletal protein in neurons normally exhibiting structural plasticity. In this hypothesis, certain proteins providing cytoskeletal stabilization are negatively affected, whereas normally labile proteins remain active. The result of this process is postulated to be a cascade of neural abnormalities, reactive gliosis, and eventual neural degeneration. Thus, the putative breakdown in plasticity components and loss of effectiveness of stable cytoskeletal proteins leads to the occurrence of neurofibrillary placques and tangles in AD brains, which are associated with resultant cognitive loss. From this perspective, NGF therapy could exacerbate the abnormal growth, and drugs that block NGF synthesis or NGF receptors would be more beneficial in the early stages of AD. These ideas can be taken to suggest that treatments entirely appropriate for one type of injury, such as trauma, or at one stage of development (e.g., young adults) might be completely contraindicated for treatment of other diseases, such as degenerative disorders, or under other conditions (e.g., aged subjects).

Despite the clear need for caution in extrapolating from preclinical studies to the human patient, there are several promising lines of research on the use of trophic factors to promote functional recovery from a variety of traumatic brain injuries. For example, in our laboratory, we have identified and employed experimental substances that: (a) are effective in the early stages of the injury process; (b) are naturally occurring substances that do not appear to have toxic side effects, even at relatively high doses; (c) can pass the BBB, and thus can be repeatedly administered systemically rather than intracerebrally; and (d) have identifiable physiological or histological/anatomical correlates that can be measured and quantified.

In addition to the use of alpha tocopherol and EGb 761, we have also used a synthetic portion of the peptide hormone ACTH as treatment for brain injury. Adrenocorticotropin plays a role in stimulating the adrenal gland to produce corticosteroids, which, in turn, affect vital functions such as energy metabolism, fluid regulation, and response to stress. ACTH fragments also have been used to enhance cognition and reverse deficits after brain damage (De Weid, 1966; Wolterink, Van Zanten, Kamsteeg, Radhakishun, & Van Ree, 1990a, 1990b). At the physiological level, Richter-Landsberg, Bruns, and Flohr (1987) showed that ACTH fragments promote neurite growth in vitro, so it was reasonable to suppose that a similar compound might protect neurons that would ordinarily die as a consequence of frontal cortex lesions. Further, Strand, Rose, King, Segarra, and Zuccarelli (1989) found that different ACTH analogs had the ability to facilitate the regeneration of peripheral nerve, offering the possibility that these compounds could initiate repair in the damaged CNS. We reasoned further that such protection would also result in behavioral recovery on a spatial learning task, where severe impairment is shown after frontal cortex injury. In our experiments, we used BIM-22015 (which is a structural analog of ACTH$_{4-10}$), injected subcutaneously. Our research indicated that BIM-22015 increased the rate of behavioral recovery on a spatial learning task, and the improved performance was accompanied by the sparing of cholinergic neurons in the nucleus basalis magnocellularis (Attela, Hoffman, Pilotte, & Stein, 1992). Positive behavioral effects of other ACTH analogs were also demonstrated by Wolterink et al. (1990a, 1990b) after chemical lesions to the nucleus accumbens. Their results indicated that the behavioral recovery was not a function of increased activity in the dopaminergic system, but rather of the increased sensitivity of dopamine receptors, which increased the efficiency of the remaining synapses. Recently, Goldman, Morehead, Hazlett, and Murphy (1992) reported that their analog GMM$_2$ increased cerebral blood flow and decreased vascular permeability, thus decreasing intracranial pressure after closed-head injury in rats. However, all of these studies support a role for ACTH analogs in the treatment of head injury, but, as in the case of vitamin E, the beneficial effects of ACTH analog therapy were more pronounced when the treatment was given soon after the injury.

Our laboratory has also utilized ganglioside GM1, an endogenous glycolipid, in treatment for several types of brain injury. Systemic injections of gangliosides to rats with lesions of the caudate nucleus resulted in a significant reduction of impairment in a battery of behavioral tests designed to reveal the deficits shown by untreated rats with this injury (Sabel, Slavin, & Stein, 1984a). Anatomical analysis of these subjects revealed early enhancement of neuronal reorganization with treatment (Sabel, Dunbar, & Stein, 1984b), a finding similar to the results of GM1 treatment after nigrostriatal lesion, where reduction of neuronal degeneration was seen (Sabel, DelMastro, Dunbar, & Stein, 1987). Systemic administration of GM1 has been shown to ameliorate behavioral deficits after discrete lesion of a diverse number of brain regions (Elliot, Garofalo, & Cuello, 1989; Schengrund, 1990; Walsh, Emerich, & Schmechel, 1989; Weihmuller, Hadjiconstantinou, Bruno, & Neff, 1988). In an exciting recent finding, GM1 treatment was given to nonhuman primates with 1-methyl-4-phenyl-1,2,3,6-tetrahydropyridine (MPTP)-induced parkinsonian syndrome (PS; Schneider et al., 1992). Not only were dopaminergic levels significantly increased over untreated animals, but also the acute motor problems characterizing PS were ameliorated.

Although an understanding of the mechanisms of gangliosides' action in normal and in injured tissue is not yet complete, they have been implicated in a number of roles. A partial listing includes modulation of neural regeneration (Feeney & Sutton, 1987; Sabel et al., 1984b), possible inhibition of lipid peroxidation (Tyurin, Tyurina, & Avrova, 1992), membrane stabilization (Fass & Ramirez, 1984; Karpiak, 1983), and protection of ion pumps and channels found in the cell membrane (for reviews, see Karpiak, Mahadik, & Wakade, 1990;

Schengrund, 1990). Additionally, current research is exploring a possible involvement of gangliosides in modulation of endogenous growth factors, such as NGF or epidermal growth factor (EGF; Bremer, Schlessinger, & Hakomori, 1986; Di Patre, Casamenti, Cenni, & Pepeu, 1989; Schengrund, 1990).

Because the injury cascade takes place over time and always in the context of the organism's environment, health status, individual learning, and emotional history, these variables, in addition to pharmacologic treatment, will play an important role in determining the success or failure of any medical or psychological therapy. It is also becoming increasingly clear that gender may be a significant contributing factor to the processes of cerebral plasticity and any concomitant recovery that can occur in response to brain damage. Gender considerations may also be important in determining the appropriate course of pharmacological therapy for brain damage because the response to drug/hormone interactions may be very different for males and females or for pre- or postmenopausal females. There are virtually no clinical studies in this area, although gender-related differences in response to injury have been shown (Loy & Milner, 1990; Wan-Hua, 1982), and a relationship between the hormonal status of females at the time of brain injury and the severity of the deficit has been demonstrated (Attella, Nattinville, & Stein, 1987).

As researchers have learned more about the complexity of the injury–recovery cycle, awareness of the injury continuum has been growing. Especially in CNS injury, an initial insult has not only immediate consequences, but also results in differing morphological and chemical alterations at later stages after injury. Thus, researchers have begun to focus on the different stages of the injury process to determine which specific agents might be most effective in blocking neuronal loss and functional impairments and when they need to be administered. As mentioned earlier, a substance indicated for treatment in an early stage of the injury process might be ineffective, or actually counterproductive, at a later stage. For example, the potential for survival of striatal transplants into damaged cortical tissue coincides with the period of peak, endogenous, trophic factor expression (Nieto-Sampedro, Manthrope, Barbin, Varon, & Cotman, 1983). Recent research also speaks to the issue of importance of matching administration of treatment to the stage of injury. When diazepam (a GABAergic agonist) was given to rats for several weeks after specific brain injuries, neural degeneration was markedly enhanced and no behavioral recovery could be observed at any time during the testing period, whereas animals not given diazepam were able to show normal recovery within a week after injury (Schallert, Hernandez, & Barth, 1986; Schallert,

Jones, & Lindner, 1990). Importantly, continued administration of diazepam for 3 weeks, begun immediately after injury, prevented behavioral recovery for 3 months (the length of the experiment), although the treatment had been discontinued (Schallert et al., 1986). It is quite possible that diazepam begun later in the continuum of the injury would have a differing effect. It is worthwhile noting that diazepam or its related compounds are often given to patients with stroke or CNS trauma, immediately after injury, to reduce postinjury agitation and to help "stabilize" them. Therefore, we must consider that proper treatments require more complex tailoring to the individual needs of the subject. We must consider not only the type of injury, but also its projected time course and the pharmacological consequences of multiple, successive CNS alterations.

In discussing trends and developments in research on recovery of function, we must also mention the worldwide interest in experiments using fetal brain tissue grafts to enhance recovery from CNS injury (there are many reviews available for the reader to consult; e.g., Bjorklund, 1991; Bjorklund & Gage, 1985; Buzsaki & Gage, 1988). Although the use of embryonic brain-tissue grafts has a long history (see Bjorklund & Stenevi, 1985 for details), the major developments in this area began in the late 1970s. The method is attractive in its initial simplicity, as embryonic brain cells can be harvested in solid pieces or in suspensions and then placed directly into the host's zone of injury. Both cell suspensions and solid blocks of fetal tissue will survive in the host brain for extended periods (McLoon, McLoon, Chang, Steedman, & Lund, 1985; Bredesen et al., 1990). Although in some cases "similar" membrane properties and "near normal" patterns of synaptic activity have been reported (Clarke, Nilsson, Brundin, & Bjorklund, 1990; Mudrick, Bainbridge, & Peet, 1989), in most cases the reciprocal connections established do not replicate normal cytoarchitecture (Mufson, Labbe, & Stein, 1986; Stein & Mufson, 1987).

Within the last 5 years, a large number of reports have been published in which the neuroanatomy and neurochemistry of the graft–host interactions have been examined. In animal models, embryonic brain-tissue grafts have been successful, for the most part, in reducing (but not completely eliminating) sensory, motor, and cognitive deficits caused by traumatic injury to the adult brain. For example, our laboratory showed that, in contrast to brain-injured rats without grafts, implants of fetal frontal cortex into the damaged medial frontal cortex grew successfully during the course of the experiment and significantly reduced the number of trials needed to attain criterion in a spatial learning task (Labbe, Firl, Mufson, & Stein, 1983).

Transplant research captured the public's attention when neurosurgeons attempted to use implanted portions of a patient's own adrenal gland to supply a precursor of dopamine and thus reduce some of the symptoms associated with Parkinson's disease. Later, Scandinavian and Mexican physicians (Backlund, Granberg, & Hamberger, 1985; Madrazo, Drucker-Colin, & Diaz, 1987) used human fetal tissue in an attempt to ameliorate the rigidity seen in the later stages of this disorder. Attempts to use grafts as potential therapy have continued, although the results have been very mixed and follow-up studies generally have been of rather short duration (Freed, Poltorak, & Becker, 1990; Goetz, Olanow, & Koller, 1989; Lindvall et al., 1990; Madrazo et al., 1987). In the United States, there is a great deal of controversy concerning the use of fetal tissue in research, particularly against the use of aborted fetuses for the purposes of obtaining tissue for any treatment conditions.

As a result of adverse publicity and the current lack of U.S. government support for fetal research, investigators have turned to the use of genetically engineered cells, as mentioned earlier, in connection with NGF therapy. Such research, employing state-of-the-art techniques in molecular biology, attracts considerable interest in the biotechnology community because of the commercial potential of developing patentable (and perhaps profitable) cells for clinical use. Although genetically engineered cells circumvent some of the problems involved in finding suitable fetal tissue, they are subject to several risks inherent in transplant work. The possibilities of tumorigenicity and/or the immune rejection of tissue placed into the compromised (damaged) brain are still present.

As a spin off of the fetal tissue research, investigators are now seeking ways to encapsulate cells (neurons, glia, or fibroblasts) that have been engineered to produce substances needed for repair (Hoffman, Wahlberg, & Aebishcher, 1990). The encapsulation in special kinds of plastic polymers allows for the slow release of small molecules from the grafts into the host brain, which could provide a steadier, more quantifiable application, and, in the absence of introduced cells, be less susceptible to an immune response. These techniques are not yet available for clinical use, and they still pose more of a risk than any systemic administration of pharmacological agents. Nonetheless, this work represents an exciting marriage between biotechnology and basic neuroscience. Even though there are considerable clinical problems to face, the use of grafts as research tools can result in a better understanding of (a) how the damaged brain attempts to repair itself, (b) what signals are necessary to initiate the process, and (c) what processes determine the growth and guidance of immature cells placed into the damaged adult brain.

CONCLUSIONS

Defining Recovery

Although we have learned a great deal about the cascade of events and processes we now call "brain injury," and although we have made great strides in developing new pharmacological agents to modify and control these events, there are still considerable gaps in our knowledge of functional recovery.

Although much has been written about functional recovery, workers in this field still do not have a clear and precise definition of what is meant by this term. This was true at the time of the last Copenhagen meeting, and it is still true now. Because the time course of functional recovery may be very long, or the functional recovery may be incomplete or result in different behaviors than in the premorbid state, who should define *recovery* and what criteria should be used? Physicians, social workers, the families of patients, insurers, and employers will all have their own standards for recovery, based on different needs. In deciding the criteria for adequate functional recovery, optimum medical practice may be overshadowed by economic, political, and social considerations.

Defining the Injury

As we noted previously, there is a complex series of events that occur following brain injury. However, the nature of these events may differ in a variety of ways from one type of injury to another. For example, some injuries, like contusions, may cause extensive disruption of the BBB (e.g., closed-head injury) and may leave the brain open to immunological attack. This immunological response can result in increased edema, demyelination, and neuronal death. In those injuries that leave the BBB more or less intact, as is the case with excitotoxic lesions, there may be a cascade that is less diffuse and extensive, consequently producing a more localized injury requiring less complex or extended treatment. The type of injury sustained will determine what specific pharmacologic agents should be used, and when they should be employed in the injury–recovery cycle. Case management in the early stage must include a careful and detailed evaluation of the injury, and define the most effective treatments to employ.

Evaluating the Outcome of Rehabilitation and Therapy

Whether rehabilitation therapy takes the form of pharmacological manipulation of the CNS, behavioral modification techniques, or some combination of both, there must be detailed and comprehensive follow-up evaluations of functional outcomes. Carefully planned studies should be developed in collaboration with the various specialists involved in the therapeutic program. It is necessary to compare distinct components of the treatments to determine which are most effective and which can be eliminated. Standards for measurement of clinical outcomes should be agreed on by the rehabilitation community and applied in a manner that can demonstrate that the techniques do, in fact, improve functional outcome, and that they meet the criteria for reliability (replicability) and validity (can be shown to make a difference).

The question of validating treatment methods is related to the issue of developing meaningful and consistently employed measures of functional recovery—issues that have yet to be resolved by rehabilitation specialists. Given the high costs of extended treatment for the brain-injured patient, it is unlikely that social agencies or companies providing payment for services will continue to do so unless they can be assured that the professional medical/rehabilitation program works better than some nonprofessional services that are far less costly (e.g., using paramedical or social work staff).

When Is It Appropriate to Begin Treatment?

If we have learned anything about treating brain injury over these last years, it is that therapy to promote functional recovery must begin as soon as possible after the initial trauma. Delaying the course of treatment to observe how much "spontaneous recovery" is likely to occur, will, in most cases, result in permanent impairments. For example, inflammatory reactions, edema, production of free radicals, and excess excitatory amino acids must be eliminated before growth-promoting and regenerating factors can take effect. At the same time, psychological and social rehabilitation should begin as soon as the patient can tolerate this type of environmental stimulation.

What Is the Appropriate Course of Therapy?

There is a principle in neuroscience that states that unless recovery occurs within a relatively short time after injury, there will be no recovery at all. Unless one is very fortunate, it is also the case that combinations of therapeutic agents will be needed to treat the various syndromes that are produced by traumatic brain injury. In the research laboratory, we examine single agents to determine what specific physiological mechanisms are associated with the functional recovery. As different pharmacological agents are identified, it may be necessary to combine agents to produce maximum beneficial effects. Additionally, as more is learned about the continuum of changes that occur after an initial insult to the CNS, we will be better able to alter treatment to coincide with a "window of efficacy." These fields of research have yet to be adequately developed.

Although it is true that a long course of medical and psychosocial therapy may be expensive, it may nonetheless be necessary if true functional recovery is the goal. Such therapy must be conducted in a positive, caring, and enriched environment. Close cooperation and coordination of treatments among neurologists, physiatrists, and rehabilitation psychologists should be the norm and the standard in the field of restorative neurology. Based on what we know from experiments in laboratory animals (Finger, 1978; Finger & Stein, 1982; Held, Gordon, & Gentile, 1985; Kelche, Dalrymple-Alford & Will, 1988; Will, Rosenzweig, Bennett, Hebert, & Morimoto, 1977), environmental enrichment, coupled with appropriate pharmacological treatments, may hold out the best hope for functional recovery in severely brain-injured patients, but only if one is prepared to invest the necessary time and effort to accomplish this goal.

In conclusion, there is no doubt that those concerned with basic research in restorative neuroscience have made great progress in opening new lines of inquiry and developing a better understanding of the injury and recovery process. Following the great strides in molecular biology, many research laboratories and pharmaceutical companies are identifying or developing new agents capable of protecting the nervous system. To paraphrase a famous Dane, we are closer than ever before to protecting brain-injured patients from "the slings and arrows of outrageous fortune" to which they are often heir.

REFERENCES

Attella, M. J., Hoffman, S. W., Pilotte, M. P., & Stein, D. G. (1992). Effects of BIM-22015, an analog of $ACTH_{4-10}$, on functional recovery after frontal cortex injury. *Behavioral and Neural Biology, 57*, 157–166.

Attella, M. J., Hoffman, S. W., Stasio, M. J., & Stein, D. G. (1989). Ginkgo biloba extract facilitates recovery from penetrating brain injury in adult male rats. *Experimental Neurology, 105*, 62–71.

Attella, M. J., Nattinville, A., & Stein, D. G. (1987). Hormonal state affects recovery from frontal cortex lesions in adult female rats. *Behavioral and Neural Biology, 48*, 352–367.

Auburger, G. R., Heumann, R., Hellweg, S., Korsching, S., & Thoenen, H. (1987). Developmental changes of nerve growth factor and its mRNA in the rat hippocampus: Comparison with choline acetyltransferase. *Developmental Biology, 120*, 322–328.

Backlund, E.-O., Granberg, P.-O., & Hamberger, B. (1985). Transplantation of adrenal medullary tissue to striatum in parkinsonism. First clinical trials. *Journal of Neurosurgery, 62,* 169–173.

Barde, Y.-A. (1989). Trophic factors and neuronal survival: Review. *Neuron, 2,* 1525–1534.

Barres, B. A. (1991). New roles for glia. *Journal of Neuroscience, 11,* 3685–3694.

Bjorklund, A. (1991). Neural transplantation—an experimental tool with clinical possibilities. *Trends in Neuroscience, 14,* 319–322.

Bjorklund, A., & Gage, F. H. (1985). Neural grafting in animal models of neurode generative diseases. *Annals of New York Academy Science, 457,* 53–81.

Bjorklund, A., & Stenevi, U. (1985). Intracerebral neural grafting: A historical perspective. In A. Bjorklund & U. Stenevi (Eds.), *Neural grafting in the mammalian CNS* (pp. 3–14). New York: Elsevier.

Boast, C. A., Gerhardt, S. C., Pastor, G., Lehmann, J., Etienne, P. E., & Liebman, J. M. (1988). The N-methyl-D-aspartate antagonists CGS 19755 and CPP reduce ischemic brain damage in gerbils. *Brain Research, 442,* 345–348.

Brailowsky, S., Montiel, T., Hernandez-Echeagaray, E., Flores-Hernandez, J., & Hernandez-Pineda, R. (1991). Effects of a Ginkgo biloba extract on two models of cortical hemiplegia in rats. *Restorative Neurology and Neuroscience, 3,* 267–274.

Braquet, P., Esanu, A., Buisine, E., Hosford, D., Broquet, C., & Koltai, M. (1991). Recent progress in ginkgolide research. *Medical Research Reviews, 11,* 295–355.

Bredesen, D. E., Hisanaga, K., & Sharp, F. R. (1990). Neural transplantation using temperature-sensitive immortalized neural cells: A preliminary report. *Annals of Neurology, 27,* 205–207.

Bremer, E. G., Schlessinger, J., & Hakomori, S.-I. (1986). Ganglioside-mediated modulation of cell growth. Specific effects of GM3 on tyrosine phosphorylation of the epidermal growth factor receptor. *Journal of Biological Chemistry, 261,* 2434–2440.

Butcher, L. L., & Woolf, N. J. (1989). Neurotrophic agents may exacerbate the pathologic cascade of Alzheimer's Disease, *Neurobiology of Aging, 10,* 557–570.

Buzsaki, G., & Gage, F. H. (1988). Mechanisms of action of neural grafts in the limbic system. *Canadian Journal of Neurological Science, 15,* 99–105.

Chen, L. S., Ray, J., Fisher, L. J., Kawaja, M. D., Schinstine, M., Kang, U. J., & Gage, F. H. (1991). Cellular replacement therapy for neurologic disorders: Potential of genetically engineered cells. *Journal of Cellular Biochemistry, 45,* 252–257.

Chollet, F., DiPiero, V., Wise, R. J. S., Brooks, D. J., Dolan, R. J., & Frackowiak, R. S. J. (1991). The functional anatomy of motor recovery after stroke in humans: A study with positron emission tomography. *Annals of Neurology, 29,* 63–71.

Clarke, D. J., Nilsson, O. G., Brundin, P., & Bjorklund, A. (1990). Synaptic connections formed by grafts of different types of cholinergic neurons in the host hippocampus. *Experimental Neurology, 107,* 11–22.

Clifton, G. L., Lyeth, B. G., Jenkins, L. W., Taft, W. C., DeLorenzo, R. J., & Hayes, R. L. (1989). Effect of D,alpha-tocopheryl succinate and polyethylene glycol on performance tests after fluid percussion brain injury. *Journal of Neurotrauma, 6,* 71–81.

Cooper, J. R., Bloom, F. E., & Roth, R. H. (1986). *The biochemical basis of Neuropharmacology.* New York: Oxford University Press.

Cotman, C. W., & Nieto-Sampedro, M. (1985). Progress in facilitating the recovery of function after central nervous system trauma. *Annals of New York Academy of Science, 457,* 83–104.

De Weid, D. (1966). Inhibitory effects of ACTH and related peptides in extinction of conditioned avoidance behavior in rats. *Proceedings for the Society of Experimental Biology and Medicine, 122,* 28–36.

Di Patre, P. L., Casamenti, F., Cenni, A., & Pepeu, G. (1989). Interaction between nerve growth factor and GM1 monosialoganglioside in preventing cortical choline acetyltransferase and high affinity choline uptake decrease after lesion of the nucleus basalis. *Brain Research, 480,* 219–224.

Elliott, P. J., Garofalo, L., & Cuello, A. C. (1989). Limited neocortical devascularizing lesions causing deficits in memory retention and choline acetyltransferase activity—effects of the monosialoganglioside GM1. *Neuroscience, 31,* 63–76.

Faden, A. I., Demediuk, P., Panter, S. S., & Vink, R. (1989). The role of excitatory amino acids and NMDA receptors in traumatic brain injury. *Science, 244,* 799–800.

Fagan, A. M., & Gage, F. H. (1990). Cholinergic sprouting in the hippocampus: A proposed role for IL-1. *Experimental Neurology, 110,* 105–120.

Fass, B., & Ramirez, J. (1984). Effects of ganglioside treatments on lesion induced behavioral impairment and sprouting in the CNS. *Neuroscience Research, 12,* 445–458.

Feeney, D. M., & Sutton, R. L. (1987). Pharmacology for recovery of function after brain injury. *Critical Reviews in Neurobiology, 3,* 135–197.

Finger, S. (1978). Environmental attenuation of brain lesion symptoms. In S. Finger (Ed.), *Recovery from brain damage: Research and theory* (pp. 297–329). New York: Plenum.

Finger, S., & Stein, D. G. (1982). Fast- versus slow-growing lesions and behavioral recovery. In *Brain damage and recovery: Research and clinical perspectives* (pp. 153–173). New York: Academic Press.

Freed, W. J., Poltorak, M., & Becker, J. B. (1990). Intracerebral medulla grafts: A review. *Experimental Neurology, 110,* 139–166.

Gage, F. H., Kawaja, M. D., & Fisher, L. J. (1991). Astrocytes are important for sprouting in the septohippocampal circuit. *Experimental Neurology, 102,* 2–13.

Gage, F. H., Olejniczak, P., & Armstrong, D. M. (1988). Astrocytes are important for sprouting in the septohippocampal circuit. *Experimental Neurology, 102,* 2–13.

Goetz, C. G., Olanow, C. W., & Koller, W. C. (1989). Multicenter study of autologous adrenal medullary transplantation to the corpus striatum in patients with advanced Parkinson's Disease. *New England Journal of Medicine, 320,* 337–341.

Goldman, H., Morehead, M., Hazlett, J., & Murphy, S. (1992). An ACTH analog minimizes brain injury in a rat model. *Journal of Neurotrauma, 9,* 60.

Hall, E. D. (1991). Inhibition of Lipid peroxidation in CNS trauma. *Journal of Neurotrauma 8*(1), 31–41.

Hefti, F., Hartikka, J., & Knusel, B. (1989). Function of neurotrophic factors in the adult and aging brain and their possible use in the treatment of neurodegenerative diseases. *Neurobiology of Aging, 10,* 515–533.

Held, J. M., Gordon, J., & Gentile, A. M. (1985). Environmental influences on locomotor recovery following cortical lesions in rats. *Behavioral Neuroscience, 99,* 678–690.

Hoffman, D., Wahlberg, L., & Aebishcher, P. (1990). NGF released from a polymer matrix prevents loss of ChAT expression in basal forebrain neurons following a fimbria fornix lesion. *Experimental Neurology, 110,* 39–44.

Kandel, E. R., Schwartz, J. H., & Jessell, T. M. (1991). *Principles of neural science (3rd ed.).* New York: Elsevier.

Karpiak, S. E. (1983). Ganglioside treatment improves recovery of alternation behavior after unilateral entorhinal cortex lesion. *Experimental Neurology, 81,* 330–339.

Karpiak, S. E., Mahadik, S. P., & Wakade, C. G. (1990). Ganglioside reduction of ischemic injury. *Critical Reviews in Neurobiology, 5,* 221–237.

Kelche, C., Dalrymple-Alford, J. C., & Will, B. (1988). Housing conditions modulate the effects of intracerebral grafts in rats with brain lesion. *Behavioral Brain Research, 28,* 287–295.

Korsching, S. (1986). The role of nerve growth factor in the CNS. *Trends in Neuroscience, 9,* 570–573.

Kromer, L. F., & Cornbrooks, C. J. (1987). Identification of trophic factors and transplanted cellular environments that promote CNS axonal regeneration. *Annals of New York Academy of Science, 495,* 207–225.

Labbe, R., Firl, A., Jr., Mufson, E. J., & Stein, D. G. (1983). Fetal brain transplants: Reduction of cognitive deficits in rats with frontal cortex lesions. *Science, 221,* 470–472.

Lindvall, O., Brunden, P., Widner, H., Rehncrona, S., Gustavii, B., Frackowiak, R., Leenders, K. L., Sawle, G., Rothwell, J. C., Marsden, C. D., & Bjorklund, A. (1990). Grafts of fetal dopamine neurons survive and improve motor function in Parkinson's disease. *Science, 247,* 574–577.

Loy, R., & Milner, T. A. (1990). Sexual dimorphism in extent of axonal sprouting in rat hippocampus. *Science, 208,* 1282–1284.

Madrazo, I., Drucker-Colin, R., & Diaz, V. (1987). Open microsurgical autograft of adrenal medulla to the right caudate nucleus in two patients with intractale Parkinson's Disease. *New England Journal of Medicine, 318,* 51.

Martin, D. L. (1992). Synthesis and release of neuroactive substances by glial cells. *Glia, 5,* 81–94.

McCall, J. M., Braughler, J. M., & Hall, E. D. (1987). Lipid peroxidation and the role of oxygen radicals in CNS injury. *Acta Anaesthesiology (Belgium), 38,* 373–379.

McIntosh, R. K., Vink, R., Soares, H., Hayes, R., & Simon, R. (1990). Effect of non-competitive blockage of N-methyl-D-aspartate receptors on the neurochemical sequelae of experimental brain injury. *Journal Neurochemistry, 55,* 1170–1179.

McLoon, L. K., McLoon, S. C., Chang, F.-L. F., Steedman, J. G., & Lund, R. D. (1985). Visual system transplanted to the brain of rats. In A. Bjorklund & U. Stenevi (Eds.), *Neural grafting in the mammalian CNS* (pp. 267–283). New York: Elsevier.

Mudrick, L. A., Bainbridge, K. G., & Peet, M. J. (1989). Hippocampal neurons transplanted into ischemically lesioned hippocampus: Electroresponsiveness and reestablishment of circuitries. *Experimental Brain Research, 76,* 333–342.

Mufson, E. J., Labbe, R., & Stein, D. G. (1986). Morphologic features of embryonic neocortex grafts in adult rats following frontal cortical ablation. *Brain Research, 401,* 162–167.

Nieto-Sampedro, M., Manthrope, M., Barbin, G., Varon, S., & Cotman, C. W. (1983). Injury-induced neuronotrophic activity in adult rat brain: Correlation with survival of delayed implants in the wound cavity. *Journal of Neuroscience, 3,* 2219–2229.

Oberpichler, H., Sauer, D., Rolfberg, C., & Mennel, H.-D. (1990). PAF antagonist ginkgolide B reduces postischemic neuronal damage in rat brain hippocampus. *Journal of Cerebral Blood Flow and Metabolism, 10,* 133–135.

Olney, J. W. (1978). Neurotoxicity of excitatory amino acids. In E. G. McGeer, J. W. Olney, & P. L. McGeer (Eds.), *Kainate as a tool in neurobiology* (pp. 95–121). New York: Raven.

Phelps, C. H., Gage, F. H., Growdon, J. H., Hefti, F., Harbaugh, R., Johnston, M. V., Khachaturian, Z., Mobley, W., Price, D., Raskind, M., Simplins, J., Thal, L., & Woodcodk, J. (Ad Hoc Working Group on Nerve Growth Factor and Alzheimer's Disease). (1988). Potential use of nerve growth factor to treat Alzheimer's Disease. *Science, 243*, 11.

Richter-Landsberg, C., Bruns, I., & Flohr, H. (1987). ACTH neuropeptides influence development and differentiation of embryonic rat cerebral cells in culture. *Neuroscience Research Communications, 1*, 153–162.

Rosenberg, M. B., Friedmann, T., Robertson, R., Tuszynski, M., Wolff, J. A., Breakefield, L. O., & Gage, F. H. (1988). Grafting genetically modified cells to the damaged brain: Restorative effects of NGF expression. *Science, 242*, 1575–1578.

Sabel, B. A., DelMastro, R., Dunbar, G. L., & Stein, D. G. (1987). Reduction of anterograde degeneration in brain damaged rats by GM1-gangliosides. *Neuroscience Letters, 77*, 360–366.

Sabel, B. A., Slavin, M. D., & Stein, D. G. (1984a). GM1 ganglioside treatment facilitates behavioral recovery from bilateral brain damage. *Science, 225*, 340–342.

Sabel, B. A., Dunbar, G. L., & Stein, D. G. (1984b). Gangliosides minimize behavioral deficits and enhance structural repair after brain injury. *Journal of Neuroscience Research, 12*, 429–443.

Schallert, T., Hernandez, T. D., & Barth, T. M. (1986). Recovery of function after brain damage: Severe and chronic disruption by diazepam. *Brain Research, 379*, 104–111.

Schallert, T., Jones, R. A., & Lindner, M. D. (1990). Multilevel transneuronal degeneration after brain damage: Behavioral events and effects of anticonvulsant gamma-aminobutyric acid-related drugs. *Stroke, 21* (Suppl. III), 143–146.

Schengrund, C.-L. (1990). The role(s) of gangliosides in neural differentiation and repair: A perspective. *Brain Research Bulletin, 24*, 131–141.

Schneider, J. S., Pope, A., Simpson, K., Taggart, J., Smith, M. G., & DiStefano, L. (1992). Recovery from experimental parkinsonism in primates with GM1 ganglioside treatment. *Science, 256*, 843–846.

Stein, D. G. (1988). Contextual factors in recovery from brain injury. In A. Christensen & B. Uzzell (Eds.), *Neuropsychological rehabilitation* (pp. 1–18). Copenhagen: Munksgaard.

Stein, D. G., Halks-Miller, M., & Hoffman, S. W. (1991). Intracerebral administration of alpha-tocopherol-containing liposomes facilitates behavioral recovery in rats with bilateral lesions of the frontal cortex. *Journal of Neurotrauma, 8*, 281–292.

Stein, D. G., & Mufson, E. J. (1987). Morphological and behavioral characteristics of embryonic brain tissue transplants in adult, brain-damaged subjects. *Annals of the New York Academy of Science, 495*, 444–465.

Strand, F. L., Rose, K. J., King, J. A., Segarra, A. C., & Zuccarelli, L. A. (1989). ACTH modulation of nerve development and regeneration. *Progress in Neurobiology, 33*, 45–85.

Teichberg, V. I. (1991). Glial glutamate receptors: Likely actors in brain signaling. *FASEB, 5*, 3086–3091.

Tyurin, V. A., Tyurina, Y. Y., & Avrova, N. F. (1992). Ganglioside-dependent factor, inhibiting lipid peroxidation in rat brain synaptosomes. *Neurochemistry International, 20*, 401–407.

Walsh, T. J., Emerich, D. F., & Schmechel, D. E. (1989). GM1 ganglioside attenuates the behavioral deficits but not the granule cell damage produced by intradentate colchicine. *Brain Research, 478,* 24–33.

Wan-Hua, A. Y. (1982). Sex difference in the regeneration of the hypoglossal nerve. *Brain Research, 238,* 404–406.

Warner, M. A., Neill, K. H., Nadler, J. V., & Crain, B. J. (1991). Regionally selective effects of NMDA receptor antagonists against ischemic brain damage in the gerbil. *Journal of Cerebral Blood Flow and Metabolism, 11,* 600–610.

Weihmuller, F. B., Hadjiconstantinou, M., Bruno, J. P., & Neff, N. H. (1988). Administration of GM1 ganglioside eliminates neuroleptic-induced sensorimotor deficits in MPTP-treated mice. *Neuroscience Letters, 92,* 207–212.

Weiller, C., Chollet, F., Friston, K. J., Wise, R. J. S., & Frackowiak, R. S. J. (1992). Functional reorganization of the brain in recovery from striatocapsular infarction in man. *Annals of Neurology, 31,* 463–472.

Whitaker-Azmitia, P. M., Ramirez, A., Noreika, L., Gannon, P. J., & Azmitia, E. C. (1987). Onset and duration of astrocytic response to cells transplanted into the adult mammalian brain. *Annals of New York Academy of Science, 495,* 10–23.

Will, B. E., Rosenzweig, M. R., Bennett, E. L., Hebert, M., and Morimoto, H. (1977). Relatively brief environmental enrichment aids recovery of learning capacity and alters brain measures after postweaning brain lesions in rats. *Journal of Comparative Physiological Psychology, 91,* 33–50.

Wolterink, G., Van Zanten, E., Kamsteeg, H., Radhakishun, F. S., & Van Ree, J. M. (1990a). Functional recovery after destruction of dopamine systems in the nucleus accumbens of rats: II. Facilitation by the ACTH4-9 analog ORG 2766. *Brain Research, 507,* 101–108.

Wolterink, G., Van Zanten, E., Kamsteeg, H., Radhakishun, F. S., & Van Ree, J. M. (1990b). Functional recovery after destruction of dopamine systems in the nucleus accumbens of rats: III. Further analysis of the facilitating effect of the ACTH4-9 analog ORG 2766. *Brain Research, 507,* 109–114.

Zivin, J. A., & Choi, D. W. (1991, July). Stroke therapy. *Scientific American, 265,* 56–63.

CHAPTER THREE

Head Trauma Destiny: Interactions of Neuropharmacology and Personality

D. Nathan Cope

ABSTRACT

Much progress has occurred in the past 5 years in understanding the indications for and responsiveness to psychopharmacologic agents in the rehabilitation of traumatic brain-injured patients. There are definite therapeutic uses for these agents in a variety of syndromes, which have been thoroughly reviewed elsewhere. To date no formal integration of this technology advance into the overall rehabilitation plan has been made. This chapter presents such an integration and suggests that a more active role for psychopharmacologic agents is appropriate for multiple indications. Particularly overlooked in clinical practice is the use of these agents for disturbances of cognition. It is important to distinguish three distinct clinical phases of treatment of TBI: (a) emergent, (b) acute recovery, and (c) long-term or chronic phase. Each has its own risk–benefit aspects that must be considered in the decision to utilize psychopharmacologic approaches.

In keeping with the theme of a 5-year reappraisal of the state of traumatic brain injury (TBI) treatment, I begin by noting that in all significant cases, the patient is still consistently left with major functional disabilities despite the most aggressive treatment and the most optimal outcome. It is likely that some form of permanent residual also persists for minor brain injuries (which do not now routinely come to the attention of rehabilitation professionals) to some extent, although these disabilities are more subtle.

If the position of intervention, in its broadest sense, in the rehabilitation of TBI is acknowledged, is there a place for psychopharmacologic treatment? Conceptual thinking in psychopharmacologic approaches has recently come a substantial distance. Approximately 5–10 years ago, it was difficult to discern a coherent general philosophy of drug treatment in the clinical literature. Such treatment as was being provided appeared random in patient choice, confused in theoretical basis, and methodologically chaotic in application. Drugs were basically seen as agents of last resort in behavioral emergencies or extremes, not as a planned component of a rational rehabilitation program. To some extent, this still characterizes much of the pharmacologic care these patients receive when they come under the treatment of unsophisticated physicians. For those physicians who are students of this condition, however, there now are emerging clear initial nosologies of the various TBI syndromes correlated with their responsiveness to psychopharmacologic intervention. Specific clinical indications, drugs of first choice, dosage ranges, and side effects are all being increasingly delineated. Thus, a certain degree of consensus has developed over the past 5 years regarding appropriate indications for psychopharmacologic intervention in TBI. We are the initial stage of such scientific understanding, and a number of comprehensive reviews of these indications have recently appeared in the literature (Bleiberg, Cope, and Spector, 1989; Cassidy, 1990; Cope, 1989, 1990; Gualtieri, 1988, 1991; Zasler, 1992). This discussion does not intend to recapitulate the arguments and evidence presented in these very adequate surveys. A simple tabulation of the major current indications for psychopharmacologic treatment in TBI patients drawn from them is given in Table 3.1; reference to the original works is suggested for the interested clinician.

Rather, the point to be made in this discussion is one of appropriately integrating the clinical application of this emerging pharmacologic technology within the context of our current rehabilitation environment (i.e., technical, fiscal, administrative, and regulatory). No one disputes that drug treatments should always be undertaken only after consideration of this entire patient–environment context, yet, to my knowledge, to date no thorough consideration has been given in the literature to the specific implications of this interrelationship in today's health-care conditions.

The specific details of the discussion that follows are based on aspects of health-care delivery in the United States. To this extent, conclusions need careful interpretation by readers from other countries. However, the underlying conflicts between resource utilization and optimum,

TABLE 3.1
Clinical Indications for Psychopharmacologic Agents in TBI

Low Arousal
Aggression
Affective Disorders
  depression
  bipolar illness
  emotional incontinence
Psychoses
Frontal Syndrome(s)
General Cognitive Impairment
Amnestic Syndromes
Anxiety Disorders
Atypical Seizure Syndromes
Miscellaneous
  neurologic disorders
  appetite disturbances
  sexual disturbances

efficient patient care transcend national boundaries, thus the discussion should prove of interest to any reader with concern about high-quality, cost-effective care of these conditions.

INDICATIONS FOR PSYCHOPHARMACOLOGY

This fundamental problem of the proper "integration" of psychopharmacologic treatments into the overall rehabilitation context remains largely unexplored. Rehabilitation clinicians have historically had a fairly strong negative attitude toward the use of psychopharmacologic agents in the treatment of TBI. The potential for negative side effects and toxicities are certainly well appreciated. Many of the "targets" of psychopharmacologic intervention are traditionally viewed as secondary phenomena or consequent to the various "primary" functional losses and disabilities. Thus the proper rehabilitation management of a "depressed" TBI patient would be the fullest restoration of lost abilities and the psychologic reconstruction of an acceptable self-image and gratifying lifestyle. These goals are seen as being primarily achieved by the full application of rehabilitation and counseling techniques. It is only failing these remedies that antidepressants are felt to constitute a secondary treatment option. The behaviorally disordered (aggressive) patient is usually seen as responding to a confusing and often uncomfortable or even painful environment. Management is directed toward simplification and clarification of the environment (orientation programs, more simple repetitive communications, nonfrustrating demands, etc.). In fact, it is with some pride that sophisticated TBI programs declare that they do not have to "rely" on drugs to manage their difficult cases. It is only with the failure of these environmental or behavioral interventions that pharmacologic management is felt justified in most instances. In some of the most sophisticated behavioral management programs in the United States, many months, or even a year or more, will not uncharacteristically be spent in nonpharmacologic approaches to these problems before a pharmacologic alternative is ventured. For the most common and most disabling of TBI deficits, cognitive loss, the clinical standard is even more unidimensional in its reliance on "psychological" or "cognitive-retraining" approaches. Remediation of cognitive loss with drugs is essentially not ventured at all except in certain clearly experimental research settings.

In summary, when considering where research is currently regarding the treatment of cognitive, behavioral, and personality deficits following TBI, it is apparent that psychological treatment is the integral, and perhaps even the quintessential, feature of TBI treatment. This is without argument. The preponderance of rehabilitation treatment efforts are principally based on interventions at the level of "mind and experience," rather than directly on the altered neurophysiology of TBI. If we accurately describe the current status of psychopharmacologic treatment, although it is now accepted in concept and a variety of approaches or options are clearly known to exist for many TBI deficits, psychopharmacologic treatment is largely considered a secondary, or backup, option. Rather than being integrated into treatment planning, current psychopharmacologic treatments are afterthoughts. This limited application of psychopharmacologic treatment is curious, given the fundamentally organic or physiologic basis of TBI deficits, and it is the contention of this writer that this limited application is not what current evidence and logic would indicate most appropriate. There is no question that the deficits of TBI reflect altered neurophysiology rather than maladaptive experience. In addition to the obvious anatomical lesions of TBI, it is also known that there are long-standing alterations in major central nervous system neurotransmitter systems following TBI. One has only to contrast this withholding of serious neurophysiologic (pharmacologic) treatments with currently accepted approaches to other major mental or behavioral conditions (with even less evidence of fundamentally disordered underlying physiology; i.e., schizophrenia, major depression, obsessive–compulsive syndromes, and panic/anxiety disorders). In these conditions, treatment with psychoactive drugs is routine. Indeed, for most clinicians, the failure to appropriately utilize psychoactive agents in these situations would meet severe criticism on both clinical and economic (cost-efficiency) grounds, and can be the basis for malpractice action.

Consider the possible reasons why there has been and continues to be this lack of integration of pharmacologic measures into rehabilitation treatment approaches to TBI. First, the general effects of psychotropics are complex, and it is difficult to specify with certainty what the results of treatment in an individual patient may be. Second, there are clearly significant negative side effects and toxicities that may occur with drug use. Third, in the strictest scientific sense, data regarding efficacy are inadequate and, it could be argued, noncompelling; there simply are no large-scale, randomized, double-blinded studies of TBI populations such as characterize studies of conditions such as primary depression or bipolar illness. Fourth, there is the heightened litigiousness of our era, in which any innovation in treatment exposes the practitioner to legal suit. Major indications for drug use in other conditions were developed in a much more benign legal environment. Fifth, there is a clear lack of expertise by the physicians usually involved with TBI care. Rehabilitation physicians do not routinely have knowledge of psychopharmacologic techniques; psychiatrists and neurologists, who do have such expertise, do not usually become involved in, nor are they sensitive to, the functional recovery processes (the rehabilitation issues) of TBI. Beyond these distinctions among physician specialities and expertises lies the "dissonance" between medical and psychologic perspectives upon TBI care. Now only the physician possesses the knowledge and right to prescribe medication for these problems, whereas historically and in practice it has been the discipline of psychology that has led the way in the description and treatment of the cognitive and behavioral consequences of TBI. Given this scenario, it is perhaps not surprising that drugs have not been given a prominent place in treatment approaches to date. Of course, in considering this persistent absence of integration of pharmacologic treatments into TBI care, despite the numerous and increasing reports documenting the "positive" effects of psychopharmacologic interventions, it is also possible that the general treating physician and the patients (and patients' families) do not in actual practice find the benefits of drug treatment nearly so impressive and helpful as the research clinician and published reports would have us believe.

At this point, special mention should be made of the particular disregard that presently characterizes approaches to drug treatments for the "cognitive" disturbances of TBI. Cognitive deficits are most obvious in severe injuries, but mild–moderate injuries also create substantial cognitive deficits. In fact, these frequently are the only deficits. There is evidence that these milder patients would benefit from pharmacologic treatment as well. For example, Gualtieri (1988) opined about stimulant usage in these populations:

> Research has not advanced to the point where it is possible to predict *which* TBI patients should be treated with stimulant drugs. It is the authors' clinical impression, however, that the best response occurs in relatively high-level, mild to moderately impaired patients, with relatively circumscribed deficits in attention, memory, organization or initiative, and stimulants are currently indicated for TBI patients who have prominent symptoms of: (1) attention deficit/hyperactivity . . . (2) anergia/ apathy . . . (3) the frontal lobe syndrome. . . . (p. 106)

However, it appears justified to state that the magnitude of the consequences of cognitive deficits following TBI are underestimated by physicians, and therefore treatment for it is correspondingly undervalued. Although not as dramatic as behavioral disorders, cognitive disorders are the central issue in TBI rehabilitation. The numbers of patients involved and the disabilities caused by cognitive deficits are probably orders of magnitude greater than for behavior disorders. At any level of severity of injury other than the totally dependent patient, the cognitive disturbances are usually the most disabling. The conclusion is clear that the single most disabling deficit of TBI is loss of these cognitive capabilities. Nevertheless, pharmacologic treatments to remediate cognitive loss are much rarer than interventions for disordered behavior or depression. Probably even more nihilism exists in regard to medications for this treatment indication. It is also a simple fact that cognitive losses are negative symptoms and are not as demanding of treatment as an assaultive or suicidal patient. As Cope (1990) phrased it, "understandably, cognitive dysfunction may appear to be less significant or critical to the treating physician and therefore innovative pharmacological treatments are more easily deferred or disregarded pending better 'scientific' evidence of efficacy" (p. 251).

PROPOSED PLACE IN TREATMENT

It is now appropriate to consider what might be the logical place of psychopharmacologic treatment in TBI management today. First, clear rationales exist for such treatment. For example, Gualtieri (1988) pointed out,

> Profound deficits in monoaminergic neurotransmission are seen in TBI
> patients [12] presumably as a consequence of shear damage to axial
> brain structures, where the monoamines are concentrated. The admin-
> istration of monoaminergic drugs such as stimulants is, in this context,
> "rational pharmacotherapy," that is drug therapy intended to correct an
> underlying neurochemical deficit. (p. 105)

Additionally, whereas the dementias (the major diagnoses studied for
pharmacologic cognitive enhancement) are progressive neurologic
conditions with increasingly severe underlying neuropathology, in TBI
one is dealing with a recovering or stable base of neurologic function.
Thus, a more modest pharmacologic effect may have a much more
significant clinical result because it is not eroded over time with
natural progression of the disease.

Psychopharmacologic intervention should be dependent on the
course of recovery. If a continual and satisfactory recovery trend is
evident, no psychopharmacologic interventions are normally indicated.
Psychopharmacologic treatment cannot, and must not, take the place
of appropriate established psychotherapeutic/rehabilitation interventions. Rather, psychopharmacologic intervention, from an early stage,
should be considered one integral component of a comprehensive rehabilitation program, not as a backup or last resort resource. Physicians also must take a more aggressive role in developing and
monitoring the entire course of rehabilitation of each patient, and
resist becoming passive "on-call" consultants to nonmedical rehabilitation clinicians once the "medical" phase of rehabilitation is over.
They must actively consider at each stage whether and to what degree
appropriate psychopharmacologic interventions have acceptable risk–
benefit characteristics and act on this deliberation by prescribing
medications when indicated. Physicians must understand the nuances
of use of these drugs to choose and utilize them appropriately and
safely. For example, they must know what might be the most likely
therapeutic drug choice among the multiple available. They must be
aware of an individual drug's contraindications and side effects, and
use them wisely.

It must also be recognized that the appropriateness of a specific
treatment plan is contingent on what resources are available.
Frequently, an appropriate treatment plan may be one that is "forced"
along by early use of psychotropic medications due to limited
resources. No mistake should be made, due to any desired theoretical
"purity" about keeping the traditional rehabilitation program separate
from "experimental" psychopharmacologic treatments. The simple
reality for each patient is that if all moneys or reimbursement sources

are exhausted in futile or simply inefficient traditional interventions, there will be no backup treatments at all. Taking the foregoing into account, in each TBI case the rehabilitation physician should develop a logical plan to integrate both traditional rehabilitation and psycho-pharmacologic approaches.

In applying neuropharmacologic interventions, however, the problem of such drug use interfering with potential neurologic recovery is a special consideration. Management of this concern is aided by the recognition of three clear phases of treatment: (a) emergent, (b) acute recovery, and (c) chronic (fixed deficit). Each phase has its own implications in regard to psychopharmacologic treatment.

EMERGENT: IMMEDIATE POSTINJURY PHASE

It is in the immediate postinjury phase, in the hours and days immediately following the insult, that effective interventions in promoting increased neurologic survival and recovery are sought (Sabel & Stein, 1986). A number of potential pharmacologic entities are currently promising in this regard, including gangliosides, lazeroids, steroids, anticholinergics, alpha-adrenergic stimulants, as well as the avoidance of cholinergic stimulation and adrenergic blockade. Nearly all work in this area is with animals, although much more human clinical trial efforts are needed. However, as this period of care is under the purview of neurosurgeons, neurologists, and other inten-sivists and does not routinely enter into the formulation of rehabilitation plans, a full discussion of these options is not central to this chapter.

ACUTE: ACTIVE RECOVERY PHASE

This is the period classically considered to encompass "active rehabilitation" interventions. It roughly continues as long as there is discernible ongoing recovery and continued improvement in function. During this period, a guarded optimism in the use of psychopharma-cologic agents is appropriate. It may be clear, due to manifest failure of traditional rehabilitation interventions, that drugs need to be used for the obvious clinical reasons: depression, seizures, uncontrollable behavior, and so on. This has been an accepted role of drug management for some time. However, psychopharmacologic interven-tion may also be indicated in this phase because of considered judgment that drugs have a substantial likelihood to increase the rate of response and recovery or to increase the patient's ability to benefit from traditional rehabilitation interventions (which practically speaking are only available over a limited period postinjury). Because there is no absolute way to make such a judgment, this is perhaps the most difficult clinical phase in determining appropriate drug interventions. Because of previously mentioned concerns over blocking underlying neurologic recovery processes (which are, to some extent, still active concerns in this period), or because of concern about impairing a patient's ability to participate in conventional rehabilitation programs, strong conservative attitudes prevail today, with drugs held as treatment of last resort. If such clinical issues were the only real concern, there would perhaps be no major problem with this conservative approach. However, increasingly severe limits are being placed on the absolute quantity of resources that may be available for an individual patient's rehabilitation. It is no longer sufficient, in a rehabilitation program, to simply say that an intervention may be of benefit to be allowed to continue providing treatment; insurance and government coverages are adopting increasingly stringent financial limitations on rehabilitation benefits.

However, in this environment, it is increasingly appropriate to utilize, even as a first-stage intervention, a combination of both traditional rehabilitation techniques and psychopharmacologic treatments if such intervention can significantly accelerate the rehabilitation process. Some clear examples can be given to illustrate the point. The patient who is too agitated or aggressive to participate fully in rehabilitation should also begin psychopharmacologic treatment at the earliest point that indicates nonresponse to environmental interventions. It is nonsensical to take months to bring a patient's aggression under control with behavioral techniques (currently a common practice), while leaving him with inadequate or no residual insurance/financial coverage to address the myriad of remaining cognitive and functional deficits that are necessary to manage to keep the patient out of long-term institutional care. A second clear example would be the patient who has obvious or strongly suggestive elements of the "depressive" syndrome. This patient should be aggressively treated with appropriate antidepressant medications even while pursuing improvement through rehabilitation and counseling. A final example is the patient who is not showing evidence of progressive recovery after a meaningful (but limited) period of observation. This patient may remain in persistent vegetative state, or in an "abulic," anergic, amotivational condition. This patient should be given thorough trials of stimulants and other dopaminergic agents to augment his or her impaired arousal and initiative, and to allow him or her the fullest possible participation in the rehabilitation program.

CHRONIC: FIXED-DEFICIT PHASE

There is a point in every case when residual losses can be accurately gauged and where little reasonable expectation remains of further spontaneous gain. Current rehabilitation practice considers this point reached at approximately several years postinjury. At this point, the long-term deficits are essentially obvious to all concerned, and their relative contribution to disability and handicap are discernible. It may be an engineer or accountant who is mildly cognitively impaired and is only marginally able to return to his or her career; or it may be a homemaker of similar injury who has great difficulty with the demands of parenting and household management. Alternatively, it may be a patient with emotional incontinence or behavioral aggressivity. It is also customary to end active treatment at this point and begin "maintenance care." Physicians' interest in these patients has characteristically lapsed at this point. Further care has been turned over to counselors, vocational specialists, and so on. It is also at this point that a large percentage of medical insurance coverage in the United States for TBI treatment tends to severely limit or end benefits. I propose that there is a further contribution that active medical intervention can make to these patients' recovery, which is currently nearly totally overlooked. To put this thought in perspective, however, a number of points must first be clearly and strongly stated.

First, TBI is not a "self-limiting condition"—the consequences of brain trauma are lifelong in effect. Remaining residual deficits are in all likelihood going to persist indefinitely, probably for the lifetime of the patient. These TBI deficits are not "cosmetic" problems or "inconveniences"; one must not undervalue or dismiss the importance of these issues to the patient. They are central to the ability to live a meaningful and satisfying life (for the patient and his or her family). The cumulative effect of even so-called "mild" disabilities (i.e., "minor" memory loss or inability to concentrate) can be catastrophic for that patient's life history. One only has to imagine how these "minor" deficits in memory, attention, or irritability would impact our own personal lives and careers if they were visited upon us.

Second, TBI is not an "agonal" event. A TBI patient's life is not at an end essentially (although the suspicion justifiably exists that, at some "preconscious" level, many physicians consider the [meaningful] life of the TBI patient to have ended). Rather, TBI survivors are principally young adults and children who face an essentially normal life expectancy. This means each of these patients has up to and beyond 50 years of further struggle coping with these "minor" deficits. These deficits may deny them adult roles in society, meaningful vocations, or satisfying interpersonal relationships—the very stuff of which a fruitful life is made. To deny these survivors the benefit of potentially helpful methods of care is to consign them to a lifetime of possibly unnecessary need and suffering.

I propose that we are scientifically and clinically at a point where there is a strong argument for more aggressive psychopharmacologic interventions at this chronic stage of TBI. I emphasize that this is an *additional* step in treatment that is not currently the standard of practice, but that has a great deal of logical merit to support it. Although the large-scale, blinded, placebo-controlled studies are not available to definitively demonstrate the benefit of many of the pharmacologic interventions available, there is little prospect of such studies being done in the appreciable future due to heavy costs and lack of interest by pharmaceutical firms. Even if many newer agents have the potential of being useful, they have not been investigated for TBI.

Many individual case reports, many with sophisticated A-B-A-B designs, support the proposition that individual TBI patients obtain benefit, and sometimes dramatic benefit, from use of various agents. I propose that after proper education regarding evidence of risks and potential benefits, patients who give informed consent should be allowed the opportunity to benefit from access to these potentially life-altering therapies. Most of the drugs proposed for trial in these patients are well known through years of use in other conditions. The side effects are understood. Most of the drugs are relatively benign in this respect as well, although serious side effects, up to and including death, are possible. It is also evident that if no therapeutic result were demonstrated in any particular case, that drug would be discontinued (i.e., no long-term exposure would be undertaken without clear evidence of significant benefit for that patient). This requirement for demonstrated benefits would also limit concerns of long-term complications of the "plastic" variety (e.g., tardive dyskinesia, dystonias, supersensitivity psychoses, etc.). The risk of these complications is minimal, whereas the benefits are potentially enormous. Even a modest amount of resolution of symptomatology could be expected to make substantial improvements in quality of life for many of these patients. Taking the preceding points in sum, it seems apparent that the risk–benefit aspects of this type of intervention are clearly acceptable.

PROBLEMS WITH IMPLEMENTATION

What might prevent or impede the implementation of these suggestions? First and foremost is the problem of educating and convincing those professionals responsible for carrying out the rehabilitation programs about the validity and importance of these new possibilities. As the limitations of current rehabilitation treatments are becoming more evident with the accumulation of various outcome studies, a less antagonistic attitude toward psychopharmacology interventions seems to be emerging. Clinicians who initially felt that medications merely served to suppress a patient's behaviors now seem to be open to considering them as part of a balanced treatment plan. Of course this is augmented by clinicians' growing awareness of increasing limitations on the funds available to treat any given patient. Another barrier is the necessity to develop the expertise in these psychopharmacologic treatments by rehabilitation physicians currently involved with their treatment, or to invite physicians with such expertise onto the rehabilitation team. Perhaps a new integral member of the rehabilitation team is necessary, the physician-neuropharmacologist, to fully implement these psychopharmacological approaches in collaboration with traditional rehabilitation methods.

One danger in moving more aggressively toward a "pharmacological" component of treatment is the possibility of creating a dichotomy of "medical" versus "rehabilitation" treatments, where prescribing drugs is equated with medical care, whereas other aspects of treatment, such as counseling or cognitive retraining, are equated with "psychological" or "rehabilitation" care. It is increasingly apparent, however, that these distinctions have more to do with administrative issues in cost containment and reimbursement than with any meaningful clinical incompatibility or conflict in the two approaches. There is a long history of administrative regulations differentiating "rehabilitation" and "mental-illness" care from basic medical care, and of placing specific, more restrictive reimbursement parameters on the former.

Paradoxically, another problematic issue is that as the science of psychopharmacologic research and treatment has become more rigorous (with demands for large-scale objective studies with blinded, random-patient assignment, etc.), the flexibility in clinical practice and innovation has become concretized and constrained. Ayd (1991) has convincingly argued that clinical advances have significantly diminished under this modern, strictly "scientific" approach. Historically, the initial investigations of nearly all currently utilized classes of medications occurred during the 1950s and 1960s. These studies were characterized by great methodological imprecision. Their eventual psychiatric usage was not the one originally predicted for them by these early investigators. The eventual indications for each class of drug initially came from the observations of an astute clinician upon a few patients, and clinicians were allowed access to these drugs for application in a variety of clinical situations (Ayd, 1991).

Today, however, much more stringent standards are held by reviewing agencies in the demonstration of new indications for drugs, which inevitably involve large-scale, double-blinded, prospective, placebo-controlled studies. These are very expensive and, as mentioned previously, insofar as TBI is concerned, appear quite unlikely to be done in the foreseeable future. One example of this modern, more methodologically stringent process's inhibiting influence upon potentially helpful drug's appropriate clinical use in TBI illustrates the point. Bupropion, although an otherwise very promising drug for treatment of TBI depression, is essentially not available for use in TBI because of the drug's documented "seizure risk." This risk was discovered during early development trials on non-TBI populations. Only recently has evidence appeared that the risk of seizures for this antidepressant is no greater than for other "acceptable" antidepressants (i.e., in a recent 102-center prospective, the seizure risk with use of Bupropion was found to be 0.40%; the generally accepted rate for more usual antidepressants ranges from 0.1% to 1.0%; Johnson et al., 1991).

Thus, today clinicians face a situation where nearly none of the proposed uses of the multiple psychoactive drugs felt useful in TBI is an "indicated" usage in the U.S. Food and Drug Administration (FDA) terminology. In fact, most official (FDA-sanctioned) psychoactive drug usage guidelines specify brain injury or seizures as relative contraindications to use. Therefore, treatment of TBI patients with nearly all drugs reviewed here are "off-label" uses, and this "off-label" usage has significant implications.

Physicians are also constrained in their use of psychoactive interventions in TBI patients by the primitive state of outcome instruments (dependent measures) available to assess the results of their pharmacologic interventions. The neuropsychological, cognitive, and behavioral deficits of TBI are subtle and difficult to quantify. Thus, clinical response to drug intervention is frequently difficult to reliably evaluate in the individual case. There are no rehabilitation corollaries to analogous psychiatric/psychological instruments (e.g. Brief Psychiatric Rating Scale [BPRS] MMPI, Hamilton/Beck Depressive Rating Scales, etc.) adequate for TBI where measures of memory (visual, auditory, etc.), attention, judgment, executive functioning, and so on are required. Due to the demands of monitoring patient response over time, these instruments must also have the capability to repeat measurement—a definite problem with current neuropsychological tests. It is not yet clear whether measures from psychiatry can be directly adapted to the requirements of monitoring TBI patients (e.g., would the overt aggression scale [Silver & Yudofsky, 1991] be adaptable or useful for behaviorally disturbed TBI patients?). A more thorough discussion of these issues has been given by Cope (1990).

How does one proceed given these clinical and scientific uncertainties and conflicting economic and administrative trends? One proposed solution, which may provide guidance for TBI care, is derived from a similar dilemma arising out of the clinical need, and patient demand, for access to "unproven" treatments for acquired immune deficiency syndrome (AIDS) and conventionally untreatable cancers. These situations—where the clinical need is great and the drug development process is slow and unlikely to benefit current victims of the diseases in question—have led to the recent concept of "parallel tracking" in the utilization of unproved drug treatments. Such parallel tracks are described as allowing both rigorous research and appropriate, potentially life-saving clinical pharmacologic care to be pursued simultaneously. Scientific data are collected as usual in rigorous experimental clinical trials, while promising therapies are made available and clinically utilized through simultaneous release of experimental drugs in exchange for an agreement by physicians that some data are to be collected (Skerrett, 1990). This same concept can be logically applied to a condition such as TBI rehabilitation, where there is no proved treatment that totally restores these patients to preinjury function, and where the deficits, if not eventually fatal (although one should not forget the increased accidental and suicidal death rates associated with TBI), are surely of major importance: If untreated, they can be expected to permanently impair that patient's function and quality of life.

CONCLUSIONS

Hayes, Stonnington, and Lyeth (1987) editorialized,

> There are currently no demonstrably effective treatments for head injury. . . . There is . . . preliminary evidence that a number of drugs could potentially prove extremely beneficial in the treatment of human head injury . . . the medical community has not attended sufficiently to the clinical potential of the drugs. . . . However, no systematic studies have exploited these laboratory findings. . . . In conclusion . . . an extremely promising approach to the treatment of head injury lies before us. The rational application of pharmacological management of head injury shows great promise . . . the implementation of clinical trials represents major commitments . . . we believe the time for such commitment is now. (p. 2)

Rehabilitationists face challenges in developing a comprehensive theoretical and treatment framework in their approaches to traumatic brain-injured patients. Historically, psychological explanations and treatments have dominated the rehabilitation approaches of these patients. Psychopharmacologic approaches have been neglected and relegated a secondary role. It is physicians' current challenge even if the integration of the two methodologies for the betterment of patients may be difficult to achieve.

Although there is almost certainly a bright and promising road for physicians to follow in their attempts to aid the TBI survivor with his or her disabilities, current economic trends in health care are threatening to block significant progress down this road. Physicians who care for the TBI victim and survivor must become aggressive in their support of these new options. They must push aggressively forward on this task because their ability as professionals to develop such innovative treatment integration in the future appears to be coming under increasing constraints. There may not be much opportunity to do so later if the present chance is lost. If physicians are successful in taking up this challenge, the next decade should provide increased recovery and promise for victims of this terrible malady: traumatic brain injury.

REFERENCES

Ayd, F. J., Jr. (1991). The early history of modern psychopharmacology. *Neuropsychopharmacology, 5,* 71–84.

Bleiberg, J., Cope, D. N., & Spector, J. (1989). Cognitive assessment and therapy in traumatic brain injury. *Physical Medicine and Rehabilitation: State of the Art Reviews, 3,* 95–121.

Cassidy, J. W. (1990). Pharmacological treatment of post-traumatic behavioral disorders: Aggression and disorders of mood. In R. L. I. Wood (Ed.), *Neurobehavioral sequelae of traumatic brain injury* (pp. 219–249). London: Taylor & Francis.

Cope, D. N. (1989). Legal and ethical issues in the psychopharmacologic treatment of traumatic head injury. *Journal of Head Trauma Rehabilitation, 4,* 13–21.

Cope, D. N. (1990). Psychopharmacology for behavioral deficits: Disorders of cognition and affect. In R. L. I. Wood (Ed.), *Neurobehavioral sequelae of traumatic brain injury* (pp. 250–273). London: Taylor & Francis.

Gualtieri, C. T. (1988). Review: Pharmacotherapy and the neurobehavioral sequelae of traumatic brain injury. *Brain Injury, 2,* 101–129.

Gualtieri, C. T. (1991). The psychopharmacology of traumatic brain injury. In *Neuropsychiatry and behavioral pharmacology* (pp. 37–88). New York: Springer-Verlag.

Hayes, R. L., Stonnington, H. H., & Lyeth, B. G. (1987). Editorial: Pharmacological treatment of head injury—a new challenge. *Brain Injury, 1,* 1–2.

Johnson, J. A., Lineberry, C. G., Ascher, J. A., Davidson, J., Khayrallah, M. A., Feighner, J. P., & Stark, P. (1991). A 102-center prospective study of seizure in association with Bupropion. *Journal of Clinical Psychiatry, 52,* 450–456.

Sabel, B. A., & Stein, D. G. (1986). Pharmacologic treatment of central nervous system injury. *Nature, 323,* 493.

Silver, J. M., & Yudofsky, S. C. (1991). The Overt Aggression Scale: Overview and guiding principles. *Journal of Neuropsychiatry, 3,* S22–S29.

Skerrett, P. J. (1990). Parallel track: Where should it intersect science? *Science, 250,* 1504–1505.

Zasler, N. D. (1992). Review: Advances in neuropharmacological rehabilitation for brain dysfunction. *Brain Injury, 6,* 1–14.

CHAPTER FOUR

Some Pathophysiological Aspects of Chronic Organic Brain Syndrome Illustrated by the Use of Brain-Imaging Techniques

Tom G. Bolwig

ABSTRACT

A review of brain-imaging techniques, with some of their advantages and limitations, is given, and perspectives of their use to understand pathophysiology related to brain damage are discussed. It is emphasized that although these technologies have yielded an enormous amount of information concerning brain structure and brain physiology, the application of them should hardly be used routinely, but rather as a research tool. Although imaging techniques are different in nature and applicability, they complement each other and do not represent redundancy.

The last few decades have witnessed an explosion of knowledge concerning how the brain works under normal and pathological conditions. During the 19th century, neurologists and psychiatrists were excited at the possibility of learning more about the brain, because at that time techniques for studying neuropathology were being developed using new stains such as the Nissl or Golgi stains. However, it soon became clear that examining neuronal structure alone would not suffice. Examination of brain structure, even at the cellular level, did not yield adequate power to resolve such difficult functions as thinking, feeling, and believing. Further, postmortem techniques have many inherent limitations, such as (a) artifactual effects of the death process, (b) the necessity to study predominantly elderly individuals, and (c) a scarcity of informative sample brain tissue. For that reason, during most of the 20th century, clinicians in psychiatry, neurology, and neuropsychology retreated from the study of the brain because suitable techniques were not available.

The situation during the past several decades has changed dramatically, and one of the major reasons for this is the development of brain imaging.

Brain imaging refers to a related group of techniques that permit one to study the structure and function of the human brain in people while they are still living. These techniques are not invasive. Some, such as computed tomography (CT) or nuclear magnetic resonance imaging (MRI), are similar to a simple X ray from the patient's point of view, although the MRI does not require the use of ionizing radiation. Positron emission tomography (PET), the most complicated and demanding, still only requires an intravenous injection. The oldest of these techniques to enjoy wide clinical use, CT, was first performed in 1971 and became available for clinical use over the next decade. Techniques and applications for the others are still in their infancy. Prior to CT, doctors were able to see only the skull with X ray techniques, and at best to obtain an outline of the ventricles to make inferences about the brain through the complicated process of pneumoencephalography. Now they can actually obtain clear pictures of the structures of the brain and observe it as it thinks and solves problems.

One can divide brain-imaging techniques into two broad categories: structural and dynamic or functional. The two major structural techniques are CT and MRI. Both are useful in visualizing brain anatomy. CT is useful for observing cortical atrophy, ventricular enlargement, tumors, and strokes. Because CT is limited to visualizing structures seen in a transverse plane, its application for constructing three-dimensional anatomy is limited. MRI has some advantages over CT: It does not use ionizing radiation, it permits visualization in a variety of planes (including coronal and sagittal, in addition to transverse), and is exquisitely sensitive for detecting white-matter lesions such as multiple sclerosis plaques. CT has already proved useful in exploring brain abnormalities in conditions hitherto not considered organic, such as the major psychoses, and MRI promises to have a similar, and perhaps better, application as well.

Although CT and MRI permit only the study of structure of anatomy, the dynamic or functional techniques allow us to observe the brain in action. The three major functional techniques are computerized mapping of the electrical activity of the brain, in the following referred to as quantitative topographic electroencephalography (QTEEG); regional cerebral blood flow (RCBF), which is based on single photon emission computerized tomography (SPECT); and positron emission tomography (PET). Each of these techniques allows us to examine brain metabolism and regional variations in brain activity.

QTEEG mapping techniques are limited to observing changing patterns in the frequency of brain waves, whereas both SPECT and PET permit a direct observation of cerebral performance and metabolic activity. In addition, PET currently permits study of neurotransmitter systems and the effect of drugs on chemical activity, and SPECT has a promising potential for this as well. These functional techniques permit the observation of cognitive activation, especially through stimulation with tasks designed to activate such cognitive functions (e.g., verbal memory). Clearly, such techniques have great promise for mapping cognitive function, both in normal individuals and patients suffering from organic brain damage as well as mental illness.

Not surprisingly, the rapid development of these techniques has attracted a tremendous interest both for basic scientists and for clinicians. We are only at the beginning of a development, and no decisive step in the therapy of behavioral disturbances has yet been made on the basis of this exciting technology.

With respect to rehabilitation from stroke or brain trauma, the techniques have proved useful for the localization of an injury only in the course of events, whereas their use in monitoring programs has had some, yet limited, value. As emphasized in chapter 2, these techniques may focus on the tree instead of the forest, and therefore may not yield great information concerning the more systemic change taking place throughout the brain as it undergoes the process of reorganization and repair.

With these words of caution about relying solely on brain-imaging techniques to understand and monitor changes of brain structure and activity during rehabilitation, I emphasize their overall importance. These techniques are important tools for diagnosing the localization of changes in the brain and for studying ways in which a malfunction adjacent to or remotely situated from a lesion can help in the study of structure and biological function of discrete brain areas.

In the following, I briefly mention some fundamental characteristics of each of these techniques and give examples of their usefulness in relation to the topic of this book.

CT AND MRI

Both of these techniques are standard equipment in numerous hospitals today. For further description, which is outside the scope of this book, I refer to a recent book edited by Nancy C. Andreasen (1989), which gives both principles and practical applications relevant for the clinician and the researcher.

MR imaging is a structural technique, although it may eventually have dynamic capacities. The most relevant comparisons of its strengths and weaknesses at this moment are with CT scanning, the other major structural imaging technique. MRI is superior to CT and is likely to substitute for this technique eventually. One major asset is the strikingly improved tissue resolution. Grey- and white-matter structures are precisely imaged and differentiated. This capacity makes MRI particularly preferable for studies of brain anatomy. Its capacity to image in various planes (i.e., coronal and sagittal, in addition to transverse) also makes MRI superior to CT in anatomical studies. Further, MRI signals contain far more information than do CT signals. Although CT indicates attenuation of X rays through tissue, MRI provides information about proton density, the interaction of protons with their environment, and the interaction of protons with other protons—the so-called T1 and T2, respectively. Thus, in clinical practice, MRI is clearly superior for studying demyelinating diseases, and is also superior for identification of tissue abnormalities in regions such as the basal ganglia or the periventricular area.

When MRI is compared with RCBF, SPECT, and PET, its major limitation, of course, is currently its inability to measure dynamic functions. However, some of these applications may be available for MRI research and clinical studies during the years to come.

Of future interest is the use of magnetic resonance spectroscopy. Spectroscopy has moved magnetic resonance (MR) into the functional area, and it allows study of metabolic processes in order to assess both normal and abnormal tissue function. Recently, techniques have been proposed that use high-field strength magnets for measuring N-acetylaspartate, GABA, lactate, and phosphocholine (Luytens & den Hollander, 1986). Sodium imaging has been used to explore vasogenic edema and stroke (Turski et al., 1986). Phosphorus-31 is a potentially informative nucleus in human biology because of its importance in energy metabolism. High-field strength magnets can also be used to examine concentrations of various phosphorus containing metabolites, such as adenosine triphosphate, phosphocreatine, or inorganic phosphate (Bottomley et al., 1984; Cohen, Pettigrew, Kopp, Mimshew, & Glomek, 1984). At present, these techniques measure activity from the whole brain and are used as an index of general brain metabolism. Refinements under development will permit the study of small subregions.

These highly promising possibilities of studying at the same time structure and function of brain tissue, alongside estimating neuropsychological measures, may become highly relevant for assessment of neuropsychological and/or drug intervention in chronic organic syndrome.

COMPUTERIZED EEG
AND EVOKED POTENTIAL MAPPING

The use of topographic techniques to display data derived from electroencephalograph (EEG) or evoked potential recordings has been under development for three decades. However, recent advances in solid-state electronics and computer-software development have revolutionized this approach.

Since 1929, when psychiatrist Hans Berger in Germany first recorded electrical activity from the human brain, the measurement of cerebral electrical activity has been refined and developed into the field of electroencephalography. It also has been extended into sleep studies (Kupfer, Foster, & Detre, 1973), telemetry (Stevens & Livermore, 1982), spectral analysis (Itil, Saletu, & Davis, 1972), and evoked potentials (Buchsbaum, 1977; Roth, 1977; Shagass, Roemer, Stravmanis, & Amadeo, 1979, 1980). What began as a research tool has now been integrated into medicine for the assessment of the clinical situations ranging from a multitude of neuro- psychiatric disorders to the determination of brain death. Over the years, new modifications have appeared (for review, see Morihisa, 1989).

A fundamental problem with the many approaches that yield increasing amounts of data was a difficulty in developing satisfactory quantitative analysis for information generated visually by this technique. With the effective application of digital computers, the basic direction of research as well as the shaping of the manner in which data could be presented were influenced enormously.

One of the greatest strengths of a computer is not that it can accomplish mathematical calculations beyond human conception, but that it can compress the time that is required for the computation of an extraordinary amount of information. The human brain, although without question the most versatile computer known, has certain basic limitations. Of particular importance to this field of study is the brain's limit concerning how many different pieces of novel mathematical data may be recorded, manipulated, and compared at any given time. A computer is ideally suited for the acquisition, analysis, and presentation of massive amounts of data in relatively short time periods, and this allows two fundamental processes. First, the data can be acquired from the physiological experiment, then categorized and compared in the mathematical fashion desired. Second, the data and compared in the mathematical fashion desired. Second, the data may then be condensed and summarized in the manner most amenable for human assimilation. The brain can analyze and interpret known pictorial representations such as photographs with a speed and flexibility far beyond the capability of most computers presently available. Computers with sophisticated pattern-recognition software are able to detect small differences or similarities between separate events, but they cannot begin to approach the human mind's ability to interpret along multiple divergent lines of inquiry and derive meaning from these similar or disparate patterns. The utility of brain electrical mapping techniques derives from the successful marriage of these two sets of formidable strengths.

Along with the proliferation of this technology, however, are controversies concerning various aspects of the methodology and its application (Duffy, 1989; Fisch & Pedley, 1989; John, 1989). These issues relate to data acquisition techniques, the physiological significance of the variables derived from spectral analysis, the spatial relationship between scalp potentials and cortical generators, the limitations of topographic mapping, and the appropriate statistical analysis of the multiple variables derived from quantitative electrophysiology. (For a recent review, see Zappulla, LeFever, Jaeger, & Bilder, 1991).

CLINICAL APPLICATIONS

Although QTEEG has a chronologic resolution several orders of magnitude greater than the PET scan, and the measurement of cerebral blood, its limitation is that it reflects only events taking place at the cortical surface of the brain. However, QTEEG's usefulness has been shown in some studies on strokes relative to language performance. These findings validate this tool for investigation of a brain function. Using the Classification and Regression Trees (CART) Breiman, Friedman, Olshen, and Stone (1984) found that the combined power of QTEEG and CART yielded objective electrophysiological methods to predict aphasia that rival the reliability of the language examination (Finitzo, Pool, & Chapman, 1991).

Thatcher, Cantor, McAlaster, Geisler, and Krause (1991) used a number of variables to study the development of prognostic equations for patients with closed-head injury. There were 162 patients studied early after injury with power spectral analyses of EEG recorded from 19 scalp locations and brain-stem, auditory-evoked potentials. These measures were made along with CT scan, Glasgow Coma Score (GCS) at time of admission, and EEG tests, and the functional outcome at 1 year postinjury was measured using the Rappaport Disability Rating Scale (DRS). The ability of the different diagnostic measures to predict outcome at 1 year postinjury was assessed using (a) stepwise discriminant analyses to identify patients in the extreme outcome categories of complete recovery versus death and (b) multivariate regression analyses to predict patients with intermediate outcome scores. The best predictors of outcome in both the discriminant analyses and the regression analyses were EEG measures (coherence and phase).

REGIONAL CEREBRAL FLOW STUDIES (SPECT)

SPECT determines the three-dimensional distribution of a radiotracer within a human body. The radiotracer can be as simple as a radioactive element (e.g., Xenon-133) or as complicated as a labeled neurotransmitter agonist (e.g., I-133-3-Quinuclidinyl 4-iodobenzilat, or QNB). Radiopharmaceuticals for SPECT are distinguished from those used in PET. The former emit a single gamma ray, whereas PET radiopharmaceuticals emit two gamma rays simultaneously in exactly opposite directions, following a nihilation of the emitted positron with a nearby electron. This distinction in gamma ray emissions leads to the distinction in instrumentation between SPECT and PET.

Today SPECT is capable of measurements of regional cerebral blood flow (rCBF) and of the muscarinic cholinergic receptor system. Measurements of dopaminergic and adrenergic receptor systems should be possible within the next few years. Although no radiopharmaceutical related to glucose metabolism exists yet, it should be remembered that rCBF and glucose metabolism are tightly coupled in the brain under most circumstances, therefore rCBF measurements reflect neuronal metabolism.

Radiopharmaceuticals for SPECT imaging fall into four categories: (a) diffusible indicators, (b) I-133-labeled lipophilic agents, (c) Tc-99-m-labeled lipophilic agents, and (d) I-133-labeled neuroreceptor ligands.

Diffusible tracers do not chemically interact with brain parenchyma and freely traverse the blood-brain barrier (BBB). For SPECT imaging, only Xenon-133 is routinely available. This isotope of the noble gas Xenon has been used routinely for more than two decades for two-dimensional measurements of rCBF using probe systems and the Kety–Schmidt model (Devous, 1989).

The strength of SPECT is that it is a three-dimensional method, as compared to the earlier modification using the Kety–Schmidt principle. For a detailed description of the principles, technology, radioligands, strengths, and limitations of SPECT, readers are referred to Devous (1989).

SPECT is available in many hospital facilities, is less expensive than PET technology, and commercially available radiopharmaceuticals can be applied.

CLINICAL APPLICATIONS

Because of the coupling of flow and metabolism, SPECT has yielded a wealth of information concerning the working brain. Looking at the chronic organic syndrome, SPECT has proved useful in distinguishing between vascular dementia and Alzheimer's disease (Waldemar, Larsson, Lassen, & Paulson, 1991a). Using a radiotracer (9mTc-HMPAO) that freely passes the BBB and then is "trapped" in the brain, measurements of events taking place at the time of injection can be estimated several hours later. SPECT technology has been elegantly used for the demonstration of brain function and normal aging (Waldemar et al., 1991b). The power of the technology in studying a neuropsychological function such as "working memory," using the Wisconsin Card Sorting Test, has been demonstrated by several groups (Berman, Zec, & Weinberger, 1986; Rubin et al., 1991; Weinberger, Berman, & Zec, 1986). All groups have clearly demonstrated a deficient function of the prefrontal-limbic network in schizophrenia.

Other studies of responses to cognitive activation using both two-dimensional and three-dimensional (SPECT) measurements of regional cerebral blood flow (rCBF) have shown that the left posterior inferior frontal region (Broca's area) undergoes increased CBF during speech in right-handed volunteers, whereas the posterior regions of the right hemisphere show similar increases during visual/spatial problem solving (Halsey, Blauenstein, Wilson, & Wills, 1977; Risberg, Maximilian, & Prohovnik, 1977). In addition, Meyer (1978) found that anterior frontal regions, particularly those of the left hemisphere, undergo rCBF increases during concentration, attention, and apprehension. This is particularly marked when solving a new task, whereas habituation to such tasks blunts the response (Risberg et al., 1977). Finally, SPECT measurements of rCBF have been performed by Devous (1989) to examine normal volunteers' responses to a variety of cognitive states. The Wisconsin Card Sorting Test, Simple Arithmetic Problem Solving, and Word Finding in Prosodic/Aprosodic readings were also performed. Results of the Wisconsin Card Sorting Test in schizophrenic patients have already been mentioned: There was a mild left activation during the various medic task, whereas little response was observed in the Prosodic/Aprosodic study. The use of SPECT in studying other pathological conditions such as affective disorder have yielded conflicting results.

It may be concluded that SPECT can be a useful technology to measure both the resting and activated state during various forms of stimulation. At least in the study of schizophrenia (which in some cases seems to belong to a condition with chronic organic syndrome character), SPECT has helped to formulate promising hypotheses regarding the relation between prefrontal and subcortical brain structures. A highly interesting use of SPECT is the study of epilepsy with complex partial symptomatology—the so-called temporal lobe epilepsy. This condition may show a great variety of psychological dysfunctions and may be difficult to detect using conventional or computerized EEG even with the use of depth electrodes (sphenoidal leads). In such cases where a chronic lesion is the background of disease that may develop into a state of dementia, SPECT studies have shown an interictal area of hypoperfusion (and probably also hypometabolism) that resembles similar zones seen with PET technology (Lee et al., 1986; Rowe, Berkovic, Austin, McKay, & Bladin, 1991). The same areas can be shown to display hyperperfusion during fits (Andersen et al., 1990). The method is highly relevant for diagnosing localization of one-sided foci, which may be removed surgically if the condition is difficult to control pharmacologically.

POSITRON EMISSION TOMOGRAPHY (PET)

With PET, a higher power of resolution is available than with SPECT. Both SPECT and PET provide the clinical neurobiologist with quantitative, physiologically relevant information concerning the regional chemical composition and metabolic activity of the brain in the context of complex behavioral and pharmacological conditions, which may be elucidated with the aid of these techniques. With PET, it is possible to generate metabolic activity maps of the brain in association with sensory cognitive motor and pharmacological interventions. Further, measurements and characterization can be made of a variety of neuroreceptor systems with and without agonist/antagonist blockade. This includes dopamine (DA), serotonin, acetylcholine, benzodiazepine, and opiate binding sites. Clinical brain imaging, especially using PET, is a product of a highly productive marriage between technologies of digital image acquisition, metabolic modeling, biochemistry, nuclear chemistry, physiology, and neuroscience.

The original PET studies applied the deoxyglucose method, which was developed to measure rates of glucose utilization simultaneously in all structural and functional components of the central nervous system in conscious animals. Although the purpose was to measure the local rates of glucose utilization, the analog of glucose-2-deoxy-D-glucose (DG), rather than glucose itself, was selected as a labeled precursor. Its biochemical properties make it easier to adhere to the essential biochemical principles for the measurement of a biochemical process in vivo by autoradiography or in emission tomographic techniques. For a further review, see Holcomb, Links, Smith, and Wong (1989).

The neuroreceptor studies have been reviewed by Sedvall, Farde, Persson, and Wiesel (1986). Their monograph provides a useful guide to this new approach. It explains that the optimal selection of ligands is one of the crucial steps in the successful development of a receptor-imaging protocol.

Briefly, neuroreceptor studies have been used to study (a) aging process, (b) schizophrenia, (c) Parkinson's disease, (d) Alzheimer's disease, (e) Huntington's disease, and (f) other neuropsychiatric disorders. Many of the findings are conflicting except those that point to the effect of various neuroleptic drugs. Again, a further description of this rich area of research is outside the scope of this chapter.

AN OVERALL VIEW

I have briefly discussed some of the current aspects of brain imaging. I have tried to look at their relative relevance to an understanding of brain structure and function.

Among the different methodologies used for the study of dynamic functional aspects of brain function, I find that MR spectroscopy represents perhaps the most promising area. The combination of MRI and spectroscopy allows the simultaneous study of structure and function of the living brain. QTEEG's advantage is the powerful time resolution. Further, it is a relatively cheap technology that, unfortunately, needs careful neurophysiological skill. The strength of PET and SPECT is their strong spatial power of resolution. However, they will hardly ever be used routinely, like QTEEG, because their applications demand a physiological steady-state situation. The pictures they give are pictures of a state, rather than of a rapidly changing situation.

Together these techniques have brought new insight to how the brain's various regions cooperate. They supplement each other and do not represent redundancy. Although brain-imaging techniques yield a great amount of information concerning both focal and ramified activity in the brain, they represent studies of gross changes. In the future, with the advent of MR spectroscopy and further development of PET and SPECT, studies of receptors in the brain, neural substrate, neuronal plasticity, and neuropharmacology will be brought much closer together than they are today.

REFERENCES

Andersen, A. R., Waldemar, G., Dam, M., Fuglsang-Frederiksen, A., Herning, M., Kruse-Larsen, C., & Lassen, N. A. (1990). SPECT and EEG in focal epilepsy with and without normal CT and MRS scans. A preliminary study of 28 cases. In M. Baldy-Moulinier, S. Askenazy, N. A. Lassen, & J. Engel (Eds.), *Focal epilepsy, clinical use of emission tomography* (pp. 97–106). London: John Libbey.

Andreasen, N. C. (Ed.). (1989). *Brain imaging. Applications in psychiatry.* Washington, DC: American Psychiatric Press.

Berman, K. F., Zec, R. F., & Weinberger, D. R. (1986). Physiological dysfunction of dorsolateral prefrontal cortex in schizophrenia: II. Role of medication, attention, and mental effort. *Archives of General Psychiatry, 43,* 126–135.

Bottomley, P. A., Hart, H. R., Jr., Edelstein, W. A., Schenck, J. F., Smith, L. S., Leme, W. M., Mueller, O. M., & Redington, R. W. (1984). Anatomy and metabolism of the normal human brain studied at 1.5 Tesla. *Radiology, 150,* 441–446.

Breiman, L., Friedman, G. H., Olshen, R. A., & Stone, C. J. (1984). *Classification and regression trees.* Belmont, CA: Wadsworth.

Buchsbaum, M. S. (1977). The middle evoked response components and schizophrenia. *Schizophrenia Bulletin, 3,* 93–104.

Cohen, M. M., Pettigrew, J. W., Kopp, S. J., Mimshew, N., & Glomek, T. (1984). P-31 nuclear magnetic resonance analysis of brain: Normoxic and anoxic brain slices. *Neurochemical Research, 9,* 785–801.

Devous, M. D., Sr. (1989). Imaging brain function by single-photon emission computer tomography. In N. C. Andreasen (Ed.), *Brain imaging. Applications in psychiatry* (pp. 147–235). Washington, DC: American Psychiatric Press.

Duffy, F. H. (1989). Comments on quantified neurophysiology: Problems and advantages. *Brain Topography, 1*(3), 153–155.

Finitzo, T., Pool, K. D., & Chapman, S. B. (1991). Quantitative electroencephalography and anatomoclinical principles of aphasia. A validation study. *Annals of the New York Academy of Sciences, 620,* 57–72.

Fisch, B. J., & Pedley, T. A. (1989). The role of quantitative topographic mapping or "neurometrics" in the diagnosis of psychiatric and neurological disorders. *Electroencephalography and Clinical Neurophysiology, 73,* 5–9.

Halsey, J. H., Blauenstein, U. W., Wilson, E. M., & Wills, E. L. (1977). The rCBF response to speaking in normal subjects and the time course of alterations in patients recovering from left and right hemisphere stroke. *Neurology, 27,* 351–352.

Holcomb, H. H., Links, J., Smith, C., & Wong, D. (1989). Positron emission tomography: Measuring the metabolic and neurochemical characteristics of the living human nervous system. In N. C. Andreasen (Ed.), *Brain imaging. Applications in psychiatry* (pp. 235–370). Washington, DC: American Psychiatric Press.

Itil, T. M., Saletu, B., & Davis, S. (1972). EEG findings in chronic schizophrenics based on digital computer period analysis and analog power spectra. *Biological Psychiatry, 5,* 1–13.

John, E. R. (1989). The role of quantitative EEG topographic mapping or "neuro metrics" in the diagnosis of psychiatric and neurological disorders: The pros. *Electroencephalography and Clinical Neurophysiology, 73,* 2–4.

Kupfer, D. H., Foster, F. G., & Detre, T. P. (1973). Sleep continuity changes in depression. *Diseases of the Nervous System, 34,* 192–195.

Lee, B. I., Markand, O. N., Siddiqui, A. R., Park, H. M., Mock, B., Wellman, H. H., Worth, R. M., & Edwards, M. K. (1986). Single photon emission computed tomography (SPECT) brain imaging using N,N,N'-trimethyl-N'-(2-hydroxy-3-methyl-5-^{123}I-iodobenzyl)-1,3-propanediamine 2 HC1 (HIPDM): Intractable complex partial seizures. *Neurology, 36,* 1471–1477.

Luytens, P. R., & den Hollander, J. A. (1986). Observation of metabolites in the human brain by MR spectroscopy. *Radiology, 161,* 795–798.

Meyer, J. S. (1978). Improved methods for non-invasive measurement of regional cerebral blood flow by 133-Xenon inhalation: part II. Measurements in health and disease. *Stroke, 9,* 205–210.

Risberg, J., Maximilian, A. V., & Prohovnik, I. (1977). Changes of cortical activity patterns during habituation to a reasoning test: A study with the 133-Xe inhalation technique for measurements of regional cerebral blood flow. *Neuropsychologia, 15,* 793–798.

Roth, W. T. (1977). Late event related potentials and psychopathology. *Schizophrenia Bulletin, 3,* 105–120.

Rowe, C. C., Berkovic, S. F., Austin, M. C., McKay, W. J., & Bladin, P. F. (1991). Patterns of postictal cerebral flow in temporal lobe epilepsy: Qualitative and quantitative analysis. *Neurology, 41,* 1096–1103.

Rubin, P., Holm, S., Friberg, L., Videbech, P., Andersen, H. S., Bendsen, B. B., Strømsø, N., Larsen, J. K., Lassen, N. A., & Hemmingsen, R. (1991). Altered modulation of prefrontal and subcortical brain activity in novel diagnosed schizophrenia and schizophreniform disorder: A regional cerebral blood flow study. *Archives of General Psychiatry, 48,* 987–995.

Sedvall, G., Farde, L., Persson, A., & Wiesel, F. A. (1986). Imaging of neurotransmitter receptors in living human brain. *Archives of General Psychiatry, 43,* 995–1005.

Shagass, C., Roemer, R. A., Straumanis, J., & Amadeo, M. (1979). Temporal variability of somatosensory, visual and auditory evoked potentials in schizophrenia. *Archives of General Psychiatry, 36,* 1341–1351.

Shagass, C., Roemer, R., Straumanis, J., & Amadeo, M. (1980). Topography of sensory evoked potentials in depressive disorders. *Biological Psychiatry, 15,* 183–207.

Stevens, J. R., & Livermore, A. (1982). Telemetered EEG in schizophrenia: Spectral analysis during abnormal behavior episodes. *Journal of Neurology, Neurosurgery and Psychiatry, 45,* 385–395.

Thatcher, R. W., Cantor, S., McAlaster, R., Geisler, F., & Krause, P. (1991). Comprehensive predictions of outcome in closed head-injured patients. The development of prognostic equations. *Annals of the New York Academy of Sciences, 620,* 82–101.

Turski, P. A., Perman, W. H., Hald, J. K., Houston, L. W., Strother, C. M., & Sacket, J. F. (1986). Clinical and experimental vasogenic edema: In vivo sodium MR imaging. *Radiology, 160,* 821–825.

Waldemar, G., Larsson, H. B., Lassen, N. A., & Paulson, O. B. (1991a). Tomographic measurements of regional cerebral blood flow by SPECT in vascular dementia. In A. Hartmann, W. Kuschinsky, & S. Hoyer (Eds.), *Cerebral ischemia and dementia* (pp. 310–315). Berlin, Heidelberg: Springer-Verlag.

Waldemar, G., Hasselbalch, S. G., Andersen, A. R., Delecluse, F., Petersen, P., Johnsen, A., & Paulson, O. B. (1991b). 99mTc-d,I-HMPAO and SPECT of the brain in normal aging. *Journal of Cerebral Blood Flow and Metabolism, 11,* 508–521.

Weinberger, D. R., Berman, K. F., & Zec, R. F. (1986). Physiological dysfunction of dorsolateral prefrontal cortex in schizophrenia: I. Regional cerebral blood flow (rCBF) evidence. *Archives of General Psychiatry, 43,* 114–125.

Zappulla, R. A., LeFever, F. F., Jaeger, J., & Bilder, R. (1991). Windows on the brain. Neuropsychology's technological frontiers. *Annals of the New York Academy of Sciences, 620,* 253.

CHAPTER FIVE

The Value of Regional Cerebral Blood Flow Measurements in Neuropsychological Rehabilitation

Jarl Risberg and Lise Randrup Jensen

ABSTRACT

Measurement of the regional cerebral blood flow (rCBF) is one way of imaging the function of the cerebral cortex. Such measurements might be helpful in the evaluation of the consequences of brain damage for the function of the brain, as well as for elucidating how different rehabilitation methods utilize its preserved potentials. In this chapter, two illustrative cases are described in which the rCBF measurements helped to understand the functional consequences of the brain disorder, as well as helped to supply information of value for the rehabilitation process.

One of the major issues in aphasia rehabilitation concerns theory and method in language therapy: How do we diagnose and describe specific aphasic disturbances for rehabilitation purposes by reference to models of brain-language functioning, and what is the rationale behind specific methods employed in aphasia rehabilitation? Modern methods for imaging of the function of the brain might be helpful tools in the elucidation of these issues. In numerous investigations, rCBF has been shown to be a sensitive indicator of brain function, and several methods of measurement are available. Concerning diagnosis, rCBF may be important for inferences of brain-language relationships based on aphasic symptoms by virtue of providing information about the functional consequences of a structural lesion. For example, localization of linguistic functions to subcortical areas based on the occurrence of aphasic symptoms in patients with exclusively subcortical lesions on CT scans may be erroneous. Using the rCBF technique, it has been shown that such patients also show reduced blood flow in cortical language areas (Skyhøj Olsen, Bruhn, & Öberg, 1986).

In the area of treatment methods, the rCBF technique may also make important contributions to advances by providing a window on changes in the spatial distribution of brain activity associated with different methods for assisting linguistic functioning of aphasic patients. We have earlier presented one case where, utilizing rCBF measurements in an aphasic patient, melodic speech training was shown to engage the right hemisphere to a greater extent than ordinary speech training (Christensen, Jensen, & Risberg, 1990). In the present chapter, two other cases are reported.

The question was whether the results of functional imaging by recording of rCBF would be consistent with the neuropsychological and neurolinguistic diagnoses of the patients. Furthermore, the measurements were undertaken to investigate whether changes in rCBF would be associated with specific rehabilitation methods, which had proved efficient in clinical training sessions in improving patients' ability to speak or comprehend language.

CASE 1

CP was a 22-year-old right-handed man who had not suffered from any prior illness. He was studying for a college entrance exam when he collapsed due to an apoplectic attack. He was taken to the hospital where a CT scan showed a left-sided intracerebral hematoma. Angiography revealed no aneurysms or other malformations, and the hemorrhage was attributed to high blood pressure with possible renovascular etiology. A second CT scan showed that the hematoma had subsided and no surgical intervention was necessary.

Initial Symptoms

CP initially presented right-sided hemiplegia, right homonymous hemianopia, and aphasia for both speech and comprehension. Furthermore, he complained of hearing problems. Audiometric tests were difficult to carry out because of CP's apparent problems in understanding the task, but tentatively showed a 60-decibel (dB) hearing loss on both ears. The hearing impairment quickly improved, and a pure-tone audiogram 5 months postinjury showed a fairly uniform loss across all frequencies of 10–20 dB on the left ear and 20–30 dB on the right ear. Brain-stem audiometry showed normal hearing on both sides and no indication of retrocochlear pathology. Likewise, motor functions improved so that only a mild right-sided weakness was evident in his walking, and slight fine motor control disturbances could be detected in his right hand. Only mild expressive aphasic problems remained. Despite the improvement in auditory sensitivity, CP remained unable to understand spoken language with any consistency, and his family had to communicate with him in writing.

Admission

CP was referred 18 months postonset to the rehabilitation program at Center for Rehabilitation of Brain Injury for treatment of severe auditory comprehension problems and social readjustment. He was evaluated by a neuropsychologist and a speech therapist for diagnosis and treatment planning.

Neuropsychological Examination

On Luria's Neuropsychological Investigation (Christensen, 1975), CP did not show any abnormalities of fine motor control or kinesthetic functioning. However, acoustic functions were found to be disturbed, such that CP only succeeded in making gross discriminations of rhythm and vocal pitch. Auditory speech comprehension, both at the level of discriminating phonemes and understanding words and sentence material, was severely affected. However, speech was well preserved, as were writing and reading. Learning and memory were within normal limits except in memory tests requiring intact auditory comprehension. Thus, his auditory retention span was severely reduced, and he had difficulties learning a list of orally presented words. Intellectual functioning evaluated with Raven's Advanced Matrices (Set 1) and Wechsler Adult Intelligence Scale (WAIS) was found to be normal or slightly above normal.

Logopedic Evaluation

Logopedic evaluation with a Danish translation of the Boston Diagnostic Aphasia Examination (Goodglass & Kaplan, 1983; see Fig. 5.1) confirmed these findings. CP's speech was rated as normal, except for a slight dysarthria and occasional problems with pitch control. Auditory comprehension was severely disturbed. The auditory problems were found to extend also to nonspeech environmental sounds, such as discriminating the sound of a door bell from the sound of a telephone.

SUBTEST SUMMARY PROFILE

NAME: C P   DATE OF EXAM:

		0	10	20	30	40	50	60	70	80	90	100
PERCENTILES:		0	10	20	30	40	50	60	70	80	90	100
SEVERITY RATING			0	1				2 ·		3	4	5
FLUENCY	ARTICULATION RATING		1	2	4	5	**6**		7			
	PHRASE LENGTH			1	3	4	5	6	**7**			
	MELODIC LINE		1	2	4		6	⊘				
	VERBAL AGILITY		0	2	5	6	8	9	11	13	14	
AUDITORY COMPREHENSION	WORD DISCRIMINATION	0	15	25	**37**	46	53	60	64	67	70	72
	BODY-PART IDENTIFICATION	0	1	5	10	**13**	15	16	17	18		20
	COMMANDS	**0**		3	4	6	8	10	11	13	14	15
	COMPLEX IDEATIONAL MATERIAL		0	**2**	3	4	5	6	8	9	11	12
NAMING	RESPONSIVE NAMING			0	1	5	10	15	20	24	27	30
	CONFRONTATION NAMING		0	9	28	43	60	72	84	94	105	114
	ANIMAL NAMING				0	1	2	3	4	6	9	23
ORAL READING	WORD READING			0	1	3	7	15	21	26	30	
	ORAL SENTENCE READING					0	1	2	4	7	9	10
REPETITION	REPETITION OF WORDS			0	**3**	5	7	8		9	10	
	HIGH-PROBABILITY				0	**1**	2	4	5	7	8	
	LOW-PROBABILITY					**0**		1	2	4	6	8
PARAPHASIA	NEOLOGISTIC	40	16	9	4	2	1		0			
	LITERAL	47	17	12	9	6	5	3	2	1	0	
	VERBAL	40	23	18	15	12	9	7	4	3	1	0
	EXTENDED	75	12	5	3	1	0					
AUTOMATIC SPEECH	AUTOMATIZED SEQUENCES			0	1	2	3	4	6	7	8	
	RECITING				0	1				2		
READING COMPREHENSION	SYMBOL DISCRIMINATION	0	2	5	7	8	9	**10**				
	WORD RECOGNITION	0	1	3	4	5	6	7		**8**		
	COMPREHENSION OF ORAL SPELLING				0	**1**		3	4	**6**	7	8
	WORD-PICTURE MATCHING			0	1	4	6	8	9	**10**		
	READING SENTENCES AND PARAGRAPHS		0	1	2	3	4	5	6	7	8	10
WRITING	MECHANICS	1		2		3		4			**5**	**47**
	SERIAL WRITING			0	7	18	25	30	33	40	43	**46**
	PRIMER-LEVEL DICTATION			0	1	4	6	9	11	13	14	**15**
	SPELLING TO DICTATION					0	1	2	3	5	7	10
	WRITTEN CONFRONTATION NAMING				0	1	2	3	6	7	9	10
	SENTENCES TO DICTATION						0	1	3	6	8	12
	NARRATIVE WRITING			0	1			2		3	4	5
MUSIC	SINGING			0	1	2						
	RHYTHM			0	1			2				
SPATIAL AND COMPUTATIONAL	DRAWING TO COMMAND	0	6	7	8	9	10	11	12		13	
	STICK MEMORY	0	3	4	6	7	8	9	10	11	13	14
	3-D BLOCKS			0	2	4	5	6	7	8	9	10
	TOTAL FINGERS	0	54	70	81	93	100	108	120	130	141	152
	RIGHT-LEFT	0	1	3	4	6	8	9	11	14	16	
	MAP ORIENTATION	0	2	5		6	9	11	13		14	
	ARITHMETIC			0	2	4	8	11	14	17	21	32
	CLOCK SETTING	0	3	4	6		8	9	10	12		
		0	10	20	30	40	50	60	70	80	90	100

FIG. 5.1. Patient CP's subtest summary profile on the Boston Diagnostic Aphasia Examination.

His repetition was very poor as could be expected from his problems with auditory analysis. Reading and writing were not disturbed.

Diagnostic Conclusion

Based on these investigations, it was concluded that CP presented basic disturbances of acoustic processing that could be characterized as word deafness, with some associated symptoms of general auditory agnosia.

Rehabilitation Methods

CP participated in the 4-month rehabilitation program at the Center, during which time he received speech therapy, training of cognitive and social skills, individual and group psychotherapy, as well as physiotherapy. Initially, speech training included attempts to restore phonemic discrimination and stable word perception on an auditory basis. However, CP did not make significant progress in basic acoustic processing. Consequently, the main effort of therapy was directed toward helping him bypass his deficit in the perception and comprehension of speech. Speech training included:

1. compensating for defective auditory analysis through lip reading and intellectual knowledge of the phonemic system;
2. exploitation of CP's remaining auditory abilities by teaching him to pay attention to information conveyed by intonation, stress patterns, and number of syllables, and maximizing use of context to infer meaning; and
3. general coping strategies for listening and communication, including pragmatic knowledge of the structure of conversations, awareness of strategies for interacting with others in different communicative settings, and attention to body language and facial mimicry.

rCBF Method

The rCBF was measured by the Xenon-133 inhalation method using a high-resolution equipment with 254 stationary scintillation detectors (Cortexplorer, Scan. Detectronic Inc., Hadsund, Denmark). The gamma emitting tracer was inhaled during 1 minute followed by 10 minutes of breathing of ordinary air according to principles described by Obrist, Thompson, Wang, and Wilkinson (1975). The arrival and disappearance of the tracer was recorded and formed the basis for calculation of different flow parameters. In this chapter, the Initial Slope Index (ISI), a flow measure dominated by cortical perfusion, is used (Risberg, Ali, Wilson, Wills, & Halsey, 1975). Repeated flow measurements were performed with approximately 20-minute intervals between recordings, with correction for remaining activity as described by Risberg (1980). Further details about the hardware and software of the Cortexplorer system were given in Risberg (1987). The activation tasks lasted for 6–8 minutes, with the start of presentation 1 minute before inhalation of [133]Xenon.

rCBF Activation Tasks

The rCBF study was carried out in cooperation with Niels Reinholdt, Institute of Phonetics, University of Copenhagen. The flow measurements were undertaken to compare the diagnosis of word deafness with the functional consequences of CP's brain lesion, and to see how his brain was activated in response to the basic compensatory strategy of lip reading, which had proved helpful to him in the training sessions. The following tasks were used:

1. recognition task with videotaped spoken words—sound alone;
2. recognition task with videotaped spoken words—lip reading alone;
3. recognition task with videotaped spoken words—sound and lip reading; and
4. recognition task with videotaped orofacial gestures—no sound (nonverbal task).

Each of the three speech recognition tasks consisted of a videotaped presentation of a woman (LRJ, CP's therapist) saying the 10 numbers from the two-times multiplication table (8, 4, 20, 12, etc.) in repeated presentations and random order. The patient was asked in each of the three speech recognition tasks to recognize and keep track of how many times the number *20* occurred. To check that he was carrying out the task as instructed, he was asked afterward to report the number of 20s he had perceived. In the first activation task, the screen was turned off so that CP had to perceive the spoken numbers based on auditory input alone. In the second activation task, the sound was turned off so that CP had to perceive the spoken numbers from lip reading alone. In the third run, both sound and lip reading were available to CP.

In the last nonverbal task CP saw a videotape with the same woman making 10 different orofacial gestures repeated in a random order (e.g., puffing out the cheeks, smiling, opening and closing the mouth, pouting, pursing the lips, etc.). CP's task was to count the number of occurrences of pursing of lips—an orofacial gesture that was perceptually highly similar to the lip movements in saying *tyve* (pronounced [ty:ve])—the Danish equivalent of *twenty*. Thus, the nonverbal task was designed to differ as little as possible in perceptual and general cognitive requirements from the speech lip-reading task, so that any differences in blood-flow distribution could be attributed to the linguistic or nonlinguistic nature of the task.

Results and Discussion

Figure 5.2 (inserted after p. 80) shows the rCBF results from the measurements during sound alone and sound and lip reading. The flow level is within the normal range, with a slight asymmetry of the hemispheric means, lower on the left side as expected. Focal flow decreases were seen in the temporal and temporo-parieto-occipital parts of the left hemisphere. Comparing activation by sound only with sound and lip reading showed higher values in left temporal and right occipital-temporal areas when lip reading was added. The addition of lip reading improved CP's recognition. With this, improved performance temporal speech areas of the left hemisphere were activated together with posterior regions of the right hemisphere possibly engaged in visuospatial processing.

The activation by orofacial gestures was also compared to lip reading without sound (not illustrated). An evident asymmetry with mimicry, causing much more right-hemisphere activation than lip reading was seen.

These results illustrate that the therapeutic strategy of lip reading gives added engagement of areas involved in comprehension of speech, and that perception of nonverbal facial movements is processed in a different, more right-lateralized way.

CASE 2

The second case, JN, was a 35-year-old nurse, mother of a child of 5, who suddenly collapsed during physical exertion with loss of consciousness. She was taken to the hospital, where a CT scan revealed a subarachnoid hemorrhage, with a small hematoma in the left Sylvian fissure. Angiography showed hemorrhage from a middle cerebral artery (MCA) aneurysm and revealed another aneurysm of the bifurcation of the internal carotid artery, which had not hemorrhaged. She was operated on, and both aneurysms were ligated.

Initial Symptoms

Postoperatively, JN had right-sided hemiplegia, global aphasia, alexia, and agraphia. Her motor function showed good remission so that she regained full function of the right arm and leg, and she was able to write with her right hand and to resume jogging as a means of exercise. One and a half years after the hemorrhage, a control scan confirmed the suspicion of two more aneurysms on the right side (located to the right MCA). She chose surgery, and the aneurysms were successfully ligated without any neuropsychological disturbances.

Admission

JN was admitted to the Center for Rehabilitation of Brain Injury 26 months postonset. Prior to admission, she had received speech training at a speech therapy institute, and she had worked intensively with her husband on her own rehabilitation.

Luria's Neuropsychological Investigation

JN was examined with Luria's Neuropsychological Investigation to identify and evaluate the disturbed elements of psychological and linguistic functioning and to develop a rationale for a treatment program. The neuropsychological investigation revealed sensorimotor disturbances of the right hand, including mild sequencing difficulties. There was a marked disturbance of kinesthetic and stereognostic functions. Similar disturbances were found for the mouth, as well as ideopractic disturbances of complex oral movements. There was a tendency to echopraxia, which the patient attempted to correct herself. Spatial organization of movement appeared to be intact.

Perception of rhythm and pitch was intact. However, JN had some difficulties discriminating consistently between similar-sounding phonemes or words. Comprehension appeared to be intact for single words and simple sentences, but lengthy or complex materials could not be grasped. Learning and memory appeared to be well preserved. Intellectual functioning evaluated with Raven's Advanced Matrices (Set 1) was within normal limits, as was the performance part of the WAIS. On the verbal part of the WAIS, JN's scores were low due to her aphasia.

Logopedic Examination

Evaluation with the Boston Diagnostic Aphasia Examination showed that JN's spontaneous speech consisted predominantly of single words put together in telegram style (see Fig. 5.3). She appeared to have learned a vocabulary of highly frequent words with simple articulatory structure by repeating these words over and over. When she tried to use less frequent words, name objects, or repeat words that were not in her automatic vocabulary, she groped at different articulatory positions, often with a clear awareness of error but an inability to correct herself.

The subtest of auditory comprehension confirmed that JN was able to understand single words, but had difficulty with more lengthy

SUBTEST SUMMARY PROFILE

NAME: JN   DATE OF EXAM:

		0	10	20	30	40	50	60	70	80	90	100
SEVERITY RATING			0	1			2			3	4	5
FLUENCY	ARTICULATION RATING		1	2	4	5	6		7			
	PHRASE LENGTH			1	3	4	5	6	7			
	MELODIC LINE			2	4		6	7				
	VERBAL AGILITY		0	2	5	6	8	9	11	13	14	
AUDITORY COMPREHENSION	WORD DISCRIMINATION	0	15	25	37	46	53	60	64	67	70	72
	BODY-PART IDENTIFICATION	0	1	5	10	13	15	16	17	18		20
	COMMANDS	0	3	4	6	8	10	11	13	14	15	
	COMPLEX IDEATIONAL MATERIAL		0	2	3	4	5	6	8	9	11	12
NAMING	RESPONSIVE NAMING			0	1	5	10	15	20	24	27	30
	CONFRONTATION NAMING			9	28	43	60	72	84	94	105	114
	ANIMAL NAMING				0	1	2	3	4	6	9	23
ORAL READING	WORD READING			0	1	3	7	15	21	26	30	
	ORAL SENTENCE READING					0	1	2	4	7	9	10
REPETITION	REPETITION OF WORDS		0	2	5	7	8		9		10	
	HIGH-PROBABILITY			0	1		2	4	5	7	8	
	LOW-PROBABILITY				0		1		2	4	6	8
PARAPHASIA	NEOLOGISTIC	40	16	9	4	2	1		0			
	LITERAL	47	17	12	9	6	5	3	2	1	0	
	VERBAL	40	23	18	15	12	9	7	4	3	1	0
	EXTENDED	75	12	5	3	1	0					
AUTOMATIC SPEECH	AUTOMATIZED SEQUENCES		0	1	2	3	4	6	7	8		
	RECITING				0	1			2			
READING COMPREHENSION	SYMBOL DISCRIMINATION	0	2	5	7	8	9		10			
	WORD RECOGNITION	0	1	3	4	5	6	7		8		
	COMPREHENSION OF ORAL SPELLING				0	1			3	6	7	8
	WORD-PICTURE MATCHING		0	1	4	6	8	9		10		
	READING SENTENCES AND PARAGRAPHS		0	1	2	3	4	5	6	7	8	10
WRITING	MECHANICS	1		2		3		4			5	
	SERIAL WRITING		0	7	18	25	30	33	40	43	46	47
	PRIMER-LEVEL DICTATION		0	1	4	6	9	11	13	14	15	
	SPELLING TO DICTATION					0	1	2	3	5	7	10
	WRITTEN CONFRONTATION NAMING				0	1	2	3	6	7	9	10
	SENTENCES TO DICTATION						0	1	3	6	8	12
	NARRATIVE WRITING		0	1			2			3	4	5
MUSIC	SINGING		0	1		2						
	RHYTHM		0	1				2				
SPATIAL AND COMPUTATIONAL	DRAWING TO COMMAND	0	6	7	8	9	10	11	12		13	
	STICK MEMORY	0	3	4	6	7	8	9	10	11	13	14
	3-D BLOCKS	0	2	4	5	6	7	8	9	10		
	TOTAL FINGERS	0	54	70	81	93	100	108	120	130	141	152
	RIGHT-LEFT	0	1	3	4	6	8	9	11	14	16	
	MAP ORIENTATION	0	2	5	6	9	11	13		14		
	ARITHMETIC		0	2	4	8	11	14	17	21	27	32
	CLOCK SETTING	0	3	4	6		8	9	10	12		
		0	10	20	30	40	50	60	70	80	90	100

FIG. 5.3. Patient JN's subtest summary profile on the Boston Diagnostic Aphasia Examination.

materials. Her repetition was severely depressed—on a par with her spontaneous language.

Reading and writing was comparatively better preserved. JN was often more successful writing a word that she could not say and then reading the word aloud. However, her spelling was faulty, suggesting a fundamental difficulty with recalling the precise phonological structure of words.

FIG. 5.2. *Maps of rCBF in the two cases.* Two measurements and the difference between them are shown for each patient using a vertex projection. The frontal pole is shown at the top and the occipital pole at the bottom. The hemispheric mean flow values (fl and ISI (2-3) flow parameter resp.) are shown in the lower part of each map. The colors represent flow distribution values (regional values in percent of hemispheric mean) as defined by the key (orange-red : high flow; green : low). The difference maps to the right are calculated by subtracting the distribution values from the first measurement from those from the second. Case 1: Note the flow increases in left temporal and right occipital-temporal regions when lip reading was added. Case 2: Note the lack of frontal flow elevations during word repetition.

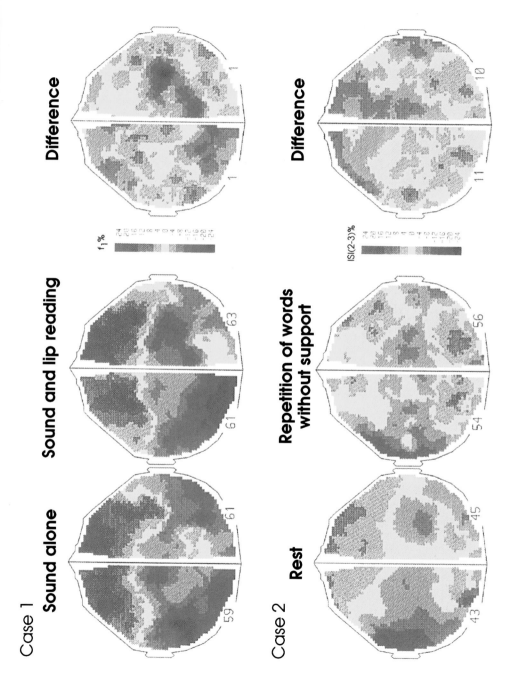

Case 1

Sound alone

Sound and lip reading

Difference

f₁%

Case 2

Rest

Repetition of words without support

Difference

ISI(2-3)%

Diagnostic Conclusions

Based on the neuropsychological and neurolinguistic evaluation, it was concluded that JN presented symptoms of both oral apraxia and aphasia. Although her profile on the Boston Diagnostic Aphasia Examination was consistent with a diagnosis of Broca's aphasia, her nonfluent speech seemed only to be (minimally) related to difficulties with initiation and transition between phonemes, which is frequent in Broca's aphasia. Rather, the aphasic symptoms were thought to be predominantly associated with disturbances of oral praxis, as well as afferent motor and acoustic-mnestic functioning. Although this diagnosis of a more posterior type of aphasia might be consistent with the absence of hemiplegia, it left some doubts as to the cause or mechanism responsible for JN's severely restricted expressive speech.

Rehabilitation Methods

JN participated in the 4-month comprehensive rehabilitation program at the Center for Rehabilitation of Brain Injury, receiving speech therapy as well as cognitive and social training, individual and group psychotherapy, and physical training. The goal of her speech training was to improve her perception of combinations of phonemes and her ability to produce or reproduce syllables voluntarily by repetition or reading. The rationale behind this was to allow her to exploit in her speech her preserved ability to recall the written form of many words she could not say. The methods employed involved (a) teaching a reduced version of the Danish phoneme inventory, (b) illustrating articulatory positions through visual diagrams, (c) guiding JN's attention to the articulatory gestures of the therapist when speaking a word, and (d) providing the orthographic word (or its phonemic transcription) for JN to have a visual representation of the phonemic structure when she was speaking. It was evident in the training sessions that articulatory modeling by the therapist, as well as the presentation of the written word, were helpful in improving JN's speech.

Another method that was only briefly explored was singing. However, although JN had a fine voice and was able to hum almost any melody, her speech did not improve with singing. This is consistent with her resemblance to other patients with oral and speech apraxia who, unlike Broca's aphasics, have been noted not to respond to Melodic Intonation Therapy (Tonkovich & Peach, 1989).

rCBF Activation Task

The rCBF measurements were undertaken toward the end of the 4-month program. The same rCBF method used in Case 1 was used in Case 2. It was of interest to (a) see how well the neuropsychological and neurolinguistic diagnosis correlated with the functional brain lesion, and (b) establish how JN's brain responded to the articulatory modeling support given by the therapist during reading of phonemic structure.

The following activations were used:

1. resting;
2. repetition of words spoken by therapist—from auditory input *with* articulatory modeling and written word support; and
3. repetition of words spoken by therapist—from auditory input alone *without* articulatory modeling or written word support.

Results and Discussion

The resting measurement (Fig. 5.2) showed a global blood-flow level within the lower part of the normal range with a lower hemispheric mean on the left side. A marked focal-flow decrease was seen temporally on the left side. Activation by repetition of words without support caused a global-flow elevation, with the largest regional flow increases in posterior areas of both hemispheres and in the left temporal lobe. There was no elevation of the flow distribution values (regional values in percentage of the global mean) in frontal areas, which is an obligatory finding in normal subjects performing tasks involving verbal production (Warkentin, Risberg, Nillson, Karlson, & Graae, 1991). Similar changes were seen when speech with articulatory modeling and written word support was compared with resting (not illustrated). Fewer words were now correctly repeated by JN, and the absence of frontal activation was clear. The lacking frontal activation was interpreted as an indication of disconnection of frontal areas, which seemed functionally disturbed despite the lack of primary frontal lesion. Such a mechanism might tentatively explain the pronounced expressive speech problems of JN.

CONCLUSIONS

The results from Cases 1 and 2 illustrate the possible value of rCBF measurements in describing the dysfunction caused by brain disorders and the way in which different therapeutic approaches utilize the remaining functional capacity of the brain. The interpretations of the present findings are tentative and speculative and should be taken as preliminary attempts to utilize a new technology. However, in view of the uniqueness of each patient, we are convinced that the present approach of "tailor-made" activations is more fruitful than trying to apply standardized activation paradigms to groups of patients.

ACKNOWLEDGMENT

Supported by the Swedish Medical Research Council (project no. 4969) and the Swedish Council for Research in the Humanities and Social Sciences.

REFERENCES

Christensen, A.-L. (1975). *Luria's Neuropsychological Investigation. Manual and Test Materials* (1st ed.). New York: Spectrum Publications.

Christensen, A.-L., Jensen, L. R., & Risberg, J. (1990). Luria's Neuropsychological and Neurolinguistic Investigation. *Journal of Neurolinguistics, 4,* 137–154.

Goodglass, H., & Kaplan, E. (1983). *The assessment of aphasia and related disorders.* Philadelphia: Lea & Febiger.

Obrist, W. D., Thompson, H. K., Wang, H. S., & Wilkinson, W. E. (1975). Regional cerebral blood flow estimated by 133-xenon inhalation. *Stroke, 6,* 245–256.

Risberg, J. (1987). Development of high-resolution two-dimensional measurement of regional cerebral blood flow. In J. Wade, S. Knezevic, V. A. Maximilian, Z. Mubrin, & I. Prohovnik (Eds.), *Impact of functional imaging in neurology and psychiatry* (pp. 35–43). London: John Libbey.

Risberg, J. (1980). Regional cerebral blood flow measurements by 133-Xe-inhalation: Methodology and applications in neuropsychology and psychiatry. *Brain and Language, 9,* 9–34.

Risberg, J., Ali, Z., Wilson, E. M., Wills, E. L., & Halsey, J. H. (1975). Regional cerebral blood flow by 133-xenon inhalation. Preliminary evaluation of an initial slope index in patients with unstable flow compartments. *Stroke, 6,* 142–148.

Skyhøj Olsen, T., Bruhn, P., & Öberg, R. G. E. (1986). Cortical hypoperfusion as a possible cause of "subcortical aphasia." *Brain, 109,* 393–410.

Tonkovich, J., & Peach, R. (1989). What to treat: Apraxia of speech, aphasia, or both. In P. Square-Storer (Ed.), *Acquired apraxia of speech in aphasic adults* (pp. 913–938). Hillsdale, NJ: Lawrence Erlbaum Associates.

Warkentin, S., Risberg, J., Nilsson, A., Karlson, S., & Graae, E. (1991). Cortical activity during speech production. A study of regional cerebral blood flow in normals performing a word fluency task. *Neuropsychiatry, Neuropsychology and Behavioral Neurology, 4,* 305–316.

CHAPTER SIX

Monitoring Behavior During Coma and Posttraumatic Amnesia

Barbara A. Wilson, Agnes Shiel,
Martin Watson, Sandra Horn,
Lindsay McLellan

ABSTRACT

This chapter is concerned with the assessment of severely head-injured people in the earliest days after insult. A set of scales for monitoring the recovery of functional skills in these people has recently been developed (the Wessex Head Injury Matrix, WHIM). The matrix is composed of 11 subscales for measuring progress in: (a) cognition, (b) self-care, (c) motor functioning, and (d) social behavior; and 1 scale for assessing posttraumatic amnesia (PTA). From the scales it is possible to (a) detect small improvements that might otherwise be missed, (b) see whether a patient is showing the typical order of recovery, and (c) pinpoint specific deficits in functioning. Observations are described in behavioral terms that enable therapists to determine steps to focus on in rehabilitation. Because this functional approach concentrates on skills required for everyday life, it has considerable implications for the care and rehabilitation of people recovering from severe head injury.

INTRODUCTION

Severity of head injury is usually judged by (a) the depth and duration of coma, and (b) posttraumatic amnesia (PTA). *Coma* has been defined as ". . . not obeying commands, not uttering words, and not opening the eyes" (Jennett & Teasdale, 1981). *Posttraumatic amnesia* has been described as ". . . a period of variable length following closed head trauma during which the patient is confused, disoriented, suffers from retrograde amnesia and seems to lack the capacity to store and retrieve new information" (Schacter & Crovitz, 1977).

The Glasgow Coma Score (GCS; Teasdale & Jennett, 1974) is frequently used to measure the depth and duration of coma. The GCS is composed of three sections involving eye opening, verbal responses, and motor responses. The original 14-point scale of the GCS, later extended to 15 points, provides an uncomplicated, easily scorable, objective measure of coma. Within each section, the worst possible response is scored 1 and the best possible response is scored 4, 5, or 6, depending on which component is being measured and which version of the test is being employed. The operational definition often used is that a combined score of 8 or less means the patient is in coma and 9 or more means the patient is out of coma.

Despite its apparent unambiguity, there are difficulties with this definition. For example, some patients with long periods of coma may fluctuate and be described as moving in and out of coma if 9 or more signifies "end of coma." Should one regard a patient as being out of coma on the first occasion a score of 9 is achieved, or should this definition be withheld until a patient scores 9 or more on three or more occasions?

The total of 9 is also questionable as a figure to distinguish noncoma from coma when one considers the component categories that make up this score. For example, spontaneous eye opening scores a 4, yet in our view such a category appears to have little relationship with end of coma. In our study, all but four of our patients, including most of those who later died, opened their eyes before the end of coma. Such a category, with its heavy loading of 4 points, could artificially inflate a total score, indicating a patient is out of coma when he or she is patently not when judged by other criteria. For example, one of our patients scored 4 for opening eyes spontaneously, 3 for flexing to pain, and 2 for incomprehensible sounds (groaning). Although these figures combine for a score of 9 on the GCS, the patient was unable to obey a command, and the team members felt it was not a true reflection of his state to say he was out of coma.

Conversely, patients may fail to score 9 yet be out of coma. Thus, although a patient with a tracheostomy tube in place, fractured limbs, and eyes swollen from bruising will not be able to speak, give a good motor response, or open his or her eyes, he or she may be able to indicate awareness by lifting of the head in response to a verbal command, suggesting the ability to process information.

This leads us to question whether it is appropriate to sum the scores from the three components. For example, a score of 7 may be achieved in numerous ways. If the scores for eyes, verbal, and motor responses are 4, 2, and 1, respectively, this reflects a different assessment of ability from someone scoring 1, 1, and 5, respectively. The authors of the GCS warn against summing scores in this way, although they do this themselves (Jennett & Teasdale, 1977). To be fair, the scale has proved useful in predicting outcome (Evans, 1981; Jennett & Bond, 1975), and it is a major improvement on personal intuition and subjective opinion. Nevertheless, summing across components leads to the loss of important information.

Despite the limitations of the GCS, it is easy to understand and, because of its wide use, it enables comparisons to be made from one center to another and from one country to another. The same cannot be said of assessments for posttraumatic amnesia (PTA), which is rarely assessed formally or objectively. When assessed at all, it is often the neurologist's subjective opinion that determines when the patient is in or out of PTA. Two standardized tests have been described: the Galveston Orientation and Amnesia Test (Levin, O'Donnell, & Grossman, 1979), and the Westmead Posttraumatic Amnesia Test (Shores, Marosszeky, Sandanam, & Batchelor, 1986). It is rare to find these employed routinely, however, despite that PTA is a useful indicator of the severity of injury (Russell, 1932, 1971) and a good predictor of outcome (Evans, 1981; Jennett & Bond, 1975; Teasdale & Mendelow, 1984).

The present study was concerned with developing functionally relevant assessment procedures for people surviving severe head injury. The procedures were designed to: (a) plot courses of recovery in motor ability, cognitive skills, self-care, and social behavior; (b) be used as outcome measures to evaluate intervention programs (e.g., sensory stimulation program); and (c) identify goals for treatment and rehabilitation.

Although there are a number of scales for monitoring recovery after coma, we believe that none of these is able to monitor recovery in fine detail and specify rehabilitation goals. The best known are the Glasgow Outcome Scale (Jennett & Bond, 1975), the Disability Rating Scale (Rappaport, Hall, Hopkins, Belleza, & Cope, 1982), the Stover and Zeiger Scale (Stover & Zeiger, 1976), the Rancho Los Amigos Scales (Hagen, Malkmus, & Durham, 1980), and the Neurobehavioural Rating Scale (Levin et al., 1987).

Perhaps the most widely used of these is the Glasgow Outcome Scale. It exists in a short (5-category) form and in two expanded (8- and 10-category) forms. Apart from the 28-item Neurobehavioural Rating Scale, the other scales consist of eight categories that, although adequate for epidemiological or large-scale studies, are too broad to detect subtle changes in recovery or to identify specific rehabilitation goals.

The established scales also cross several behavioral dimensions (e.g., motor ability, cognitive functioning, and social awareness), thus making it difficult to identify improvement in any one area. Furthermore, certain behaviors may fit into more than one category so that fine gradations of behavior are lost (Gouvier, Blounton, Laporte, & Nepomuceno, 1987).

Another limitation of these scales is that they *rate* behaviors rather than *measure* their occurrence, and thus rely on subjective interpretations that may not reflect the true level of behavior. For example, in the Disability Rating Scale, one item is concerned with employability and four ratings are permitted (0–3). The problem with this category is that one rater's idea of employability may be very different from another's.

The final criticism of the existing scales is that they do not specify the sequence of recovery in sufficient detail. For example, Item 4 on the Glasgow Outcome Scale is defined as "can travel by public transport and work in a sheltered environment and can therefore be independent as far as daily life is concerned." This begs the question of whether the ability to travel on public transport precedes, follows on, or always goes along with the ability to work in a sheltered environment.

Standardized assessments may of course be employed instead of rating scales, but these too have limitations. The relationship between performance on tests and performance in real life is far from clear. People may score normally on measures such as the Barthel Index (Mahoney & Barthel, 1965) but still have deficits such as severe memory impairments that preclude independent living. Some patients may be too impaired to participate in a particular test employed. Sensory or motor handicaps may result in underestimation of true potential. The tests typically assess what the patient is capable of doing, not what he or she actually does. Finally, tests rarely provide adequate information for designing a specific treatment program.

One way to design assessments free of these weaknesses is to adapt procedures used in the assessment of people with mental handicaps. Many of these procedures are influenced by behavioral assessment techniques, telling us what a person *does* rather than what a person *has* (e.g., "this woman asks the same question 20 times in an hour and forgets to put on her wheelchair brakes" rather than "this woman has memory problems").

It is possible to combine a psychometric and behavioral approach in one assessment procedure. For example, the Rivermead Behavioural Memory Test (Wilson, Cockburn, & Baddeley, 1985) is a standardized test that asks people to remember items analogous to those required for everyday living rather than relying on experimental items.

One procedure used as both an assessment and treatment technique for parents of preschool children with a mental handicap is Portage (Bluma, Shearer, Frohman, & Hilliard, 1976). Children are assessed initially on five developmental checklists: motor, language, self-help, socialization, and cognition. Assessment is carried out through: (a) direct observation, (b) interviews with parents, and (c) attempts to elicit behavior by presenting specified tasks. Gaps in functioning are pinpointed, and the treatment is implemented in an attempt to close the gaps. Specific objectives (ones that are almost certain to be achieved within the week) are set, and a treatment program is worked out between the home advisor and the parents. Portage has been used with brain-injured people who are too impaired for more conventional assessments, and therapists have been employed instead of parents (Wilson, 1985).

The advantages of the Portage approach include the following: (a) it is adaptable to a fairly wide range of ability levels; (b) many of its items can be completed through observation or interviews with carers, thus avoiding motivational problems or the need for parallel versions; (c) it looks at real-life skills rather than experimental material; and (d) it assesses actual performance rather than capacity. The main disadvantage is that Portage is designed for children from 0 to 6 years of age, making some of the items inappropriate for adults. More adult-orientated items can be found in measures such as Bereweeke (Felce, Jenkins, de Kock, & Mansell, 1983) and the Hampshire Assessment for Living with Others (HALO; Shackleton-Bailey & Pidcock, 1982).

Using a developmental approach to monitor recovery after head injury is not new (Eson, Yen, & Bourke, 1978), nor is it necessarily appropriate, but it posed questions that we wanted to answer in the study to be described. We planned to combine items from Portage, Bereweeke, and HALO with activities of daily-living tasks, motor skills, and tasks to measure early cognitive recovery in order to develop scales to monitor recovery and pinpoint rehabilitation goals. The pilot study is described in Wilson (1988).

DEVELOPMENT OF THE WESSEX HEAD INJURY MATRIX (WHIM)

We wanted to trace the development of recovery from severe head injury and observe changes in behavior throughout coma and beyond. Would there be a sequence of behaviors that followed from each other in some consistent order? In our attempt to answer such questions, we planned to observe severely head-injured people defined as having a GCS of 8 or less on admission and in coma for at least 6 hours. These were admitted to five district general hospitals in the Wessex region (Hampshire and Dorset). Intensive care for these people is typically good, but after intensive care they are often admitted to general wards where expertise in managing severe head injury is often lacking. From an original sample of 97 head-injured patients, 88 survived and were observed and assessed over a period of approximately 27 months. The pilot study of this project is reported by Horn, Watson, Wilson, and McLellan (1992).

Originally we intended to observe people after they emerged from coma (i.e., with a GCS of 9). However, because of the limitations outlined previously, we had to start our observations earlier while patients were in coma. We started observing as soon as the patients were no longer being ventilated, paralyzed, or sedated. We also decided to accept "ability to obey a command" as our operational definition of the end of coma. The ability to obey a command means that a message has been received, understood, and acted upon. In other words, a conscious state is present. Of course we are not the first researchers to make use of this category. Klove and Cleeland (1972); Pazzaglia, Frank, Frank, and Gaist (1975); Bricolo, Turazzi, and Feriotti (1980); Brink, Imbus, and Woo-Sam (1980); Najenson, Groswasser, Mendelson, and Hackett (1980); Mitchell, Bradley, Welch, and Britton (1990); and Newton, Pasvol, Winstanley, and Warrell (1990) have employed it.

Care has to be taken to use appropriate commands for people in or emerging from coma. For example, "open your eyes" is not a good command because a patient may be opening eyes to speech (i.e., to the sound of a human voice) rather than to the actual words spoken. Similarly, a command like "hold my hand" should be avoided because the tester may simply be activating a grasp reflex. An unequivocal response must be observed and must follow a specific request such as "lift your arm" or "move your fingers."

Given that all patients were assessed on the GCS, we noted the scores and in some analyses used both GCS and "obeying a command" as measures of coma. However, we were concerned with the abuse of the GCS (Watson, Horn, & Curl, 1992). We saw instances when the GCS was completed on the basis of previous recordings. In other instances, the sheet was not filled in at the specified time, completed incorrectly, or when the recording had been stopped too soon. One nurse confused "flexion" with "extension." Another, when asked why she had failed to score a patient correctly, said, "Because it gives too good a picture of how he's doing." On another occasion, a nurse scored the verbal section as 3 (inappropriate words) because the patient swore at her. We are not criticizing the scale here, but its misuse.

A further concern was the number of potentially avoidable complications noted in our sample. Of the first 58 patients entered into the study, 12 developed contractures, 2 developed inhalation pneumonia through being fed solids before swallowing and gag responses were established, and 7 developed behavior problems that appeared to result from overarousal (i.e., there were too many people and there was too much noise in the room) or as a signal to the staff. For example, one man attempted to hit and scratch staff immediately prior to opening his bladder or bowels. Having relieved himself, he became quiet again. Five patients had their daily calorie intake reduced in the absence of weight gain when they were already underweight. At least two of these were in danger of death from starvation.

The duration of coma of the 88 patients (73 males and 15 females) ranged from 1 day to 366 days. The median coma length was 6 days, and the age range was 14–67 years. The patients were observed at varying intervals from daily to weekly. A subgroup was observed at least once daily for periods ranging from 15 minutes to 3 hours of continuous observation. Both direct observation and video recordings were used. The main aim was to record spontaneous behavioral events, but we also elicited other behaviors, employing items from the Portage scales, the Rivermead Activities of Daily Living Scale, existing motor assessment scales, and the Cognitive Competency Test (Wang & Ennis, 1986).

Three types of responses were noted:

1. Spontaneous behavior, such as opening eyes, grimacing, lifting hand to face, and touching nasal-gastric tube.
2. Response to naturally occurring stimuli, such as looking at nurse leaving the room.
3. Responses to a standard set of stimuli, such as tracking a small pencil beam or responding to name.

Any behavior that occurred within 30 seconds of the stimulus counted as a response. This was regarded as necessary to take into account the response latency characteristic of some early head-injured people, and has been used in similar tests by others (Brinkmann, Von Cramon, & Schultz, 1976).

Ten assessment scales in four main areas were constructed from 145 items of behavior observed during different stages of recovery—from the day of trauma including the period of coma. Dates on which the items were first observed were recorded.

Not all subjects were observed on all 145 items. There were six possible reasons for this: (a) the patient died before the item was observed, (b) the recovery date of the item was missed, (c) the item was inappropriate for that patient, (d) the patient was never observed to attain the item, (e) the patient was transferred before the item was observed, or (f) the patient recovered very quickly so the item was missed. The 10 scales were: (a) early cognition, (b) communication and speech, (c) awareness, (d) concentration, (e) attention span, (f) social, (g) self-care (washing), (h) continence, (i) gross motor, (j) upper limb, and (k) feeding.

Using the operational definition of obeying a command to determine end of coma, it became apparent during the study that, in our sample, two behaviors always occurred during coma, even in those patients who later died. These were: (a) eyes opening briefly and (b) eyes open for an extended period.

Other behaviors were sometimes seen during coma and sometimes after coma. These were: (a) moving spontaneously to facilitate dressing, (b) distress caused by a cloth placed over the face, (c) removing a cloth placed on the face three consecutive times, (d) eyes following a sound source for 3–5 seconds, and (e) selectively responding to preferred person.

The cloth on face item is from the Portage Developmental Checklists (Bluma et al., 1976), and is the first of the cognitive items. Preliminary observations showed that some patients removed a cloth placed on the face while still in coma. A typical sequence was for the patient to first become quiescent when the cloth was placed on the face, later to become agitated, and finally to remove the cloth.

After these early observations, a systematic attempt was made to teach eight patients to remove the cloth by physical prompting and backward chaining. Three trials were given at each assessment. The assessments began as soon as the patient's eyes were open for an extended period. The number of prompts per trial was six. Scores were recorded as "the number of prompts required to learn to remove the cloth." The operational definition of *success* was "removal of the cloth without any prompt on three consecutive occasions." Five patients removed the cloth before the end of coma. Since then, three other patients have been assessed on the "cloth on face" item at a much earlier stage and with much lower GCS. All three have learned to remove the cloth during coma, and two have demonstrated learning on other tasks.

Boyle and Greer (1983) tried to teach three patients with protracted coma to comply to a verbal request. Only one patient demonstrated learning (the only head-injured patient). Such studies are very rare despite their theoretical and practical potential. Theoretically, they can throw light on the relevance of conscious awareness for learning, and practically they may enable us to avoid or reduce complications such as contractures.

In the immediate postcoma period, patients may demonstrate a limited repertoire of responses. Hence, to elicit behaviors, it may be necessary to use stimuli of an unusual or innovative nature. For example, one head-injured patient who showed very little response to most stimuli and who remained sluggish for 91 days since the end of coma, reacted promptly and accurately when offered a £10 note. Another man who had been interested in motor cars prior to his head injury showed no response for several months postinjury, and he always kept his head turned to the left. However, when a motor car magazine was held open and within reading distance on his right side, he turned his head toward the magazine. He appeared to be looking at the magazine for several minutes. Any turning back to his preferred side could be altered by turning the page of the magazine. In both these cases, once responses were initiated the patients went on to respond to a greater variety of stimuli (Watson & Horn, 1991).

Because there were different numbers of observations for each patient, we used the "paired-preference technique" as the main measure in the analysis. This is similar to the "paired-comparisons method" (Allen & Yen, 1979) and was further developed by Watson and Horn (1992). All variables were compared with all other variables in terms of order of recovery to establish a hierarchy. This was achieved by paired comparisons, each pairwise comparison measuring which one of the two behaviors tended to recover first (i.e., recovers first more than 50% of the time). The percentage of wins in the resultant matrix could be used to generate a hierarchy of order of recovery. Individual scales were constructed by this means, as well as an overall battery of 50 items selected as possible key events. Spearman's rho was used to calculate correlations between the proposed order of recovery from the matrix, and the median rankings of recovery in a core group of 16 patients for whom there was the most complete data, to verify the suggested order of recovery of items (rho = .866, $p < .01$, two-tailed test). Apart from 10 items judged not to have developmental equivalents, the remaining 40 items were ranked developmentally by members of the child health-care team. The correlation between their rankings and ours was .746 ($p < .01$).

We also used two other analyses: mean recovery curve for each variable, and mean rank for each item in each subscale. The correlation between mean recovery curve and the order determined by the paired-preference technique was .92 ($p < .0001$), and the

TABLE 6.1
Typical Order of Recovery of Awareness

1. Eyes open briefly
2. Eyes open for extended period
3. Eyes open and move, but do not focus
4. Attention held momentarily by dominant stimulus*
5. Looks at person briefly
6. Eyes follow person moving in line of vision
7. Tracks for 3 to 5 seconds
8. Makes eye contact for over 5 seconds
9. Tracks a source of sound
10. Looks at object when requested
11. Looks at and apparently explores TV, picture, etc.
12. Switches gaze from one person to another
13. Can attend, but is vulnerable*
14. Momentarily distracted by stimulus*
15. Able to ignore distraction*

*Items from the Concentration scale.

correlation between mean rankings and paired-preference technique was .92 ($p < .0001$).

Table 6.1 provides an example of the order of recovery for the Awareness scale (with four items from the Concentration scale included). Table 6.2 shows the typical order of recovery of upper limb movement. The developmental order of this ranking is shown in Table 6.3.

TABLE 6.2
Recovery of Upper Limb Movement

1. Movement of any kind
2. Takes hand to mouth
3. Crosses mid-line
4. Holds with a mass grasp
5. Scratches self
6. Raises arm beyond shoulder line
7. Removes nasal-gastric tube
8. Reaches out and uses mass grasp
9. Handles other arm or hand
10. Holds with a pincer grip
11. Reaches out with a pincer grip
12. Puts pen to paper and marks
13. Transfers from one hand to the other
14. Puts pen to paper and writes
15. Weight bears on forearm
16. Reaches out and takes object with both hands

TABLE 6.3
Ranking of Upper Limb Items According to Development Ranking

Age	Development Ranking	Ranking(Hi)
Birth		
Movement of any kind	1.5	1
Scratches self	1.5	5
3 Months		
Weight bears on forearm	5	14
Handles other arm or hand	5	8.5
Crosses the mid-line	5	3.5
Raises arm beyond shoulder	5	6
Takes hand to mouth	5	2
6 Months		
Reaches out and uses mass grasp	9	7
Reaches out to take object with both hands	9	15
Holds and manipulates with mass grasp	9	3.5
9 Months		
Uses a fine pincer grip	11.5	8.5
Transfers from one hand to the other	11.5	12
12 Months		
Reaches out and holds with fine pincer grip	13	10
15 Months		
Pen to paper and marks	14	11
66 Months		
Pen to paper and writes	15	13
N/A		
Removes nasal-gastric tube		

Using a Spearman rank-order correlation coefficient test on the rankings ($rs = .608$, $n = 15$), a significant positive correlation between the two sets of rankings was found ($p < .05$, two-tailed test).

In addition to establishing the 11 scales, we also modified an existing posttraumatic amnesia scale—the Westmead (Shores et al., 1986). Using a subgroup of 18 patients, the modified Westmead was found to correlate with length of coma. There was closer correlation between the two measures when coma duration was equal to or greater than 6 days ($r = .684$, $p = .03$) than when coma was less than 2 days ($r = .584$, $p = .051$). Inspection of the patterns of recovery from PTA showed a typically uneven course, with brief islands of improved memory occurring before full recovery took place.

A further question that arises with patients in PTA concerns those patients whose memory problems do not resolve. When are we to regard the person as out of PTA? Wilson, Shiel, Patton, and Baddeley (1992) compared memory and attention functioning in three groups of patients: (a) those in PTA, (b) those with the amnesic syndrome, and (c) those with chronic memory impairment following severe head injury, but who were no longer in PTA. A control group of people with orthopedic injuries was also tested. Patients in PTA differed from all other groups on semantic processing, verbal fluency, and simple reaction time. The results suggested that PTA is not solely a disorder of memory and orientation as suggested by the Westmead, but includes slowness and impaired retrieval from semantic memory.

CONCLUSIONS

We have described the development of 11 scales for measuring progress of functionally relevant behaviors from the earliest days of coma in patients surviving severe head injury. We have also commented on aspects of PTA.

Because progress in the early days (particularly with long periods of coma) is often very gradual, it can easily be missed unless actively measured. When signs of progress are missed, staff may be poorly motivated and inattentive, thereby allowing potentially avoidable problems to develop. For example, behavior problems can arise because no means of communication is established in patients able to use a communication board or other signaling system. Inhalation pneumonia can arise because patients with no gag reflex are given liquids to swallow, and falls can occur because patient mobility has improved without staff being aware of it. Adequate monitoring of progress could reduce these and many other such problems.

Pinpointing the specific deficit and describing it in behavioral terms should inform therapists of the steps they need to focus on in rehabilitation. This is unlike other measures, such as MRI or CT scans. An MRI can identify the precise areas affected after brain injury, but cannot tell how the effects of the lesion are manifested when attempting to cope with real-life tasks. Nor does the MRI guide the sequence of stimulation and therapy required for rehabilitation. If we can identify a behavioral deficit, such as inability to grasp a spoon, we can try to remediate or compensate for the deficits.

REFERENCES

Allen, M. J., & Yen, W. M. (1979). *Introduction to measurement theory*. Monterey, CA: Brooks/Cole.

Bluma, S., Shearer, M., Frohman, A., & Hilliard, J. (1976). *Portage guide to early education*. Portage, WI: Co-operative Educational Service Agency.

Boyle, M. E., & Greer, R. D. (1983). Operant procedures and the comatose patient. *Journal of Applied Behavior Analysis, 16,* 3–12.

Bricolo, A., Turazzi, S., & Feriotti, G. (1980). Prolonged post-traumatic unconsciousness: Therapeutic assets and liabilities. *Journal of Neurosurgery, 52,* 625–634.

Brink, J. D., Imbus, C., & Woo-Sam, J. (1980). Physical recovery after severe closed head trauma in children and adolescents. *Journal of Paediatricians, 97,* 721–727.

Brinkman, R., Von Cramon, D., & Schultz, H. (1976). Munich coma scale (MCS). *Journal of Neurology, Neurosurgery and Psychiatry, 39,* 788–793.

Eson, M. E., Yen, J. K., & Bourke, R. S. (1978). Assessment of recovery from serious head injury. *Journal of Neurology, Neurosurgery and Psychiatry, 41,* 1036–1042.

Evans, C. D. (1981). *Rehabilitation after severe head injury.* Edinburgh, Scotland: Churchill-Livingstone.

Felce, D., Jenkins, J., de Kock, U., & Mansell, J. (1983). *The Bereweeke Skill-Teaching system: Assessment checklist.* Windsor: NFER-Nelson.

Gouvier, W. D., Blounton, P. D., Laporte, K. K., & Nepomuceno, C. (1987). Reliability and validity of the Disability Rating Scale and the Levels of Cognitive Functioning Scale in monitoring recovery from severe head injury. *Archives of Physical Medicine and Rehabilitation, 68,* 94–97.

Hagen, C., Malkmus, D., & Durham, P. (1980). Levels of cognitive functioning. In C. A. Downey (Ed.), *Rehabilitation of head injured adults: Comprehensive management* (pp. 87–88). Los Angeles: Association of Rancho Los Amigos Hospital.

Horn, S., Watson, M., Wilson, B. A., & McLellan, D. L. (1992). The development of new techniques in the assessment and monitoring of recovery from severe head injury: A preliminary report and case history. *Brain Injury, 6,* 321–325.

Jennett, B., & Bond, M. (1975). Assessment of outcome after severe brain damage: A practical scale. *Lancet, 1,* 480–484.

Jennett, B., & Teasdale, G. (1977). Aspects of coma after severe head injury. *Lancet, 1,* 878–881.

Jennett, B., & Teasdale, G. (1981). *Management of head injuries.* Philadelphia: F. A. Davis.

Klove, H., & Cleeland, C. S. (1972). The relationship of neuropsychological impairment to other indices of head injury. *Scandinavian Journal of Rehabilitation Medicine, 4,* 55–60.

Levin, H. S., High, W. M., Goethe, K. E., Sisson, R. A., Overall, J. E., Rhoades, H. M., Eisenberg, H. M., Kaliszky, Z., & Gay, H. E. (1987). The Neurobehavioural Rating Scale: Assessment of the behavioural sequelae of head injury by the clinician. *Journal of Neurology, Neurosurgery and Psychiatry, 50,* 183–193.

Levin, H. S., O'Donnell, V. M., and Grossman, R. G. (1979). The Galveston orientation and amnesia test. A practical scale to assess cognition after head injury. *Journal of Nervous and Mental Diseases, 167,* 675–684.

Mahoney, D. W., & Barthel, F. I. (1965). Functional evaluation: The Barthel index. *Maryland State Medical Journal, 14,* 61–65.

Mitchell, S., Bradley, V. A., Welch, J. L., & Britton, P. G. (1990). Coma arousal procedure: A therapeutic intervention in the treatment of head injury. *Brain Injury, 4,* 273–279.

Najenson, T., Groswasser, Z., Mendelson, L., & Hackett, P. (1980). Rehabilitation outcome of brain damaged patients after severe head injury. *International Journal of Rehabilitation Medicine, 2,* 17–22.

Newton, C. R. J. C., Pasvol, G., Winstanley, P. A., & Warrell, D. A. (1990). Cerebral malaria: What is unrousable coma? [Letter]. *Lancet, 335,* 472.

Pazzaglia, P., Frank, G., Frank, F., & Gaist, G. (1975). Clinical course and prognosis of acute post-traumatic coma. *Journal of Neurology, Neurosurgery and Psychiatry, 38,* 149–154.

Rappaport, M., Hall, K., Hopkins, K., Belleza, T., & Cope, N. (1982). Disability rating scale for severe head trauma: Coma to community. *Archives of Physical and Medical Rehabilitation, 63,* 118–123.

Russell, W. R. (1932). Cerebral involvement in head injury. *Brain, 35,* 549–603.

Schacter, D., & Crovitz, N. F. (1977). Memory function after closed head injury: A review of the quantitative literature. *Cortex, 13,* 150–176.

Shackleton-Bailey, M. J., & Pidcock, B. E. (1982). *Hampshire assessment for living with others: Users handbook.* Winchester, Hants: Hampshire Social Services.

Shores, E. A., Marosszeky, J. E., Sandanam, J., & Batchelor, J. (1986). Preliminary validation of a clinical scale for measuring the duration of post-traumatic amnesia. *The Medical Journal of Australia, 144,* 569–572.

Stover, S. L., & Zeiger, H. E. (1976). Head injury in children and teenagers: Functional recovery correlated with duration of coma. *Archives of Physical and Medical Rehabilitation, 57,* 201–205.

Teasdale, G., & Jennett, B. (1974). Assessment of coma and impaired consciousness: A practical scale. *Lancet, 2,* 81–84.

Teasdale, G., & Mendelow, D. (1984). The pathophysiology of head injuries. In D. N. Brooks (Ed.), *Closed head injury: Psychological, social and family consequences* (pp. 4–36). Oxford: Oxford University Press.

Wang, P. L., & Ennis, K. E. (1986). Competency assessment in clinical populations: An introduction to the cognitive competency test. In B. P. Uzzell & Y. Gross (Eds.), *Clinical neuropsychology of intervention* (pp. 119–133). Boston: Martinus Nijhoff.

Watson, M., & Horn, S. (1991). The ten-pound note test: Suggestions for eliciting improved responses in the severely brain-injured patient. *Brain Injury, 5,* 421–424.

Watson, M., & Horn, S. (1992). Paired preferences technique: An alternative method for investigating sequences of recovery in assessment scales. *Clinical Rehabilitation, 6*(Abstract No. 170).

Watson, M. J., Horn, S., & Curl, J. (1992). Searching for signs of revival: Uses and abuses of the Glasgow Coma Scale. *Professional Nurse, 7,* 670–674.

Wilson, B. A. (1985). Adapting "Portage" for neurological patients. *International Journal of Rehabilitation Medicine, 7,* 6–8.

Wilson, B. A. (1988). Future directions in the rehabilitation of brain injured people. In A.-L. Christensen & B. Uzzell (Eds.), *Neuropsychological rehabilitation* (pp. 69–86). Boston: Kluwer.

Wilson, B. A., Cockburn, J., & Baddeley, A. D. (1985). *The Rivermead Behavioural Memory Test.* Flempton, Bury St. Edmunds, Suffolk: Thames Valley Test Company.

Wilson, B. A., Shiel, A., Patton, G., & Baddeley, A. (1992). How does post-traumatic amnesia differ from the amnesic syndrome and from chronic memory impairment? *Neuropsychological Rehabilitation, 2,* 231–243.

CHAPTER SEVEN

Strategic Aspects of Neuropsychological Rehabilitation

Lance E. Trexler
Patrick M. Webb
Giuseppe Zappala

ABSTRACT

The experimental literature in neuropsychological rehabilitation has continued to evolve. Although empirical evidence supporting the efficacy of cognitive remediation remains discouraging, initial results for the utility and efficacy for a variety of compensatory techniques and holistic approaches to neuropsychological rehabilitation are quite encouraging. A class of neuropsychological rehabilitation interventions has emerged which focus on the development of cognitive strategies that serve to promote cognitive functioning following acquired brain damage. This chapter provides a theoretical perspective on strategic aspects of neuropsychological functioning, and reviews available assessment and rehabilitation methodologies that may lay a foundation for a heuristic assessment and intervention approach in neuropsychological rehabilitation.

HISTORY OF NEUROPSYCHOLOGICAL REHABILITATION

The field of neuropsychological rehabilitation has witnessed substantial conceptual differentiation and evolution in its precocious history. This conceptual differentiation has resulted in the development of new methods designed to ameliorate cognitive disturbances, as well as to minimize the impact of cognitive disturbances on functional

99

adaptation and environmental integration. Further, early approaches to neuropsychological rehabilitation have evolved in their methodological sophistication and have been more rigorously tested through applicable experimental designs.

Neuropsychological rehabilitation paradigms have been characterized by diverging levels of analysis (measurement methodologies) and diverging treatment methodologies (Trexler, 1987). In context of the model developed by the World Health Organization (1980), some investigations have emphasized restoration of function at the level of impairment (e.g., amnesia), whereas others have developed strategies to ameliorate deficits at the level of disability (e.g., communication) and/or handicap (employment status). These different levels of function have been addressed through different types of neuropsychological rehabilitation methodologies, including remediation, compensation, and holistic or multimodal programs of neuropsychological rehabilitation (Trexler & Thomas, 1992).

Cognitive Remediation

Cognitive remediation was described by Diller and Gordon (1981) as "procedures designed to provide patients with the behavioral repertoire needed to solve problems or to perform tasks that seem difficult or impossible" (p. 822). Remediation approaches typically target specific cognitive disabilities (impairments) as defined by psychometric measurement and through drills or exercise seeking to restore the underlying cognitive ability. However, cognitive remediation may also employ components of compensation training or teaching the patient cognitive strategies utilizing intact functions, as illustrated next.

The most researched and methodologically developed cognitive remediation techniques continue to be those utilized in a series of investigations by Weinberg and colleagues at New York University Medical Center in the treatment of spatial awareness and visuospatial organization deficits following right-hemisphere stroke. In their first landmark study, Weinberg et al. (1977) treated right-hemisphere stroke patients with neglect, utilizing both skill-training and compensatory strategies. More specifically, these investigators demonstrated that systematic cognitive remediation techniques that involved: (a) promoting the patients' awareness of their neglect, (b) providing an anchor in the left-hemispatial field, (c) training the patients to deal with visual stimuli of decreasing spatial density, and (d) training the patients to slow down scanning behavior resulted in significantly improved performances on psychometric measures of reading, writing, and arithmetic computations using paper and pencil, as well as other measures of visuospatial perception as compared with a well-matched control group of patients with right-hemisphere stroke. However, Weinberg et al. noted that the treated right-hemisphere stroke patients did not improve on measures of sensory awareness and spatial organization. Therefore, Weinberg et al. (1979) added components of skill training in sensory awareness (spatial localization of tactile stimuli) and visual organization (size estimation and visuospatial judgments) to their previous remediation paradigm for patients with right-hemisphere stroke and neglect. Results suggested more significant gains on a variety of psychometric measures of visuospatial functioning and reading-related functions as compared with the gains obtained in the original study.

Despite the effectiveness of cognitive remediation for scanning and visuospatial disturbances following right-hemisphere stroke, these investigators observed that the treated patients still lost their place when reading, had difficulties with reading comprehension, and would visually omit stimuli in the left-hemispatial field. Weinberg, Piasetsky, Diller, and Gordon (1982) hypothesized that these residual defects were attributable to an inability to actively utilize compensatory strategies for hemispatial inattention while simultaneously fulfilling other task demands (comprehension of material read). In this latter study, the investigators provided a remediation program designed to automatize the compensatory strategies for visual exploration and attention to the left-hemispatial field so that the utilization of strategies did not compete with other task demands (i.e., reading comprehension). Relative to a matched control group composed of right-hemisphere stroke patients, a rather weak treatment effect was demonstrated with reference to psychometric measures of visual analysis and organization. These investigators concluded that the training provided in the latter study had an effect on underlying cognitive skills, as measured by neuropsychological instruments. But in contrast to the previous studies by Weinberg et al., the training effect did not generalize to a wider range of cognitive functions. Further, it was thought that "while targeting training to impact a domain of functioning is a plausible goal, some specific application to individual skill areas might be necessary to achieve a more clinically significant outcome" (p. 73).

The investigations by Weinberg et al. exemplify the simultaneous utilization of skill-training and compensatory strategies targeted at the level of impairment (visuospatial disorders following right-hemisphere stroke). Training stimuli were experimental, as well as "real world" (i.e., written paragraph-length prose). Outcome measurement was performed at the level of impairment (nontreated visuospatial functions) and the level of disability (reading).

Results suggest some significant improvements on measures of reading and other academic abilities that can be compromised by visuospatial disorders associated with right-hemisphere lesions, as long as the training incorporated ecologically valid training material. These conclusions are supported by the research of Robertson, Gray, Pentland, and Waite (1990). These investigators utilized a computer-based training approach with a variety of visuospatial disorders for patients with evidence of hemispatial neglect. The training tasks emphasized skill learning as well as faded cueing to attend to the left-hemispatial field. Using randomly selected control and experimental groups, these investigators found no significant improvement in either the target functions (visuospatial and scanning performances) or on related abilities, such as reading. Therefore, one might conclude that without the specific inclusion of ecologically valid training materials (at the level of disability in this case), training of visuospatial cognitive skills (level of impairment) does not, in and of itself, generalize to target functional outcome measures.

Compensatory Techniques

In the last 5 years, significant advances have emerged with regard to the development of compensatory approaches to impairments in neuropsychological function. In general, the goal of compensatory techniques is not to restore cognitive abilities, but to enable performance of behaviors that depend on impaired cognitive functions. Therefore, by definition most compensatory interventions occur at the level of disability in the World Health Organization (1980) model. Compensatory techniques may involve task reorganization or task-substitution techniques (Trexler & Thomas, 1992). Task-reorganization techniques typically involve the infusion of a new processing component into the behavior (i.e., teaching a patient with left-hemispatial inattention to improve reading by way of placing a red line at the left side of a page to serve as a visual anchor provides for task reorganization; Weinberg et al., 1977). Task-substitution techniques refer to the acquisition of a new behavioral repertoire, often using external or "orthotic" devices that have little or no resemblance to the means used preinjury. Additionally, task-substitution approaches rely conceptually more on preserved cognitive functions following acquired cerebral lesions, more specifically the relative preservation of procedural and implicit learning and memory (Schacter & Graf, 1986; Warrington & Weiskrantz, 1974).

As an example of task substitution and external memory aids, Sohlberg and Mateer (1989) developed a systematic training procedure for the utilization of a memory notebook to compensate for defects of prospective and episodic memory. The training procedure was conceived in three phases: (a) skill acquisition, (b) application, and (c) adaptation. These investigators described behavioral procedures for training memory notebook utilization to specific criteria and methods for generalizing its utilization to nonclinical residential and specific vocational applications. Although data on only one patient were presented, the findings were persuasive. Computer-based compensatory strategies have been developed by Kirsch and co-workers (Kirsch, Levine, Fallon-Krueger, & Jaros, 1987; Kirsch, Levine, Lajiness-O'Neill, & Schnyder, 1992), where no attempt was made to modify the amnestic patient's learning and/or memory abilities. Rather, these investigators developed computer-based methodologies as "interactive task guidance" systems to promote performance of functional and vocational tasks. The interactive task-guidance system provides sequential instructions, cues, and feedback to the patient to promote performance of the target functional task, as well as timing and monitoring of task performance. Kirsch et al. (1992) demonstrated that in two of four severely amnestic patients, the interactive task-guidance methodology enabled performance of a vocational task. An absence of motivation apparently accounted for the failure of this approach in the other two patients.

Brain-injured persons' ability to learn "domain-specific knowledge" has been capitalized on in methods developed by Glisky, Schacter, and Tulving (1986a). In a series of studies with amnestic patients of various etiologies, these investigators demonstrated that, through the use of a method referred to as "vanishing cues," patients could (a) learn a new vocabulary related to the use of a computer (Glisky, Schacter, & Tulving, 1986b), (b) reliably perform data entry on a computer (Glisky & Schacter, 1987), and (c) utilize the newly learned skills in a vocational placement (Glisky & Schacter, 1989). Through computer-based training methods, the learning of new domain-specific vocational skills occurred in two phases: knowledge acquisition and skill acquisition (Glisky, 1992). Learning in both phases was accomplished through repetitive trials using the vanishing cues method, where cue density is progressively faded until the patient is able to successfully draw on implicit memory to produce the correct response without cueing. These investigations have shown considerable promise for promoting ecologically valid vocational and functional skills in persons with severe amnesia, albeit "hyperspecific" (i.e., the extent to which these patients can utilize the newly learned knowledge to solve novel problems or accommodate modifications in the domain-specific procedures is reportedly limited; Glisky, 1992).

Holistic Neuropsychological Rehabilitation

The last 5 years have also witnessed the initial experimental evaluation of more comprehensive and holistic neuropsychologically oriented rehabilitation paradigms for the treatment of the complex constellation of psychological, interpersonal, and vocational disturbances characteristic of the person with acquired brain injury. These programs typically incorporate a variety of services within the context of a day-treatment model, and often include (a) group and individual psychotherapy, (b) group therapy focusing on awareness and modification of neurobehavioral disturbances, (c) cognitive remediation, (d) exercise, and (e) functional independent living and vocational skills training.

One of the exemplary studies of holistic neuropsychological rehabilitation was performed by Ben-Yishay, Silver, Piasetsky, and Rattock (1987). These investigators studied 94 mostly traumatic brain-injured patients who were on average 3 years postinjury and had an average length of coma of 34 days. All patients were seen in a three-phase neuropsychologically and vocationally oriented program. Phase 1 was composed of a 20-week day-treatment program, where the patient received 5 hours of individual and group therapies 4 days a week. This phase was focused on cognitive remediation, as well as acceptance, social and interpersonal competence, and awareness. Phase 2 of the program provided guided occupational trials in real work situations. The duration of Phase 2 ranged from 3 to 9 months. Lastly, Phase 3 provided work placement and follow-up. Results of the 3-year follow-up demonstrate significant gains for a population of chronic, unemployed persons with traumatic brain injury. At the time that Phase 2 was completed, 84% of the patients were judged to be capable of engaging in productive activity (63% of whom were at a competitive level). At the 3-year follow-up, some regression was found, but 50% were still competitively employed and 22% were noncompetitively productive. A subgroup of eight patients was shown to be the least stable vocationally. Review of their clinical presentation suggested that social isolation, difficulties in generalizing rehabilitation strategies, and financial disincentives were the main reasons that vocational stability was not obtained.

More recently, Christensen, Pinner, Moller-Pedersen, Teasdale, and Trexler (1992) studied a heterogeneous group of patients with acquired cerebral lesions who were on average 2.9 years postinjury. All patients were treated in a neuropsychologically oriented day-treatment program that lasted for 4 months and was conducted 4 days a week, 6 hours per day. The treatment included (a) group and individual psychotherapy,

(b) physical therapy for exercise and conditioning, (c) individual cognitive remediation, and (d) individual speech and physical therapy provided as needed. The program emphasized psychosocial adjustment, awareness and social interaction, as well as neuropsychological control and regulation of cognitive–emotional functioning. Patients were followed at least bimonthly after the program, and more often if needed. On 1–2½-year follow-up, the patients demonstrated significant improvements in independent living and decreased dependence on health and home-care services. Further, significant gains were achieved with respect to leisure and recreational activities, reflecting enhanced interpersonal relationships and psychosocial adjustment. Return to competitive work was less impressive, but significant improvements were noted for overall productivity, described as work trials, competitive work, and education for the group as a whole.

This brief review of the recent history of neuropsychological rehabilitation has emphasized empirical studies, and overall significant progress has been achieved. Research in the area of cognitive remediation has been limited, and the results of empirical studies are not encouraging. In this context, it is important to remember that Diller and Gordon (1981) differentiated cognitive remediation from rehabilitation, where the former was defined as efforts to restore impaired cognitive abilities and the latter was the domain of an interdisciplinary team where a wide range of deficits and aspects of the disability were addressed. Although cognitive remediation is often embedded in more holistic programs of neuropsychological rehabilitation, the methodologies employed in these studies do not permit parceling out treatment effect attributable to specific components of the treatment program. At the very least, however, the available research would suggest that more global and multimodal rehabilitation efforts are necessary for cognitive remediation to contribute to the functional outcomes achieved through holistic neuropsychological rehabilitation.

Certainly significant advances have been achieved in the area of compensatory techniques for cognitive disorders, which are also often employed in holistic neuropsychological rehabilitation programs. As Brooks (1991) observed, there is a growing trend toward effecting and measuring outcome at the level of "real-world" behavior, as opposed to laboratory or clinical measures of "function." This trend toward the study of the ecological validity of neuropsychological rehabilitation has resulted in the development and utilization of methodologies targeted at functional adaptation. However, the work of Glisky, Ben-Yishay, and Christensen, and their respective colleagues, clearly suggests that a neuropsychological framework remains essential to obtain ecologically valid outcomes. Moreover, results obtained by Ben-Yishay et al. (1987)

and Christensen et al. (1992) corroborate the earlier work of Prigatano (1986) and empirically substantiate the benefits of holistic neuropsychological rehabilitation, with particular reference to psychosocial adaptation, social integration, independent living, and vocational adaptation.

STRATEGIC ASPECTS
OF NEUROPSYCHOLOGICAL FUNCTION

The conceptual and methodological differences between cognitive remediation and compensatory approaches seem to center on diverging levels of analysis in complex human behavior. Cognitive remediation seeks to restore cognitive functioning, assuming that with the restitution of cognitive functions performance of functional activities is possible. This assumption has not been empirically supported. In comparison, compensatory techniques strive to enable performance of functional tasks through reorganization of behavior. The intervention strategies may be based on neuropsychological theory, as in the case of Glisky et al. (1986a) and Sohlberg and Mateer (1989), or they may employ more of an environmental engineering approach (i.e., Kirsch et al., 1987). Although attempts at cognitive remediation for patients with traumatic brain injuries have not been empirically supported, studies by Weinberg et al. support that: (a) remediation can promote the reorganization of cognitive functions; and (b) these gains can generalize to target functional tasks when they are explicitly incorporated into the remediation strategy, at least in patients with focal (or relatively focal) lesions. However, the remediation techniques utilized by Weinberg et al. did not just involve repetitive drills, but incorporated a variety of techniques involving patient awareness, task reorganization, and teaching of new strategies that the patient was to actively and consciously utilize. This approach seems to be more accurately described as a strategic approach to neuropsychological rehabilitation.

In contrast, cognitive-remediation methodologies typically rely on drills or repetitive exercises that share stimulus and response properties of neuropsychological measures utilized to define the impaired cognitive function. In this context, cognitive functions are sometimes viewed as unidimensional, and cognitive deficits are strengthened analogous to muscle weakness. In this cognitive-remediation paradigm, the intervention seeks to promote the recapitulation of normal cognitive structure. Conversely, compensatory techniques seek to modify the utilization of either internal or external components

of the behavior and how the person attempts to perform the task—
essentially reorganizing multidimensional behavior with available or
preserved functions. At a neuropsychological level of analysis, we may
distinguish function (i.e., memory) from strategy (i.e., semantic
organization), and conceptually neuropsychological function and
strategy may be viewed as orthogonal dimensions of complex cognitive
functions integrated in a third dimension, namely time or temporal
sequence. Considerable experimental and clinical evidence points to
the role of the frontal cortex in the organization of complex human
behavior, and it provides for alterations in behavior according to the
external and internal contexts and desired goal attainment (Damasio,
1985; Fuster, 1980; Jouandet & Gazzaniga, 1979). The programming,
regulation, and verification of activity was attributed to the frontal
lobes by Luria (1966). Although the role of the frontal lobes in
"strategy" has not been the explicit focus of neuropsychological
research, electrophysiological data suggest that the use of elaborative
mnemonic strategy resulted in left frontal negative amplitude shifts,
regardless of whether semantic or imagery mnemonics were used (Uhl,
Lang, Lindinger, & Deecke, 1990). However, these investigators also
found that the temporal lobes served an important role in strategy.
More specifically, utilization of a semantic strategy resulted in
unilateral temporal negative amplitude shifts, whereas imagery
mnemonics resulted in bitemporal negative amplitude shifts. Certainly, functions in part subserved by the frontal and temporal lobes
are often compromised in patient populations for whom neuropsychological rehabilitation efforts are undertaken.

NEUROPSYCHOLOGICAL ASSESSMENT
OF STRATEGY

Whether we emphasize function or strategy in neuropsychological
rehabilitation depends not only on one's theoretical orientation, but
also on how, methodologically, we assess or define *cognitive functions*
in clinical populations. Specific approaches to neuropsychological
assessment have been developed that emphasize the strategies or
processes that patients utilize when performing multifactorial, complex cognitive functions. For example, Christensen (1979) expanded
the concept of a "qualitative analysis" of the defect(s) underlying
impaired performances in the neuropsychological assessment methodology developed by Luria (1973), suggesting that "we must describe
selectively the components included in the activity and analyze the
neurodynamic conditions necessary for the completion of the action"

(p. 17). The qualitative analysis was based on the view that neuropsychological function

> is, in fact, a functional system . . . directed toward the performance of a particular biological task and consisting of a group of interconnected acts that produce the corresponding biological effect. The most significant feature of a functional system is that, as a rule, it is based on a complex dynamic "constellation" of connections, situated at different levels of the nervous system, that, in the performance of the adaptive task, may be changed with the task itself remaining unchanged. (Luria, 1966, p. 22)

These views necessitated a theory-driven neuropsychological analysis of function and process, where the objective of the neuropsychological investigation was to describe the components contributing to a functional system, the dynamic changes inherent in neuropsychological functions, and the effects of an underlying defect on a functional system.

In contrast to a psychometric definition of function, where a particular task is used to measure (define) a specific cognitive function, the Luria–Christensen methodology provided for the study of individual differences and a means to describe the processes and underlying components of neuropsychological function. Similarly, Kaplan (1983) argued that an achievement approach to neuropsychological assessment, where only the overall score produced on a given psychometric task is considered, fails to differentiate underlying cognitive impairments. Kaplan provided multiple examples of how vastly different cognitive impairments can produce identical overall or globally impaired scores.

In the development of a "process approach" to neuropsychological assessment, Kaplan and co-workers provided for the quantification of processes and components of neuropsychological function through the development of new neuropsychological instruments and the modification of previously existing ones. These investigators have relied on a theoretical and experimental understanding of cerebral function in the formulation of their neuropsychological assessment strategies, but have also infused knowledge gleaned through cognitive neuroscience. More specifically, Delis, Kramer, Fridlund, and Kaplan (1990) suggested that

> the goal of the cognitive science approach to test construction is to design instruments that quantify test performances in terms of component functions that have been empirically identified in cognitive and neuropsychological research. Each task should yield multiple

scoring categories that reflect different problem-solving strategies, error types, and other cognitive mechanisms. (p. 103)

The neuropsychological assessment strategies provided by Christensen and Kaplan have provided for the qualification and quantification of individual differences in apparently similar diagnostic groups, but also go beyond the assessment of function and provide at least a tentative framework for neuropsychological assessment of relevance to planning and executing individual programs of neuropsychological rehabilitation. Strategic approaches to the assessment of neuropsychological function emphasize the analysis of differentiable syndromes of cognitive impairment according to: (a) components of cognitive function and (b) cognitive processes utilized to complete the task. Moreover, it is important to consider that cognitive processes occur in the context of biological, emotional and motivational, and environmental dynamics of the situation in which the behavior is sampled. The Boston Process Approach to Neuropsychological Assessment (Kaplan, 1988; Milberg, Hebben, & Kaplan, 1986) provides for the quantitative measurement of the patient's performance, as well as a dynamic serial "picture" of the cognitive strategies inherent in the patient's performance. This approach to assessment provides for the analysis of the compensatory strategies that are spontaneously utilized by the patient and the extent to which these strategies were effective. Strategic approaches to neuropsychological rehabilitation modify the patient's strategy to more adaptively solve a problem or complete a task, while utilizing (or better utilizing) intact cognitive functions, without necessarily assuming that underlying defects or impaired components of cognitive functions can be "remediated." In this context, strategy refers to the processes or methods of utilizing intact or available cognitive functions to reach an outcome or goal, or "perform" a meaningful and adaptive behavior.

A variety of specific instruments, developed by Kaplan and co-workers, provide for the quantification of rehabilitation-relevant strategies, as demonstrated in Table 7.1. One of these instruments is the California Verbal Learning Test (CVLT; Delis, Kramer, Kaplan, & Ober, 1987). The CVLT utilizes constructs from normal and pathological memory research for the purpose of quantifying the different strategies that individuals use in learning, storing, and retrieving material. Delis, Kramer, Freeland, and Kaplan (1988) conducted a psychometric investigation of the validity of the CVLT with 113 neurological patients and 286 normal subjects. Through the findings of factor analysis, it was discovered that Learning Strategy emerged as an apparent dimension, with loadings in semantic

TABLE 7.1
Examples of Strategic Neuropsychological Assessment

Instrument	Source	Strategies Assessed
Sorting Test	Delis, Squire, Bihrle, & Massman (1992)	1. To identify sorting rules 2. To generate accurate sorts 3. To verbalize the principles of accurate sorts performed by the subject 4. To initiate different sorts 5. To verbalize the principles of sorts performed for them by the examiner 6. To comprehend abstract cues provided by the examiner in order to identify correct sorts 7. To use explicit information provided by the examiner to generate sorts 8. To inhibit perseverative sorts 9. To inhibit the verbalization of perseverative rule names
California Verbal Learning Test	Delis, Kramer, Freeland, & Kaplan (1988)	1. Recall 2. Recognition 3. Semantic learning strategies (clustering) 4. Serial learning strategies (clustering) 5. Serial position effects 6. Learning rate across trials 7. Consistency of item recall across trials 8. Degree of vulnerability to proactive and retroactive interference 9. Retention of information over short and long delays 10. Learning errors in recall (i.e., perseverations and intrusions) 11. Learning errors in recognition (i.e., false positives)

California Discourse Memory Test	Kramer, Delis, & Kaplan (1988)	1. Recall
		  a. verbatim recall
		  b. accurate paraphrased recall
		  c. total correct recall (verbatim plus accurate paraphrase)
		  d. gist recall (five main ideas to each story)
		2. Error analysis
		  a. Semantically related intrusion
		  b. Semantically unrelated intrusion
		  c. Interstory intrusion
		  d. Contextured error
		3. Recognition—12 multiple-choice questions for each story. Foils incorporate words from different parts of the story or from the other story, whereas other foils represent responses that are semantically or phonologically related to the correct response.

(Continued)

TABLE 7.1
(Continued)

Instrument	Source	Strategies Assessed	

California Global Local Learning	Delis, Kaplan, & Kramer (1988)	Visuospatial Memory Strategies
		1. Recall
		  a. Free recall
		  b. Learning rate
		  c. Delayed free recall
			Forms that are global or local (whole vs. detail analysis)
			Forms that are linguistic or nonlinguistic
			Presented in left or right Hemispatial Field

		2. Recognition a. Signal-detection three foils (global-only correct, local-only correct, neither level correct). Provide an assessment of retrieval deficits 3. Intrusions, perseverations, omissions, and false positives are tabulated	
California Proverb Test	Delis, Kramer, & Kaplan (1988)	Verbal abstraction (ability to generate abstract thoughts in free-response format and to appreciate abstract concepts in multiple-choice format) 1. Correct abstract 2. Partial abstract (part of response is interpreted abstractly and the rest is interpreted concretely or omitted) 3. Specific instance (only a specific example of the proverb's meaning is given) 4. Correct concrete (literal meaning of proverb) 5. Correct reiteration (concrete interpretation that reports many of same words in target proverb) 6. Partial concrete (only part of proverb is interpreted correctly; rest is incorrect or omitted) 7. Incorrect responses	

clustering. Additionally, results indicated that because only semantic clustering yielded a significant positive loading on the factor of General Verbal Learning, it is a more effective learning strategy than serial clustering. The authors concluded that the results support the psychometric construction and scoring that captures the cognitive profile of each individual patient and the strategies that are utilized.

Recently, Delis, Squire, Bihrle, and Massman (1992) developed a new sorting test that was constructed to isolate and assess specific aspects of strategies utilized by patients in problem solving. For this study, four subject groups (patients with focal frontal-lobe lesions, patients with both frontal dysfunction and Korsakoff's syndrome, patients with circumscribed amnesia, and normal control subjects) were administered the new sorting test. It was found that patients with Korsakoff's syndrome and frontal-lobe lesions were impaired on eight of the nine sections of the task. However, in contrast to the existing literature, results indicated that there was not a single mechanism (such as perseveration) that led to impaired strategies of problem solving in patients with frontal-lobe dysfunction. The present study revealed that there is apparently a wide plethora of deficits in several strategies of executive order functions such as abstract thinking, concept formation, cognitive flexibility, and utilization of knowledge to regulate behavior that contribute to the impairment of problem-solving abilities in these subjects. Therefore, this new sorting task may have certain clinical utility as a neuropsychological assessment of strategy.

Further, Delis et al. (1990) recently presented an approach that they named "The California Neuropsychological System." Assessment instruments utilized for this approach include the previously described CVLT (Delis et al., 1987), the California Discourse Memory Test (CDMT; Kramer, Delis, & Kaplan, 1988), the California Global–Local Learning Test (CGLT; Delis, Kaplan, & Kramer, 1988), the California Proverb Test (CPT; Delis et al., 1988), and the California Finger Tapping Test (CFTT; Friedlund & Delis, 1987). This approach dictates that each assessment instrument be constructed to perform the following functions: (a) enumerate and measure multiple cognitive strategies, processes, and errors that reveal the method that an individual utilizes to solve a task; and (b) provide for microcomputer analysis to yield cost-effective, yet rigorous assessment. For a detailed review of this approach, the reader is invited to peruse the book chapter by Delis et al. (1990). Thus, we are in an exciting era for neuropsychology. Although the literature in the domain of neuropsychological assessment of strategy is limited, there are several approaches that are promising. In the next few years, as the level of accountability for outcome increases, neuropsychological assessments may be linked with neuropsychological rehabilitation interventions to provide for more successful outcomes. Therefore, diagnostic information on individualized strategies will be essential.

STRATEGIC APPROACHES
TO NEUROPSYCHOLOGICAL INTERVENTIONS

Research in the area of strategic neuropsychological intervention has begun to emerge in the last few years. Although there have been reports of studies on neuropsychological intervention that possess heightened methodological rigor, a lack of a unifying theoretical approach to strategy continues to persist. In reviewing the existing empirical studies that address strategic rehabilitation interventions in neuropsychology, the authors have observed that, although there are many impressive findings, there exists no theoretical framework to focus the individualized strategies that were utilized. Additionally, few of the studies in neuropsychological rehabilitation utilize strategies examined in research conducted with normal populations in the derivation of rehabilitation strategies for brain-injured subjects. We present the empirical strategic intervention studies conducted with normal adult populations, and then shift to a summarization of the empirical research investigating strategic interventions for brain-injured and learning-disabled adult populations.

Strategic Intervention Studies for Normal Adult Samples

Cognitive strategy has been examined with normal adult populations (see Table 7.2). Seamon and Gazzaniga (1973) measured the effects of relational imagery and rehearsal coding strategies on a short-term recognition memory task. Utilizing six right-handed university students as the subject sample, it was found that the rehearsal coding strategy led to faster response rates for probes in the left hemisphere than for probes in the right hemisphere. The results were reversed when the relational imagery strategy was employed. These findings suggest a hemisphere preference for type of strategy. Shaver, Pierson, and Lang (1974) investigated the impact that strategies incorporating linguistic principles and visuospatial imagery have on problem solving. These researchers stated that future problem-solving research should address the individualization of strategy choices for problem solving.

Anecdotally, it would seem from these two studies that the type of strategy that an individual employs will most likely lead to different effects as tasks are encountered. Recently, in a very important series of experiments conducted by Reder (1987), this concept of "strategy selection" was investigated as a strategy. Over the course of six experiments, the selection of strategy to answer questions was examined, with 278 undergraduates comprising the subject sample. Results indicated that specific contextual variables can affect the selection of strategy (e.g., plausibility of the question, task requirements). Further, it was found that "question evaluation" is a strategy. Therefore, individualized strategy selection may warrant future research because it has apparently emerged as an important component of cognitive processing.

TABLE 7.2
Strategy Intervention Studies for Adult Normals

Source	Target Function	Strategy	Sample	Findings
Speth & Brown (1990)	Approach to studying, gender, type of examination	Test preparations "Approaches to Studying Inventory Scales": a. Meaning orientation b. Strategic orientation c. Reproducing orientation d. Nonacademic orientation	125 male and 258 female undergraduates	When sources on the time-effort, integration, selection, and cognitive monitoring subsoules were used in a MANCOVA (cluster × gender × type of test), it was discovered that Ss using different approaches reacted differently to multiple-choice or essay tests, and the patterns differed by strategy. Females felt multiple-choice tests were more challenging, requiring more time and effort than males in the same clusters.
Speth & Brown (1988)	Comparison of inventories tapping into three strategies	1. Cognitive processes (Inventory of Learning Processes) 2. Approaches to learning (Approaches to Studying Inventory) 3. Autonomous studying (Cognitive Transformational activities and self-management activities	383 U.S. undergraduates	The following strategies emerged as a result of a series of factor analyses that revealed that they transcended differences in theoretical background and terminology: 1. effort-intensive organized study 2. intention to understand, personalize, and integrate the information being learned 3. strategic or context-sensitive study behavior 4. unselective intention to reproduce information, impervious to external cues, and without personal involvement. The best perspective for understanding the other two functions (cognitive processes and autonomous learning)

Reference	Task	Variable	Subjects	Results
Reder (1987)	Question–answering	Selection of strategy to answer questions (It is reported that there is a specific strategy selection component)	278 undergraduates in six experiments	Experiments I–III: Ss have strategic control over the strategy selection: Ss were sensitive to extrinsic factors when selecting a strategy. Experiments IV & V: Ss "evaluated" sentences quickly enough for initial evaluation of a question to be an aspect of the strategy selection process. Experiment VI: The recency of exposure to words influences Ss "feeling of knowing" process involved in strategy selection. Model is consistent with processing strategies in domains other than question-answering (i.e., dual-task monitoring in divided attention tasks).
Shaver, Pierson, & Lang (1974)	Problem solving (three term-series problems)	Linguistic principles and visuospatial imagery (organize and store in an efficient form information regarding the relationships among objects or people)	80 university students	Results suggested that imagery plays a functional role in problem solving because it reduces the memory load but it is not necessary. Future research on problem solving should address the diversity of cognitive representations and individualized differences in problem-solving strategy choices.
Seamon & Gazzaniga (1973)	Short-term recognition memory task	Relational imagery and rehearsal coding	6 right-handed university students	When utilizing the rehearsal strategy, Ss showed faster response rates for probes in the left hemisphere than in the right. When employing the imagery strategy, faster response rates were yielded in the right hemisphere than the left. Imagery should be used as an aspect of the visual processing system with general visual information being a coding alternative to mediation conducted verbally.

More recently, Speth and Brown (1988, 1990) engaged in a line of research investigating individualized studying and learning strategies of college undergraduates. The first of these studies examined three areas: (a) cognitive processing, (b) approaches to learning, and (c) autonomous studying techniques of 383 undergraduates. A series of factor analyses revealed the emergence of the following four strategies: (a) effort-intensive organized study; (b) motivation to understand, personalize, and integrate the information being learned; (c) context-sensitive studying behavior; and (d) an unselective motivation or intention to reproduce information impervious to external influence and without personal involvement. In a follow-up study, Speth and Brown (1990) investigated the relevance of learning style for strategy utilization in preparation for tests. The results demonstrate that differences in strategy utilization significantly affect performance on tests, depending on the task requirements. Individualization of strategy seems to emerge as an underscoring factor in each of these aforementioned studies. As stated earlier, however, the researchers do not adopt an overriding theoretical framework on which future rehabilitative interventions could be couched. The following examination of the neuropsychological rehabilitation literature similarly emphasizes a trend toward an individualization of strategy, without explicitly stating the movement toward that concept.

Strategic Intervention Studies for Brain-Injured and Learning-Disabled Samples

As incidence and prevalence rates for brain injury have continued to soar, the need for successful interventions for this population has obviously also increased. In the last few years, empirical investigations of strategic interventions have flourished in the neuropsychological literature. In this section, we present several of these studies (as summarized in Table 7.3), all of which drive toward a promising model of strategic rehabilitation intervention for neuropsychology. In an investigation utilizing 16 long-term patients with diagnoses of closed-head injury and 14 controls, Goldstein, Levin, Boake, and Lohrey (1990) discovered that induced semantic-processing strategies facilitated increases in cued recall and recognition levels for the patients, but not to the same extent as with the control subjects. Acoustic and physical processing strategies were reported as being less effective facilitators. Further, Goldstein et al. (1988) found that both list-learning strategies and face-name association strategies resulted in improved levels of recall and learning efficiency, respectively, in the sample of 10 severe head-injury subjects. Additionally, in a study conducted by Berg,

TABLE 7.3

Strategy Intervention Studies for Brain-Injured and Learning-Disabled Patients

Source	Target Function	Strategy	Sample	Findings
Goldstein, Levin, Boake, & Lohrey (1990)	Word recognition memory and cued word recall	Induced semantic processing (levels of processing paradigm involving detection of semantic [categorical], physical [letter], or acoustic [rhyme] features of to-be-remembered words)	16 long-term CHI patients and 14 controls	Induced semantic processing facilitated recognition and cued recall in CHI, but not to the same extent as for controls. Induced acoustic and physical processing were less effective. Results indicate attention to semantic features facilitates memory performance in survivors but may require greater cognitive effort.
Von Cramon, Mathes-Von Cramon, & Mai (1991)	Problem solving (psychometric and functional measures)	Problem-solving training: reduce the complexity of a multistage problem by breaking it down into more manageable portions	32 TBI patients, 2 CVA patients, and 8 others	Results indicated significant pre–post effects of the problem-solving training in the planning test scores, in all behavioral ratings, and in some intelligence subsets. For the memory training, the same tests showed only minor impairments.
Berg, Konig-Haanstra, & Deelman (1991)	Memory rehabilitation	Memory strategy training or drill and repetitive practice on memory tasks	39 severely CHI'd patients	Neither treatment method indicated significant effects on reaction time measures. Both groups subjectively rated therapy effects on their everyday memory functioning as highly positive. Only the memory strategy training group showed significant objective memory performance effects. These were most clear at 4-month follow-up.

(Continued)

117

TABLE 7.3
(Continued)

Source	Target Function	Strategy	Sample	Findings
Goldstein et al. (1988)	Memory training	List-learning technique (infusing words into high-imagery stories) Face-name association technique (used an imagery technique in which physical facial features were associated with names)	10 subjects with severe head injuries, most followed by a period of unconsciousness (persistent amnesia also)	Results indicated that Ss increased their ability to recall lengthy lists despite the changing of list items at each session during the last 7 sessions of the 15-session training course. For the face-naming technique, learning efficiency was also improved, as shown by the significant reduction in necessary trials to learn a series of eight face-name associations.
Gruneberg, Sykes, & Hammond (1991)	Face-name association	Visual mnemonic associative strategy (taking a feature of an individual's face and linking it to some concrete feature of that individual's name)	30 learning-disabled adults	Experimental condition Ss recalled names significantly more often than the control Ss. However, ecological validity was limited.

Koning-Haanstra, and Deelman (1991) with 39 subjects, it was discovered that both the memory strategy training group and the drill and repetitive practice group showed significant objective memory performance effects that were maintained at a 4-month follow-up. These investigators explicitly labeled their interventions as "strategy rehabilitation," which included a focus on ecological validity through utilizing home practice and having the patient identify the targets for memory rehabilitation. Interventions were based on the application of specific "rules" about memory functioning, which the patients were expected to learn and apply to functional situations. The approach was highly individualized, but strategies including attention control, repetition, association, and organization, among others were utilized. The study of maintenance of treatment effect through adequate follow-up measurements continues to be an important methodological requirement for neuropsychological rehabilitation research.

A strategic approach to neuropsychological rehabilitation of problem-solving deficits was utilized by Von Cramon, Matthes-Von Cramon, and Mai (1991). These investigations studied 32 subjects with traumatic brain injury, 2 subjects with cerebrovascular accident, and 8 subjects with other diagnoses, of which 20 were treated within a problem-solving group and 17 in a control group. The strategy training was designed to decrease the complexity of a multistage problem by breaking it down into smaller and more manageable components. Problem-solving training consisted of three components: (a) production of goal-directed ideas, (b) discrimination between relevant and irrelevant information, and (c) processing multiple information. The intervention's impact showed significant pre–post effects on each of the dependent measures, which included neuropsychological measures as well as behavioral ratings.

Additionally, ecological validity must have a heightened level in strategic interventions. In an investigation with a sample of 30 learning-disabled adults, Gruneberg, Sykes, and Hammond (1991) developed a visual mnemonic associative strategy that was designed to improve face-name association function by extracting a feature of an individual's name. Although experimental condition subjects recalled names at a significantly higher rate than the control subjects, the researchers noted that the study was lacking in ecological validity because it was a laboratory experiment. Individualized strategic neuropsychological rehabilitation must focus on ecological validity and generalization to "real-life" activities.

Ecological validity and generalization were addressed in a useful treatment paradigm developed by Toglia (1991). Utilizing a single-subject design, the effect of a multicontext treatment approach on treatment generalization was examined in a 30-year-old male patient with a

closed-head injury. This approach consisted of the following components designed to increase generalization of treatment: (a) use of
multiple environments; (b) task analysis and establishment of criteria
for transfer; (c) metacognitive training in self-knowledge, self-monitor-
ing, self-awareness, etc.; (d) emphasis on processing strategies (situ-
ational and nonsituational); and (e) use of meaningful activities.

The Future of Strategic Approaches
to Neuropsychological Rehabilitation

Empirically, we have observed the diversity of the various strategic
intervention studies for normal, brain-injured and learning-disabled
samples. There has been a noticeable, although unspoken, movement
toward an individualization of strategy in neuropsychological assessment and rehabilitation. Review of the rehabilitation research would
suggest that, in addition to individualization, strategic approaches to
neuropsychological rehabilitation need to incorporate meaningful, ecologically valid training tasks, as well as utilize measures of outcome
targeted at different levels of analysis. Future research will hopefully
incorporate a heuristic model of neuropsychological assessment and
rehabilitation of strategy.

ACKNOWLEDGMENT

The authors wish to express gratitude to Edith Kaplan, PhD, for her
critique of and contributions to this chapter.

REFERENCES

Ben-Yishay, Y., Silver, S. M., Piasetsky, E., & Rattock, J. (1987). Relationship
between employability and vocational outcome after intensive holistic cognitive
rehabilitation. *Journal of Head Trauma Rehabilitation, 2,* 35–48.

Berg, I. J., Konig-Haanstra, M., & Deelman, B. G. (1991). Long-term effects of
memory rehabilitation: A controlled study. *Neuropsychological Rehabilitation, 1,*
97–111.

Brooks, N. (1991). The effectiveness of post-acute rehabilitation. *Brain Injury, 5,*
103–109.

Christensen, A.-L. (1979). *Luria's Neuropsychological Investigation* (2nd ed.).
Copenhagen: Munksgaard.

Christensen, A.-L., Pinner, E. M., Moller-Pedersen, P., Teasdale, T. W., & Trexler,
L. E. (1992). Psychosocial outcome following individualized neuropsychological
rehabilitation of brain damage. *Acta Neurologica Scandinavia, 85,* 32–38.

Damasio, A. R. (1985). The frontal lobes. In K. M. Heilman & E. Valenstein (Eds.),
Clinical neuropsychology (2nd ed., pp. 360–412). New York: Oxford University
Press.

Delis, D. C., Kaplan, E., & Kramer, J. H. (1988). *The California Global-Local Learning Test*. Unpublished manuscript.

Delis, D. C., Kramer, J. H., Freeland, J., & Kaplan, E. (1988). Integrating clinical assessment with cognitive neuroscience: Construct validation of the California verbal learning test. *Journal of Consulting and Clinical Psychology, 56,* 123–130.

Delis, D. C., Kramer, J. H., Friedlund, A. J., & Kaplan, E. (1990). A cognitive science approach to neuropsychological assessment. In P. McReynolds, J. C. Rosen, & G. J. Chelune (Eds.), *Advances in psychological assessment* (pp. 101–132). New York: Plenum.

Delis, D. C., Kramer, J. H., & Kaplan, E. (1988). *The California Proverbs Test*. Unpublished manuscript.

Delis, D. C., Kramer, J. H., Kaplan, E., & Ober, B. A. (1987). *The California Verbal Learning Test-Research Edition*. New York: Psychological Corporation.

Delis, D. C., Squire, L. R., Bihrle, A., & Massman, P. (1992). Componential analysis of problem-solving ability: Performance of patients with frontal lobe damage and amnestic patients on a new sorting task. *Neuropsychologia, 30,* 683–697.

Diller, L., & Gordon, W. A. (1981). Interventions for cognitive deficits in brain-injured adults. *Journal of Consulting and Clinical Psychology, 49,* 822–834.

Friedlund, A. J., & Delis, D. C. (1987). *The California Finger Tapping Test*. Unpublished manuscript.

Fuster, J. M. (1980). *The prefrontal cortex*. New York: Raven Press.

Glisky, E. L. (1992). Computer-assisted instruction for patients with traumatic brain injury: Teaching of domain-specific knowledge. *Journal of Head Trauma Rehabilitation, 7,* 1–12.

Glisky, E. L., & Schacter, D. L. (1987). Acquisition of domain-specific knowledge in organic amnesia: Training for computer-related work. *Neuropsychologia, 25,* 893–906.

Glisky, E. L., & Schacter, D. L. (1989). Extending the limits of complex learning in organic amnesia: Computer training in a vocational domain. *Neuropsychologia, 27,* 107–120.

Glisky, E. L., Schacter, D. L., & Tulving, E. (1986a). Computer learning by memory-impaired patients: Acquisition and retention of complex knowledge. *Neuropsychologia, 24,* 313–328.

Glisky, E. L., Schacter, D. L., & Tulving, E. (1986b). Learning and retention of computer-related vocabulary in amnesic patients: Method of vanishing cues. *Journal of Clinical and Experimental Neuropsychology, 8,* 292–312.

Goldstein, F. C., Levin, H. S., Boake, C., & Lohrey, J. H. (1990). Facilitation of memory performance through induced semantic processing in survivors of severe closed-head injury. *Journal of Clinical and Experimental Neuropsychology, 12,* 286–300.

Goldstein, G., McCue, M., Turner, S. M., Spanier, C., Malec, E. A., & Shelly, C. (1988). An efficacy study of memory training for patients with closed-head injury. *The Clinical Neuropsychologist, 2,* 251–259.

Gruneberg, M. M., Sykes, R. N., & Hammond, V. (1991). Face-name association in learning-disabled adults: The use of a visual associative strategy. *Neuropsychological Rehabilitation, 1,* 113–116.

Jouandet, M., & Gazzaniga, M. S. (1979). The frontal lobes. In M. S. Gazzaniga (Ed.), *Handbook of behavioral neurobiology* (Vol. 2, pp. 25–60). New York: Plenum Press.

Kaplan, E. (1983). Process and achievement revisited. In S. Wapner & B. Kaplan (Eds.), *Toward a holistic developmental psychology* (pp. 143–156). Hillsdale, NJ: Lawrence Erlbaum Associates.

Kaplan, E. (1988). A process approach to neuropsychological assessment. In T. B. Boll & B. K. Bryant (Eds.), *Clinical neuropsychology and brain function: Research, measurement, and practice* (pp. 129–167). Washington, DC: American Psychological Association.

Kirsch, N. L., Levine, S. P., Fallon-Krueger, M., & Jaros, L. A. (1987). The microcomputer as an "othotic" device for patients with cognitive deficits. *Journal of Head Trauma Rehabilitation, 2,* 77–86.

Kirsch, N. L., Levine, S. P., Lajiness-O'Neill, R., & Schnyder, M. (1992). Computer-assisted interactive task guidance: Facilitating the performance of a simulated vocational task. *Journal of Head Trauma Rehabilitation, 7,* 13–25.

Kramer, J. H., Delis, D. C., & Kaplan, E. (1988). *The California Discourse Memory Test.* Unpublished manuscript.

Luria, A. R. (1966). *Higher cortical functions in man.* New York: Basic Books.

Luria, A. R. (1973). *The working brain: An introduction to neuropsychology.* New York: Basic Books.

Milberg, W. P., Hebben, N., & Kaplan, E. (1986). The Boston process approach to neuropsychological assessment. In I. Grant & K. M. Adams (Eds.), *Neuropsychological assessment of neuropsychiatric disorders* (pp. 65–86). New York: Oxford University Press.

Prigatano, G. P. (1986). *Neuropsychological rehabilitation after brain injury.* Baltimore: Johns Hopkins University Press.

Reder, L. M. (1987). Strategy selection in question answering. *Cognitive Psychology, 19,* 90–138.

Robertson, I. H., Gray, J. M., Pentland, B., & Waite, L. J. (1990). Microcomputer-based rehabilitation for unilateral neglect: A randomized controlled trial. *Archives of Physical Medicine and Rehabilitation, 71,* 663–668.

Schacter, D. L., & Graf, P. (1986). Preserved learning in amnesic patients: Perspectives from research on direct priming. *Journal of Clinical and Experimental Neuropsychology, 8,* 727–743.

Seamon, J. G., & Gazzaniga, M. S. (1973). Coding strategies and cerebral laterality effects. *Cognitive Psychology, 5,* 249–256.

Shaver, P., Pierson, L., & Lang, S. (1974). Converging evidence for the functional significance of imagery in problem solving. *International Journal of Cognitive Psychology, 3,* 359–375.

Sohlberg, M. M., & Mateer, C. A. (1989). Training use of compensatory memory books: A three stage behavioral approach. *Journal of Clinical and Experimental Neuropsychology, 11,* 871–891.

Speth, C., & Brown, R. (1988). Study approaches, processes and strategies: Are three perspectives better than one? *British Journal of Educational Psychology, 58,* 247–257.

Speth, C., & Brown, R. (1990). Effects of college students' learning styles and gender on their test preparation strategies. *Applied Cognitive Psychology, 4,* 189–202.

Toglia, J. P. (1991). Generalization of treatment: A multicontext approach to cognitive perceptual impairment in adults with brain injury. *American Journal of Occupational Therapy, 45,* 505–516.

Trexler, L. E. (1987). Neuropsychological rehabilitation in the United States. In M. J. Meier, A. L. Benton, & L. Diller (Eds.), *Neuropsychological rehabilitation* (pp. 437–460). London: Livingstone.

Trexler, L. E., & Thomas, J. T. (1992). Research design in neuropsychological rehabilitation. In Y. Steinbuchel, D. Y. Von Cramon, & E. Poppel (Eds.), *Neuropsychological rehabilitation.* Heidelberg: Springer-Verlag.

Uhl, F., Lang, W., Lindinger, G., & Deecke, L. (1990). Elaborative strategies in word pair learning -DC- potential correlates of differential frontal and temporal lobe involvement. *Neuropsychologia, 28,* 707–717.

Von Cramon, D. Y., Matthes-Von Cramon, G., & Mai, N. (1991). Problem-solving deficits in brain-injured patients: A therapeutic approach. *Neuropsychological Rehabilitation, 1,* 45–64.

Warrington, E. K., & Weiskrantz, L. (1974). The effect of prior learning on subsequent retention in amnesic patients. *Neuropsychologia, 12,* 419–428.

Weinberg, M. A., Diller, L., Gordon, W. A., Gerstman, L. J., Liebermann, A., Lakin, P., Hodges, G., & Ezrachi, O. (1977). Visual scanning effect on reading related tasks in acquired brain damage. *Archives of Physical Medicine and Rehabilitation, 58,* 479–486.

Weinberg, M. A., Diller, L., Gordon, W. A., Gerstman, L. J., Liebermann, A., Lakin, P., Hodges, G., & Ezrachi, O. (1979). Training sensory awareness and spatial organization in people with right brain damage. *Archives of Physical Medicine and Rehabilitation, 60,* 491–496.

Weinberg, M. A., Piasetsky, E., Diller, L., & Gordon, W. (1982). Treating perceptual organization deficits in nonneglecting RBD stroke patients. *Journal of Clinical Neuropsychology, 4,* 59–75.

World Health Organization. (1980). *International classification of impairments, disabilities, and handicaps: A manual of classification relating to the consequences of disease.* Geneva: Author.

CHAPTER EIGHT

Cognitive Training Methods in Rehabilitation of Memory

Ritva Laaksonen

ABSTRACT

This chapter deals with the application of cognitive training methods in neuropsychological rehabilitation of memory. The role and status of rehabilitation methods in relation to rehabilitation goals are discussed, as well as the factors influencing the proper choice of methods. Approaches to treatment of impaired memory are described in relation to theory and practical procedures performed in a stepwise fashion and combining individual and group techniques.

Neuropsychological rehabilitation is a specialized domain in clinical neuropsychology requiring multidisciplinary knowledge in neurosciences, cognitive and experimental psychology, as well as acquaintance with psychotherapeutic models and theory. The demand for scientifically based treatment techniques has been made by many authors during the past years (Diller & Gordon, 1981; Luria, 1963; Maruszewski, 1968; Powell, 1981; Tsvetkova, 1972; Wilson, 1987).

Tsvetkova wrote that material about rehabilitation dealt with practical problems, whereas the theoretical and scientific bases of therapeutic education were less developed. She believed that the development of theoretical foundations is an essential task for the neuropsychology, and therefore started to create specific programs along these lines. In current literature, the emphasis is on using knowledge of various branches of psychology to provide theories about

125

the nature of human memory and the methodology for treatment (Wilson, 1987).

The treatment procedures can be viewed from several angles, relating to their usefulness and to the theoretical framework from which they are designed. The methods can be viewed as ways to reach certain goals, not a cookbook collection of strategies to improve 'impaired functional abilities. The aim in Diller and Gordon's (1981) terms is to treat "real people" in the "real world." To attain this aim, several aspects must be considered. The cognitive training methods contribute to the following goals as seen in Fig. 8.1.

All of these goals are relevant whether the treatment is at outpatient polyclinics for a couple of sessions a week, or in intensive holistic programs like those discussed by Christensen and Uzzel (1987), Ben-Yishay et al. (1985), or Prigatano, Fordyce, Zeiner, Rouche, and Pepping (1984). All areas, as shown in Fig. 8.1, contribute to each other.

As for the deterioration of quality of life, there is evidence that subjectively experienced depression plays a more central role than specific disabilities. The quality of life for 46 stroke survivors under

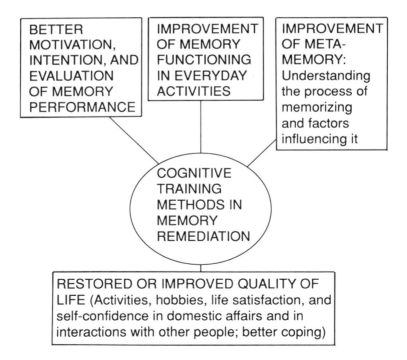

FIG. 8.1. Goals of neuropsychological rehabilitation of memory in relation to training methods.

the age of 65 was studied by the author and collaborators 4 years after onset. The results showed that, despite good recovery in terms of discharge from hospital, activities in daily living, and return to work, the quality of life of most patients (83%) had not been restored to the prestroke level. The subjective tendency to depression was found to correlate highly and negatively with the quality of life (Niemi, Laaksonen, Kotila, & Waltimo, 1988).

The findings can be interpreted as meaningful for management of depression and emotional factors after illness. The patient group in the study did not get any treatment except physiotherapy and speech therapy, so the lack of specific emotional support can be understood. Memory impairment and metamemory cannot be seen in isolation from motivation and intention. Both are also linked with domains of (a) perceived capacity, (b) experienced change, (c) task structure, (d) strategies, (e) achievement goals, (f) anxiety, and (g) locus of control (Dixon & Hultsch, 1983).

FACTORS INFLUENCING THE CHOICE OF METHODS

Diller and Gordon (1981) made a summary of critical issues for clinical psychologists to consider in the 1980s in rehabilitation practices. First, the ecologic issues should be considered, such as the meaning of deficits in everyday situations and the use of remediated skills in novel situations. Second, remediation in various populations should be considered differently whether senile, stroke, trauma, or mentally retarded. Third, attention should be paid to emotional problems and their management. Fourth, a metatheory of rehabilitation should be established with interdisciplinary knowledge concerning scientific basis of rehabilitation, as well as practical knowledge of factors influencing treatment procedures. Besides treatment methods or procedures, several factors influence the outcome. Intervention techniques should be designed in accordance with the interacting variables. The factors concerning the lesion, the patient, and the procedures are listed in Table 8.1.

Planning of treatment depends on these interactive variables. Individual factors influence treatment procedures. Worry, anxiety, or pain can make all the efforts in vain unless treated separately. Age factors must also be taken into account, particularly when setting the goals for treatment. Powell (1981) divided the mechanisms of recovery in relation to time into three categories: (a) biological, (b) reorganizational, and (c) new learning mechanisms. Biological mecha-

TABLE 8.1
Mechanisms and Factors Influencing the Outcome
of Neuropsychological Rehabilitation

Mechanisms	Factors
1. Lesion or injury	Localization
	Size
	Speed of development and mechanism
	Other specific features
2. Individual factors of the patient	General state of health
	Degree of dominance in brain functions
	Intellectual capacity
	Motivation, interests and personality
	Age
	Reactions in the process of psychic crisis at the time of treatment
	Family affairs
3. Factors concerning therapeutic procedures	Time of treatment after onset
	Therapeutic methods
	Personality and skills of the therapist
	Duration of treatment

nisms operate within a few days after the onset of illness, whereas reorganization of function is possible for longer periods of up to a year or more. On the other hand, new learning is possible as long as the patient has any intellectual or mental memory capacity left. In the behavioristic framework, new learning can be seen as a central mechanism when the aim is coping with handicap. Also, using new devices for memory problems or learning specific strategies can be considered new learning (Wilson, 1987; Wilson & Moffat, 1984). Metacognition is used to increase awareness of complex acts and behavior that were previously carried out automatically. Several studies confirm the role of metacognition (Kurtz & Borkowski, 1984; Lachman, Lachman, & Thronesbery, 1979; Schneider, Korkel, & Weinert, 1987). The nihilism against possibilities of treatment of specific deficits due to localized lesion was based on false conceptions of strict localization, heredity, stability, and global nature of functions, as well as the misconception of the mechanisms of recovery. The self-evident possibility of new learning opens more optimistic views even to nihilists.

The mechanism of reorganization of function is neuropsychologically the most interesting and challenging mechanism to consider when specific treatment procedures are designed for specific neuropsychological deficits. Reorganization as a central mechanism of recovery of function after brain injury has been well documented by Luria (1963, 1970, 1973, 1976).

ILLUSTRATIONS OF TREATMENT METHODOLOGY

The illustrations of treatment methodology aim at demonstrating how theoretical concepts can serve as guidelines. Memory is viewed from a systemic point of view having functionally different phases in time sequence (i.e., receiving or encoding, storing, and retrieving or recalling information). Luria's creative work during and after World War II formed the basis for detailed and specific methods for treatment of disabilities of brain-injured people. Luria's approach is a dynamic, systemic theory of localization of higher cortical functions. A detailed qualitative neuropsychological analysis of the basic defects and an evaluation of the preserved abilities make it possible to plan individual rehabilitation strategies and methods using the unimpaired and accessible functional properties of the patient's capacity in neuropsychological reorganization.

The reconstruction methods can be divided into two groups: (a) direct methods, which include the more mechanical training procedures and stimulations; and (b) indirect (compensatory) methods, which aim at neuropsychological reorganization of functional systems. The central mechanisms of recovery act toward reorganization of the impaired functional systems that form the psychophysiological basis of man's higher mental processes (Laaksonen, 1987).

Memory cannot be seen in isolation from other domains necessary in the process of memorizing. Adequate coding of any new material is dependent on the modally specific basic skills required in the process. One cannot learn to dance without intact voluntary motor functions or remember passages of prose without language. Poor attention and easy fatigue affect the ability to learn any new material or even recall old information.

Before treatment, it is important to note that the treatment design is based on detailed qualitative neuropsychological assessment using Luria's Neuropsychological Investigation (Christensen, 1975) and qualitative measures using the traditional psychometric memory tests. The aim is to qualify the central mechanisms of defective functioning with Luria's method. For mild memory disturbances, a short period of training (i.e., 2–3 months) is possible.

Counseling and demonstrating to the patient how memory works is of crucial importance. It is also important to emphasize the meaning of deep coding: The more the material is elaborated and deeply encoded, the better it will be remembered. Good visualization is an asset when verbal memory is poor, and structuring and rehearsal do not work as elaboration strategies. Visual imagery training can serve as the basis for memorizing things to do, appointments, or other specific verbal material. If the weaknesses are focused on visual memorizing, verbal structuring or cuing can be used. In severe memory disturbances, it is important to orient the patient to time, place, and personal matters. A diary is of use, as well as close communication with the relatives or other informants. Other memory devices (Wilson, 1987) can also be used as external memory aids. The Memory Enrichment Program (MEP; Laaksonen & Peltomaa, 1990) has proved a suitable starting method for severe memory disturbances. Theoretically, it aims at overcoming the increased inhibition of memory traces, lack of intention, and passive spontaneous coding. Linking associations with a coherent familiar framework benefits later recall, in which the framework (schema) can be used as an opening for completing previously learned associations and details. New material is added when all previous material has been accurately remembered, therefore repetition plays a role in the procedure, as well as self-control and insight. It is a time-limited procedure fitted into 3 weeks, at the minimum of two to three sessions a week. In severe cases, the time span is longer. For frontal types of memory disturbances where the encoding is poor, a stepwise program can be of use. The first stage does not involve memory tasks, but rather tasks teaching the patient "tools" necessary in memorizing. The second stage includes tasks in which the skills learned in the first stage are put to use. Clinical features during the first stage include: (a) lack of intention, (b) ability to pay attention to the essential and inhibit irrelevant stimuli, (c) unawareness, (d) poor control, and (e) evaluation of performance.

Running a memory group is a good continuation for individual therapy. In a group, patients tend to be more alert and motivated when they can share their experiences with others. They learn better ways of coping and adapt better to having residual problems in everyday life. To an open-ended question like, "What have you learned in the group?" one may get answers like, "I have learned to use my head in a different way," but the answer may also be, "I am not suicidal any more." The goal is to improve metamemory domains: (a) knowledge of change, (b) strategy, (c) importance of achievement and effort, (d) locus of control, and (e) insight into emotional factors. The effect of memory training per se is a controversial subject, but it is still listed as a goal. The group usually lasts about 3 months and meets once a week for 1½ to 2 hours. Between the sessions, the patients monitor their memory behavior and emotional reactions as a homework assignment to be discussed in the beginning of the next session. The group is run by two persons, usually a senior neuropsychologist and a student. Procedures are documented in a group diary. The stages advance from counseling to more difficult exercises. It is important to have a special structure for each session:

first to relax and then begin to work. Summaries develop metafunctions, as well as evaluate the learning process.

Although the memory training was not performed as an experimental design, it is worth noticing that improvement in test results occurred 16–17 months postonset. Previously, individually treated patients also improved after the group intervention. For future work, it would be of central importance to collect research data, as well as have theoretical foundation for treatment processes.

REFERENCES

Ben-Yishay, Y., Rattok, J., Lakin, P., Piasetsky, E., Ross, B., Silver, L., Ziele, E., & Ezrachio, O. (1985). Neuropsychologic rehabilitation: A quest for a holistic approach. *Seminar of Neurology, 5,* 252–259.

Christensen, A.-L. (1975). *Luria's Neuropsychological Investigation.* Copenhagen: Munksgaard.

Christensen, A.-L., & Uzzell, B. P. (1987). *Neuropsychological rehabilitation. Current knowledge and future directions.* Boston: Kluwer.

Diller, L., & Gordon, W. (1981). Interventions for cognitive deficits in brain-injured adults. *Journal of Consulting Clinical Psychology, 49,* 822–834.

Dixon, R. A., & Hultsch, D. F. (1983). Structure and development of metamemory in adulthood. *Journal of Gerontology, 38,* 682–688.

Kurtz, B. E., & Borkowski, J. G. (1984). Children's metacognitions: Exploring relations among knowledge, process, and motivational variables. *Journal of Experimental Child Psychology, 37,* 335–354.

Laaksonen, R. (1987). Neuropsychological rehabilitation in Finland. In M. Meier, A. L. Benton, & L. Diller (Eds.), *Neuropsychological rehabilitation* (pp. 387–395). New York: Churchill Livingstone.

Laaksonen, R., & Peltomaa, K. (1990). The memory enrichment program for severe memory disturbances. A case study. In H. Kalska, R. Laaksonen, A.-R. Putkonen, & K. Olsson (Eds.), *Neuropsychological rehabilitation* (pp. 111–117). Helsinki: Kuntoutussäätiö.

Lachman, J. L., Lachman, R., & Thronesbery, C. (1979). Metamemory through the adult life span. *Developmental Psychology, 15,* 543–551.

Luria, A. R. (1963). *Restoration of function after brain injury.* Oxford: Pergamon.

Luria, A. R. (1970). *Traumatic aphasia.* New York: Mouton.

Luria, A. R. (1973). *The working brain.* London: Allen Lane, Penquin Press.

Luria, A. R. (1976). *The neuropsychology of memory.* Washington, DC: V. H. Winston & Sons.

Maruszewski, M. (1968). A Polish-Soviet neuropsychological symposium. *International Journal of Psychology, 3,* 313–315.

Niemi, M. L., Laaksonen, R., Kotila, M., & Waltimo, O. (1988). Quality of life 4 years after stroke. *Stroke, 19*(9), 1101–1106.

Powell, G. E. (1981). Mechanisms underlying the recovery of function. In G. E. Powell (Ed.), *Brain function therapy* (pp. 1–19). England: Gover.

Prigatano, G. P., Fordyce, D. J., Zeiner, H. K., Rouche, J. R., & Pepping, M. (1984). Neuropsychological rehabilitation after closed head injury in young adults. *Journal of Neurology, Neurosurgery and Psychiatry, 47,* 505–513.

Schneider, W., Korkel, J., & Weinert, F. E. (1987). The effects of intelligence, self-concept, and attributional style on metamemory and memory behaviour. *International Journal of Behavioural Development, 10,* 281–299.

Tsvetkova, L. S. (1972). Basic principles of a theory of re-education of brain-injured patients. *Journal of Special Education, 6,* 135–144.

Wilson, B., & Moffat, N. (1984). *Clinical management of memory problems.* London: Croom Helm.

Wilson, B. A. (1987). *Rehabilitation of memory.* New York: Guilford.

CHAPTER NINE

Computers in Aphasia Rehabilitation

Franz-Josef Stachowiak

ABSTRACT

This chapter attempts to examine computer-based aphasia therapy with respect to its possibilities for training, efficacy, and role in a comprehensive therapy plan. After presenting the Lingware-STACH therapy system developed in Bonn, Germany, a review of the literature establishes the efficacy of aphasia therapy in general as a basis for examining the efficacy of supplementary computer-based therapy. With this background, a report on a randomized multicenter therapy study with 156 aphasic patients is given. The results show specific, significant supplementary effects brought about by computer training; for instance, in written language performance per aphasic syndrome and individual patients. Open questions, particularly with regard to the effects of aphasia therapy on communicative behavior, are discussed. Standardized tests measure the progress of therapy in language modalities, but do not sufficiently assess improvements relevant to daily living. In this connection the objectives and approaches in aphasia therapy, particularly symptom-oriented versus holistic, are reconsidered. On the basis of a therapy trial, suggestions are made for establishing integrated therapy plans and new evaluation schemes based on conversational analysis.

Computer-based techniques are being increasingly implemented in neuropsychological rehabilitation. For the training of basic functions such as attention, visual discrimination, spatial and sequential memory, as well as the treatment of hemianopia, computers present new treatment possibilities. Graphics and text stimuli can be presented randomly, and presentation time and the time between presentations in addition to allotted reaction time can be preset by the therapist. Many programs adjust automatically to the patient's level of performance while providing continuous feedback to support the patient and guide his or her work. The registering of the patient's performance data allows the progress made to be monitored and assists in making therapy plans. The treatment of higher cognitive functions, such as problem solving, memory disorders, and, above all, language disorders requires highly developed, interactive learning programs that go beyond simple pattern drilling. It offers patients the opportunity to train simulated, real-life situations, thereby helping to prepare them for the return to daily life.

Nevertheless, it is clear that computers cannot replace human therapists. Rather, the computer is an additional aid for patients and therapists that can increase the amount of training time and offer interesting therapy material. An important goal is also the possibility of controlled home training. Programs should be designed to allow patients to work at home, perhaps with the assistance of family members or friends. This could be used to bridge the time between periods of treatment, as well as to assist in maintaining or improving an achieved level of performance. However, this requires the programs to be neuropsychologically founded, their efficacy proved, and for therapy progress to be controlled and guided by a professional therapist. At present, only a few programs meet these requirements.

One of the principal arguments for the development of computer-based therapy programs is their contribution to cost reduction in the area of neuropsychological rehabilitation. Although this does not lead to a reduction in the number of therapists, therapy can be intensified and examined more objectively, and the rehabilitation process can be accelerated. Due to their cost-reducing potential, computer-based methods have become interesting for health-care insurance agencies and, due to the high number of patients, also have a certain commercial potential. By the same token, one can expect an increase of commercially developed programs particularly because large computer companies already produce special rehabilitation software. Nevertheless, it is important not to lose sight of ethical values and not to forget that the rehabilitation of a brain-damaged person involves more than just the restitution of specific physical and cognitive functions. The main goal is to help the handicapped person become emotionally stable, reintegrate him or her socially, and assist him or her to become as independent as possible. Therefore, computer-based methods have to be incorporated into a comprehensive treatment program and implemented to achieve the best effects possible for each individual. In the framework of a European concerted action supported by the Commission of the European Community (EC) entitled "The Evaluation of the Efficacy of Technology in the Assessment and Rehabilitation of Brain-Damaged Patients,"[1] a pool of programs for disorders in the areas of language, memory, attention, and visual neglect was established from 1990 to 1992 (Stachowiak, Willeke, Grassau, Schädler, & Rivetto, 1991). Evaluation studies were carried out to compile the scientific basis for using computers in the area of neuropsychological rehabilitation. The following presents some of the results obtained in the area of computer-assisted aphasia therapy.

EXAMPLES OF THERAPY PROGRAMS

First Developments

The first trials using computers in aphasia therapy in Europe were at the end of the 1970s in Paris (Deloche and team) and in Bristol, England, at the beginning of the 1980s (Enderby and team). In addition, work was being done on a computerized therapy system at the technical university in Delft (STAP Project), one of the main focuses being on ergonomy specifically for the handicapped. In the United States, Katz and Loverso have done prominent work in the area of computer-assisted language therapy, with the focus on treating specific disorders such as reading. The first therapy system containing comprehensive language material—based on linguistic criteria—for the treatment of all aphasic symptoms, and equipped with a special speech synthesizer developed for this purpose, was the Lingware/STACH System, a program developed in Bonn from 1983 to 1989 and funded by the German Federal Ministry For Research and Technology (BMFT).[2] At the same time, although at first not designed for IBM compatible computers, Vendrell in Barcelona developed a system that, similar to the Bonn system, combines written texts, graphics, and synthesized speech. However, the Bonn system is the only system today that has been evaluated for efficacy in a large, randomized multicenter clinical study.

During the course of the European project, versions of the Bonn program were developed in the following languages: Dutch, Swedish, English, and French. Partial versions have been developed in Spanish and Italian. A Danish version is planned. More recent programs, such as Cognisoft in Denmark and a Swedish program developed by Kitzing

---

[1]Supported by a grant from the Commission of the European Communities.
[2]Supported by the Federal Ministry for Research and Technology, Project No. 01VJ033.

and team in Malmö, with the Hypercard from Apple, also aim at constructing a comprehensive training program comprising a wide variety of exercises.

The Lingware/STACH System

The typical structure of a computer-based aphasia therapy system is illustrated using the components of Lingware/STACH (see Fig. 9.1). The DOS compatible system is composed of two elements: the therapy system containing the therapy program, and an authoring system for modifying the exercises in the therapy system or creating new exercises.

The therapy system is composed of approximately 150 exercises, each with about 50 tasks. Text, auditive speech, and graphics can be presented simultaneously to activate as many channels as possible. The program can be operated with a standard keyboard, a joystick with four keys, a mouse, or a trackerball. The auditive speech is given via an

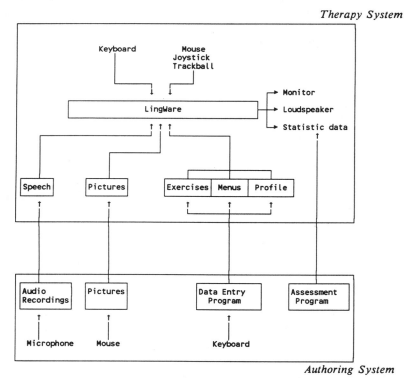

Therapy System

Authoring System

FIG. 9.1. Overview of the Lingware/STACH System.

external loudspeaker. It is also possible for the patient to use the system to record his or her own speech output and, by pressing a specific key, to have this replayed as often as desired. In this way, he or she can compare his or her own speech output to that given by the computer. There are approximately 1,000 pictures and 1,500 audio recordings of speech and sound in the program. Used daily in therapy sessions of 1 hour, the material is sufficient for 3 months of training. For patients with severe language disorders, this period may be longer. Accompanying physical handicaps (e.g., hemiplegia, hemianopia, apraxia, etc.) were taken into consideration to ensure the program's being user friendly. Special measures such as (a) text entering the screen slowly from the right, (b) operational procedure limited to a few keys with a constant order, (c) constant correlation of color to function, and (d) dialogue lines at the bottom of the screen with simplified feedback (also given auditively) help patients to quickly become familiar with the program even if they have no computer experience. Work with the computer is made easier by the use of prototypical pictures and larger fonts, which can be adjusted. The exercises can be combined as desired, depending on the therapeutical goal and the severity of the impairment. The duration of a session can also be determined individually, and breaks are always possible at any time. Following a break, whether it be a matter of minutes or days, training can be resumed at the point at which it was interrupted. The therapy system also contains an extensive statistics program to register the steps of therapy. The recording, evaluation, and graphic representation of the data for each patient provide the therapist with a quick overview of the work done and the progress made.

In comparison with most other programs created with commercially available authoring systems, Lingware/STACH has its own authoring system tailored to the needs of therapists, meaning software used to create exercises for therapy purposes. Lingware/STACH has an open-program structure that can be expanded. Using the authoring system, the therapist is able to modify and elaborate existing exercises. All of the exercise types can be used freely (create file, modify file, copy file, delete file). The other elements (menus, graphics, speech files, tasks) can also be changed. Special programming knowledge is not required. For instance, to add new pictures to the program, graphics can be made using a graphics program (PCX format), or they can be scanned and inserted into the picture database of the program. Speech files are made with the microphone, and are digitized and saved in the audio database in the computer. Picture (.pcx) and speech files (.voc; there are drivers for different speech cards) are combined by filling in the corresponding paths and names of the files desired in a control file. Then in every instance of use, the task will appear with the picture(s) and speech file(s) selected. The control file also contains the written text(s) used for a task. For example, this could be a fill-in-the-blank sentence as cue. Of course, it must contain the correct solution against which the response of the patient is checked. It also can be used as feedback to confirm the patient's response or to provide the solution after an error (error limit depends on exercises) or time limit (Griessl, Stachowiak, & Burbulla, 1992).

Examples of Exercises

There are 19 different preprogrammed open-exercise frames (i.e., exercise types) for exercise procedures in Lingware/STACH. The present version of the program contains a wide variety of exercises with different training material created with these 19 exercise types. The exercises are located in menus and submenus. To load a specific exercise, one first uses a pull-down menu in the Lingware shell, which correlates for the most part with the exercise types (name, naming, dictation, comprehension, categories, syntax, minimal pairs, numbers/letters, take notice, Token/Screening Test, and situations). This menu branches into subsequent menus as shown in Fig. 9.2. This is an example of a written naming menu. The first submenu following the main menu offers a selection of "single picture" or "scene," whereby "scene" allows the patient to select the picture segment to be named. If "single picture" is selected, a further submenu is presented that offers a selection of different operational procedures, such as typing the solution with the keyboard.

A color picture, for instance a foot or a sandal, is shown for the exercise area "Shoe Shop," in which the patient can train language material in the form of words, sentences, multiple choice, and so on all belonging to the situation "Shoe Shop" (Fig. 9.3). The task is to type the word (article is given) on the keyboard. If the patient completes the task correctly, the computer provides the oral name. A dialogue line at the bottom of the screen tells the patient to press the green key to go on to the next task. Erroneous input is signaled by a beep and is not shown on the screen. If the patient is unable to find the next letter, he or she can "request" it by pressing the space bar twice. The dialogue line provides information on the exercise (e.g., that the patient should type in the answer or, that by pressing the black key, the audio recording can be repeated). An example for the exercise type syntax is given in Figs. 9.4 and 9.5. By way of the menu (Fig. 9.4), one can call a multiple-choice exercise "Prepositions." This exercise is from the exercise area "Restaurant," in which language

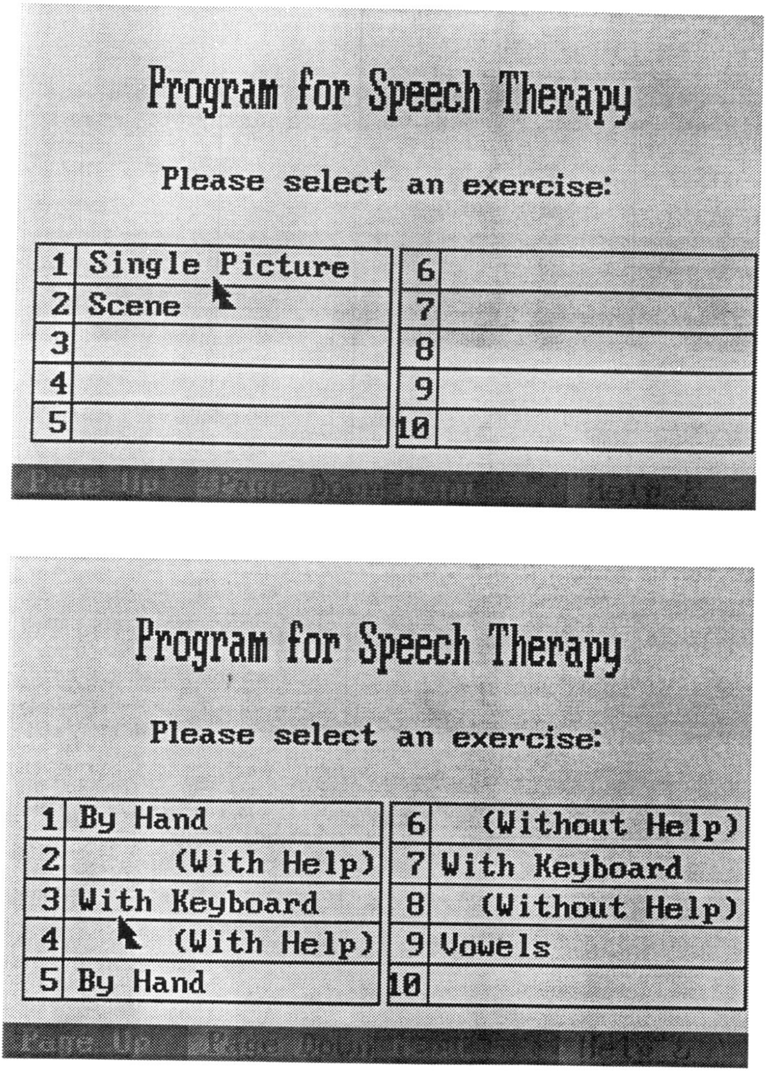

FIG. 9.2. Example of menus.

material is trained with focus on a typical restaurant situation (e.g., ordering food, paying, etc.).

Figure 9.5 shows an exercise task in which the fill-in-the-blank sentence "The plate is _____ the table" enters the screen from the right after a picture of a restaurant scene is shown. A multiple-choice selection of prepositions is given at the top of the screen. According to

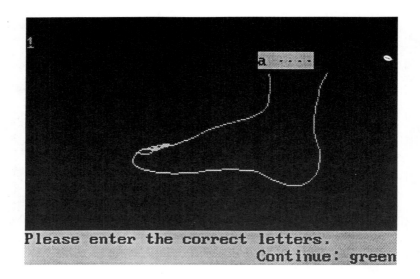

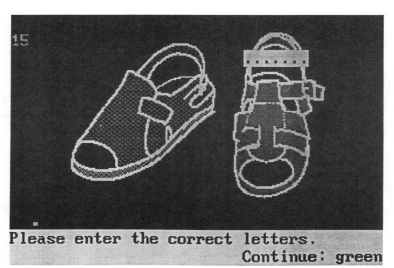

FIG. 9.3. Example of Naming tasks for the situation "Shoe Shop."

Program for Speech Therapy

Please select an exercise:

1	Name	6	Syntax	
2	Naming	7	tree	
3	Dictation	8	Text	
4	Word Formation	9		
5	Categorization	10		

Program for Speech Therapy

Please select an exercise:

1	Prepositions	6	Modal Verbs	
2	Adjectives	7		
3	Prefixes	8		
4	Verbal Inflexion	9		
5	Verb Semantic	10		

FIG. 9.4.   Example of syntax menu.

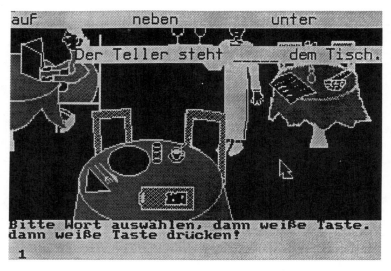

FIG. 9.5. Example of a multiple-choice exercise with prepositions.

the directions given in the dialogue line, the patient is to select the correct preposition with the cursor (controlled by the mouse or track-erball). If he or she selects the correct preposition, it automatically appears in the blank, and the corresponding digitized recording is played. By pressing the green key, the patient can then go on to the next task. Table 9.1 shows the cue scheme that has been designed for this exercise task in the case of erroneous performance.

The patient is first given a cue that uses abstract representation to illustrate the meaning of the prepositions *on*, *next to*, and *under*. After viewing this cue, he or she is presented with the original task again. Following another error, a second cue is shown that contains concrete representations with respect to the restaurant situation. If the patient is still unable to select the correct preposition, the correct solution is presented, otherwise he or she goes on to the next task.

Lingware/STACH also contains exercises that train complex and very specific linguistic structures based on a functional language model (Stachowiak, 1993). The exercises are ordered according to linguistic complexity (i.e., starting with one syllable to multisyllable words, sentences, and then advancing to texts). The exercises vary between the poles of indication (training reference) and predication. Linguistic functions such as determination (more precise definition of objects using attribute structures) have been given special attention. The exercises are in language modalities such as naming, repetition, written language comprehension, and so on. Furthermore, the program also has exercises dealing with basic functions such as memory, sequential

TABLE 9.1
Cueing Procedure for Preposition Exercise

Task 1		
	Type:	sentence completion
	Picture:	situation restaurant
	Text:	fill-in-the-blank sentence
	Multiple-choice set:	three spatial-static prepositions
	correct:	go to task 2
	incorrect:	go to cue 1
Cue 1		
	Type:	name
	Picture:	abstract presentation of spatial represen-tations
	return to task 1	
Task 1:	(see above)	
	correct:	go to task 2
	incorrect:	go to cue 2
Cue 2:		
	Type:	differences
	Picture:	concrete presentation of the prepositions corresponding to prepositional phrases
	correct:	go to task 2
	incorrect:	go to solution
Solution:		
	Type:	name
	Solution:	= original task (task 1) + correct solution (written and auditive)
	go to task 2	

memory, and attention with respect to language. Examples are also given for other exercises in the area of cognitive rehabilitation so that therapists can use them as models when creating their own exercises. In this way, exercises can be tailored to fit patients' individual needs.

An advantage of this structure is that controlled therapy trials can be carried out in which certain variables can be changed (e.g., the same task may appear with or without picture, with or without an acoustic cue, or with or without written cues). A wide variety of combinations is possible. Combined with examinations of regional cerebral blood flow (rCBF) as presented by Risberg and Jensen (chapter 5, this volume) carried out during the course of computer-based aphasia therapy, this method could provide more exact information about which areas of the brain are active during which exercise variations.

Further information about the aphasia therapy programs developed in the previously mentioned European research collaboration can be found in Stachowiak et al. (1993).

EXPERIMENTAL DATA ON THE EFFICACY OF COMPUTER-ASSISTED APHASIA THERAPY

Efficacy of Aphasia Therapy in General

Before a statement can be made about the efficacy of computer-assisted aphasia therapy, the effects of aphasia therapy in general need to be determined. Therapists working in clinics who see patients daily over months at a time report good effects of therapy. The reports required by health-care insurance agencies following treatment contain detailed information on the specific language problems addressed and the improvements made.

At our clinic, we have been able to follow cases of aphasia for periods of up to 10 years because some patients have been treated as often as seven times for a period of 3 months each time. Our department has been a sort of contact address for former patients who call when they have problems. The continuous observation of individual patients has shown that, except in extremely severe cases, there is a continual restitution of language. Following noticeable improvement in the beginning—spontaneous remission can be promoted by therapeutic measures—further restitution continues at a slower pace that is sometimes almost imperceptible for the patient and his or her relatives. However, treatment accelerates this process. Patients often gain better control of their spontaneous speech after years; they can use more words and find these more quickly. Even patients suffering from agrammatism or paragrammatism develop an acceptable sentence structure. They are able to communicate about almost all relevant topics. Usually patients acquire particular automatized phrases that help them in communication situations. Progress is not always of linguistic nature. Rather, some patients demonstrate an increased amount of flexibility with regards to communication. Despite their handicap, they are more willing to try to communicate and develop a certain level of initiative in overcoming difficulties. To achieve this, it is necessary that aphasia therapy, in the narrower sense linguistic or logopedic, be imbedded in other therapies such as ergotherapy, neuropsychological and social reintegration, sport, and so on.

Nevertheless, scientifically speaking, the clinical reports on success are unsatisfactory. Although undisputed by experts, objectiveness is lacking. Studies need to use standardized instruments to measure the effects of therapy and to determine the factors that influence the success of therapy. In looking through the literature, Horner and Loverso (1990) ascertained that out of 593 articles on aphasia therapy, only 75 were databased (i.e., only 12% of the articles contained statistics on the effects of therapy). The articles reported on only 212 aphasic patients. Several larger studies (e.g., Basso, 1987) were post-hoc studies that examined data collected in a clinic, but did not have an experimental design from the start. Several experimental studies that primarily involved nonhospitalized patients who received 2 hours of aphasia therapy a week for a short period of time did not show any effects (Lincoln, Mulley, Jones et al., 1984).

In the meantime, studies have been conducted that are adequately controlled, including the consideration of several important factors such as (a) duration of illness, (b) influence of spontaneous remission in the first 6 months, (c) type and intensity of treatment, (d) age, and (e) type of aphasia. These studies provide information about specific effects of aphasia therapy. Thus, some of the studies examine in which language modalities the improvements occur (i.e., naming, written language, language comprehension, etc.), and whether different therapy methods or occupational groups providing the treatment and the therapy material used have different effects. It is also important to examine whether the effects of training are generalizable and stable.

Three large investigations on improvement in performance were carried out using standardized aphasia batteries such as the Western Aphasia Battery. Shewan and Kertesz (1984) compared treated to nontreated aphasics and established groups of patients with different treatments. The treated patients received aphasia therapy for 1 year: One group received linguistically oriented therapy (*N* = 28); one group received therapy according to the classical stimulation approach (Schuell, 1974; Wepman, 1972; *N* = 24); a third group was supervised by psychologists and nurses who were trained for this task (*N* = 25); and a fourth group of 23 patients received no therapy. Therapy effects were measured using the Western Aphasia Battery. The test was administered initially, at 3 months, at 6 months, and following treatment. Oral and written language performances were evaluated together. The groups treated by professional speech therapists showed significantly higher effects than the untreated group. The three treated groups did not show any differences with respect to the approach used. However, this was attributed to the small number of patients. There was also no difference shown between the two therapy approaches. Gender was not a decisive factor, but age was. Patients with Broca's and global aphasias showed the most improvement. In comparison to earlier studies by Basso, Capitani, and Zanobio (1982), language comprehension did not improve more than language production.

Poeck, Huber, and Willmes (1989) examined the results of therapy of three groups of aphasic patients with the standardized Aachen Aphasia Test (AAT). One group of 23 patients was treated in the early phase following damage (i.e., 1–4 months poststroke; all patients had vascular damage); a second group of 26 patients was in a middle stage (4–12 months following onset); and a third group of 19 cases was more than 12 months postonset. All of the patients were treated for 6–8 weeks and received 9 hours of therapy a week, 4 of which were group therapy. To control the effect of spontaneous remission, the authors proceeded on the results of a study on spontaneous remission with untreated patients (Willmes & Poeck, 1984). They deducted the average improvements per AAT subtest from the scores of patients in the therapy study with duration of illness up to 1 year. The net improvements measured in testing with the AAT following therapy were examined to check whether they exceeded the critical value set in the AAT for significance. This was the case with 78% of the patients in the early phase, 46% of the patients in the middle phase, and 68% of the patients in the chronic phase. Allowance for spontaneous remission was not necessary for the last group. Influence of gender, age, location and size of lesion, and intelligence could not be proved.

My study (Stachowiak, 1989), in which more detailed information was available due to the large number of multicentric samples taken, also showed positive effects of aphasia therapy. Because the study was primarily concerned with proving the efficacy of computer-based supplementary aphasia therapy, the results are presented in more detail next.

The Efficacy of Computer-Assisted Therapy Methods

The effects of computer-assisted therapy methods have been proved in several studies. These have addressed different questions so that a more comprehensive view is emerging of how and where computers can be implemented appropriately.

Seron, Deloche, Moulard, and Rouselle (1980) were the first to show the effects of computer-based aphasia therapy. Therapy was limited to improvements in written language because at that time the computer was seen as an instrument most appropriate for text processing and calculation. Only five patients with severe writing disorders participated in the study. They were to type words dictated to them on the keyboard. The program offered assistance by showing a box for each letter of the word dictated. A major characteristic of the program was that only correct letters were shown. Incorrect entries were rejected by the computer. After training, patients were able to type more words correctly and made fewer errors per word, with the errors being more approximate to the target word. A generalization effect was found for reading.

More recent studies have also primarily used the computer for training with texts. Thus, Katz and Wertz (1992) explored the possibility of using a hierarchically structured training program to improve the reading performance of aphasic patients. The program was composed of 29 reading activities, each with eight levels of difficulty, totaling 232 different tasks. The first 10 activities (i.e., the first 80 tasks) were concerned with perceptual visual-matching tasks (e.g., matching of letters). The other tasks required reading comprehension skills. In the visual-matching tasks, the patient was to match letters, numbers, mixed letters, and numbers and words. The reading comprehension tasks focused on words, phrases, questions, and longer texts. For instance, categories, synonyms, and antonyms had to be comprehended and matched; questions about participants in a sentence such as who/what/where had to be answered; and finally training was done with attributes, comparisons, and the logic of more complex reading assignments. Only texts were displayed on the monitor. The program began with a baseline set of 20 tasks. If the patient had a performance of accuracy of at least 80%, the program automatically proceeded to the next level.

The program was evaluated for its efficacy with 43 chronic, vascular aphasic patients 2–19 years postonset. The patients were assigned to one of three conditions. Thirteen patients participated in the computer training (computer reading treatment), which was 3 hours a week for a period of 6 months; 15 patients performed other activities with the computer (computer stimulation): They worked with cognitive rehabilitation software and played computer games; and 15 patients received no therapy (no treatment). All three groups were tested initially, at 3 months, and at 6 months. The patients in the computer reading treatment group quickly became familiar with the program, and after three sessions they were able to work independently with minimal assistance from the clinician. By the end of the 6 months, most of the patients in this group had worked their way up to the more difficult tasks in the hierarchy. The average number of tasks carried out was 146. Significant improvements were seen from test to test, as measured with general, standardized tests (PICA subtests and Western-Aphasia Battery [WAB]), showing generalization effects for noncomputerized performance variables. Furthermore, it was examined whether the specific training with the computer reading treatment group lead to more improvement in performance in the tests than just computer stimulation or no treatment at all. Analyses of variance revealed that the specific training resulted in significantly better scores in the PICA "Overall Score." Computer stimulation (cognitive rehabilitation software and computer games) did not produce more effects than no treatment. However, the three groups did not differ significantly from test to test in the PICA reading test, although the absolute numbers speak for an improvement in performance in the computer reading treatment group.

In summary, it can be noted that, for the most part, the computer training was carried out independently with little assistance from therapists. There were also improvements in nontrained material; the tasks in standardized test procedures showed that the improvements were brought about by the specific language content in the training program and not by general stimulation by the computers. It was also seen that chronic aphasics benefited from the computer-based training.

Loverso, Prescott, and Selinger (1992) reported on the preliminary results of a study in which they examined the efficacy of delivery systems; clinician versus clinician/assisted microcomputer. Although it seems ethically questionable because the comparison of human therapists to computers implies that human therapists may become redundant, the results are interesting. As can be expected, human therapists were found to be superior to computers. This was particularly the case for certain types of tasks. As in the study carried out by Katz and Wertz (1992), the therapy material was hierarchically structured. For instance, in Level IA, the patients were to copy 30 verbs and, following a "Wh..?" question, repeat the actor and the action. At Level IIB, the patients were to produce an actor and an agent after being presented with a verb, a "Wh..?" question, and a set of the target and four foils. The patients remained at that level when they initially achieved 60% accuracy and progressed through the levels, starting at Level IA with an initial percentage of less than 60%. Tasks of Type A proved to be more successful with therapeutical assistance. There was no difference seen between the two forms of presentation for multiple-choice tasks. Nevertheless, this experiment shows that methodical-didactical criteria should be considered in the development of computer-assisted therapy systems, and that future studies should evaluate where the focus of computer training should be.

The degree to which aphasic patients can work independently with the computer and which exercise types are beneficial is especially important for home training. Enderby and Petheram (1992) reported positive experience in England, where home training plays an important role because long inpatient treatment for aphasia therapy is seldom possible. They installed BBC computers in the homes of 20 patients. The programs did not use graphics or speech synthesizers, but rather primarily contained written language exercises. In a second experiment (10 patients), in which self-adapting exercises were used, the average working time per task decreased by 5.72 seconds for correct answers and 4.67 seconds for incorrect answers. The average working time per task was 12.27 seconds in the first experiment compared with 6.79 in the second experiment for correct answers and for incorrect answers, and 11.03 seconds compared with 6.36 in the second experiment. The adaptiveness of the exercises had the effect that, with a moderate degree of difficulty, the patients spent more time working on the program, thus working at an appropriate level. Patient behavior revealed the following: (a) work was divided into sessions, (b) the patients worked at any time of day (including weekends), and (c) there was an even distribution of working time throughout the 6-week period with a slight peak in the first and last weeks. These data reflect the patient's motivation to work with the program. The mean average working time per session was 38.18 minutes ($N = 17$). Patients worked every day of the week and at all hours (Petheram, 1992). These results show the direction of future developments, particularly with regard to home training.

THE BONN STUDY ON SUPPLEMENTARY
COMPUTER-BASED APHASIA THERAPY

Objectives

The objective of this study was not to compare computer-based therapy with conventional therapy, nor to see whether the computer is as effective as a human therapist. Rather, the concept was to supplement conventional therapy with computer therapy, thus offering an increased amount of therapy, and then to examine whether supplementary training produces supplementary effects. A pilot study (Kotten, Stachowiak, and Willeke, 1985) with 10 patients with Wernicke's aphasia and 10 patients with Broca's aphasia had shown that a computer program that used animated graphics (e.g., the ball flying in the basket) to train the use of prepositions achieved special training effects. Graphics and speech recordings proved particularly beneficial with prepositions in achieving learning effects—more so than purely verbal stimuli and cues. Furthermore, long clinical experience had shown that few patients are able to operate cognitively more demanding interactive programs (i.e., programs requiring more than a simple stimulus–response scheme) on their own. We proceeded on the basis that a well-structured training program would not necessarily require a professional therapist to assist the patient. Help could be provided by trained nonprofessionals (e.g., family members, students and assistants who do social work as an alternative to military service, etc.). The professional therapist's work load would then be reduced, and the amount of therapy given to the patient would be increased. To reach a statistically sufficient number, the study was to be multicentered. Therefore, depending on the center, a number of different occupations were responsible for carrying out the training: logopedians, clinical linguists, and students who assisted the patients in working with the computer. It was later seen that the occupational group did not affect the results. There were no significant differences in the individual centers. Hence, the results of the study provide a representational view of inpatient aphasia therapy at 12 rehabilitation facilities in Germany.[3]

Methodology

The Biometrical Center Aachen was responsible for the experimental design and the statistical evaluation. This was funded by the German Ministry for Research and Technology (BMFT) in a separate project. All of the patient data collected were sent to the Biometric Center on disks. The patient data were then randomized and stratified. Pre- and posttesting were conducted at the participating centers, usually by therapists who were not directly involved in the study. The design was very simple: Those patients who signed a letter of consent to participate in the study were randomly assigned to one of two groups. One group of patients received the normal amount of conventional speech therapy (control group): 1 hour 5 days a week for 6 weeks. The second group of patients received the normal amount of conventional speech therapy

---

[3]Rheinische Landesklinik Bonn; Neurologisches Rehabzentrum Godeshöhe, Bonn; Universität Tübingen: Aussenstelle Ravensburg; Neurologisches Reha-Zentrum Soltau; Reha-Zentrum der Universität Köln; Lehranstalt für Logopädie, Mainz; Kliniken Schmieder, Allensbach; Hardtwaldklinik, Zwesten; Albertinen Krankenhaus, Hamburg; Neurologisches Therapiecentrum, Düsseldorf; Marcus-Klinik, Bad Drieburg; Neurologisches Reha-Zentrum, Geesthacht; and Dept. of Neuropsychology of the Erasmus University of Rotterdam.

plus 1 hour a day of supplementary computer training (computer group). The effect of these 30 hours of supplementary training was to be measured. A third control group (e.g., the computer stimulation group as in the study conducted by Katz and Wertz, 1992) was not established because a greater number of patients would have been statistically necessary and this would not have been therapeutically beneficial (compare also the results from Katz and Wertz, 1992). The results were expected to show effects of the specific content of the exercises in the program. In a post-hoc study, I examined the results of 17 patients who received the same amount of speech therapy spread over a period of 12 weeks as the total amount of speech therapy received by the computer group in the 6-week period (60 hours). These patients did not have better results than the computer group.

The computer program contained so many different exercises of varying complexity that it was possible to put together an individual training program for each patient (i.e., the assisting person selected exercises depending on the patient's needs or wishes and provided assistance when necessary). Details of every session (i.e., the exercises selected, the number of correct and erroneous responses, and the response time) were recorded by the computer. These data have not yet been evaluated statistically. However, they were controlled to ensure that every patient had actually done a certain number of exercises. The AAT was administered immediately before and following therapy. Furthermore, a computerized version of the Token Test, as well as a newly developed evaluation of spontaneous speech, was carried out. The effects of spontaneous remission were controlled by including only patients at least 4 months postonset. Exclusion criteria were: (a) 75 years or older; (b) bilateral lesions; (c) retro- and anterograde amnesia; and (d) progressive diseases such as senile dementia, inability to complete the first part of the Token Test, and failure to pass a screening test (directing cursor to circles) designed to control ability to work with computer.

Results

One hundred fifty-six patients participated in the study. In summary, 77.9% of the patients in the computer group and 77.2% of the patients in the control group had suffered vascular accidents. Traumatic lesions composed the second largest group (6.5% vs. 10.1%), with the rest having mixed etiologies. The average age was 50.7 versus 49.7 years, and the mean average length of illness was 16.5 versus 15.7 months. The proportion of men to women was 52 to 25 in the computer group and 49 to 30 in the control group. A CT scan was done on each patient.

The influence of neurological variables was determined, but this cannot be discussed in detail here (please see report by Biometric Center, Aachen). Ten patients in the computer group versus eight in the control group dropped out of the study (5 vs. 4 due to rejection of study, 1 vs. 2 due to death of patient, 3 vs. 0 due to illness, 1 vs. 2 due to earlier release). Five patients from Rotterdam who took part in the study were not evaluated continuously because the Dutch version of the AAT was not standardized at that time. Both of the groups were homogenous with respect to these parameters: (a) belonging to a center, (b) gender, (c) age, (d) duration of illness, (e) syndrome classification, (f) etiology, (g) localization of damage, (h) neurological symptoms such as paresis, and (i) performances on the AAT.

The following presents a small part of the results: Using the AAT, the percentage of patients who had improved their scores by at least one raw point in the subtests of the AAT was established (see Table 9.2).

The amount of improvement made can be presented by deducting (Token Test) or adding (other subtests) raw points in the subtests. Table 9.3 shows the median of these values for the computer and control groups, respectively.

This table illustrates a rather small range of deviation of improvements in the raw score that can be measured with the AAT. For instance, the patients in the control group (1 hour a day for 6 weeks) improved from pre- to posttesting by a medium score of 2.6 error points in the Token Test; this included only those patients who had a maximum of 40 errors in pretesting. For instance, in Written Language, there were 30 tasks with a maximum of 90 points and a minimum of 0 points. The average improvements were at a median of 7.7 points versus 4.5 points.

Figure 9.6 further breaks down the results; every point represents a patient. The small crosses represent the previously mentioned median of the raw score in the respective subtest by which the patients in the computer group improved as compared with the control group.

TABLE 9.2
Percentage of Patients with Improvements in the AAT Subtests

Subtest	Computer Group[a] (%)	Control Group[b] (%)
Token Test	71.6	67.6
Repetition	78.8	76.1
Written Language	80.3	67.6
Naming	78.8	74.6
Language Comprehension	75.8	62.0

Note. AAT subtests exclude Spontaneous Speech.
[a]$N = 67$. [b]$N = 71$.

TABLE 9.3
Median of Improvements in the AAT Subtests as Measured
According to the Minimal and Maximal Range of Improvement

Subtest	Decrease/ Increase Raw Score	Number of Test Items	Minimum-Maximum Possible Improvement
Token Test	−4.5 vs. −2.6	50	50–0 errors
Repetition	7.9 vs. 5.7	50	0–150 points
Written Language	7.7 vs. 4.5	30	0–90 points
Naming	9.2 vs. 4.9	40	0–120 points
Language Comprehension	7.4 vs. 4.5	40	0–120 points

Note. Computer group versus control group.

Every point above the zero line represents an improvement. Thus, the patient in the computer group represented by the highest point under Token Test improved 24 points in comparison with the preceding test. Tables 9.2 and 9.3, as well as Fig. 9.6, show that, on average, 77% of the patients in the computer group and 70% of the patients in the control group showed improvements in the AAT following the 6-week training period, although the figures are relatively low in comparison with the maximum number of points possible. The computer training resulted in 7% more patients showing improvement, and that the average level of improvement was almost twice as high.

If one simply looks at the raw scores, the numerical improvements appear to be low. However, it must be considered that standardized tests like the AAT represent a relatively rough instrument for measuring. Thus, the test registered only if approximation of a target item (e.g., in naming or repetition) was semantically or phonologically closer than in the preceding test. However, improvements of this kind can only serve as indicators for a trend that may be clearer in communication situations.

Communication behavior also can only be evaluated approximately with the instruments available. Thus, in the AAT Communication Behavior; Articulation/Prosody; Automatic Speech; and Semantic, Phonemic, and Syntactic Structures are rated on a scale of 0–5 points. In an evaluation sheet that I developed, Word Finding is a separate parameter, whereas Articulation/Prosody and Automatic Speech have been left out. As in the AAT, a rating scale of 0–5 was used. The evaluation criteria, in particular with respect to the Syntactic Structure, were more precisely defined. The average percentage of patients who improved by at least one point was 27.8% (AAT) and 31.5% (Stachowiak) in the computer group versus 19.8% (AAT) and 22% (Stachowiak) in the control group. Table 9.4 shows the individual scores.

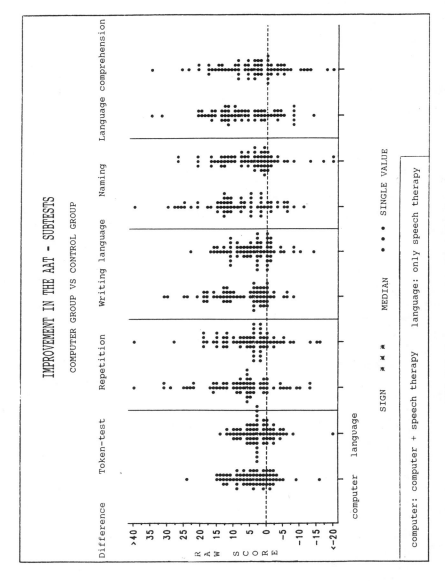

FIG. 9.6. Improvement in the AAT subtests.

TABLE 9.4
Percentage of Patients in the Computer Group and Control Group
with Improvements of at Least One Point in Spontaneous Speech
in Two Evaluation Schemes (AAT and Stachowiak)

Subtest	Computer Group		Control Group	
	AAT (%)	Stachowiak (%)	AAT (%)	Stachowiak (%)
Communication Behavior	45.3	39.0	30.4	30.4
Articulation/Prosody	20.3		11.5	
Automatized Speech	29.6		21.7	
Semantic Structure	26.5	25.0	24.6	18.8
Phonemic Structure	20.3	25.0	18.8	20.2
Syntactic Structure	25.0	34.3	11.5	21.7
Word Finding		34.3		18.8

Similar to the other subtests, even if starting at a lower level, one can see that the supplementary training led to improvements in approximately an additional 10% of the cases. The clearest supplementary effects were in syntactic structure and word finding. For these results, the rating scale in the AAT for spontaneous speech could not establish standard norms. Therefore, Poeck et al. (1989) suggested only considering improvements of at least two points as relevant. In our study, as measured in the subtests, this was the case with 4.1% of the patients in the computer group and 2.1% of the patients in the control group. It is very difficult to find suitable criteria with which to evaluate spontaneous speech, and a change in spontaneous speech within a period of 6 weeks (except in particularly impressive cases of spontaneous remission) cannot be very obvious. Even in language acquisition, 6 weeks is a short period of time to measure relevant qualitative changes such as the sudden appearance of two-word sentences. Insofar as we were able to measure a relatively steady improvement of one point in spontaneous speech with two different evaluation schemes, and given the relatively large number of patients, we can assume that our results are reliable. However, without a doubt, new methods for evaluating spontaneous speech and communication behavior have to be developed.

The results shown up to now have been raw scores. Their significance can be determined by checking if the improvements made by each individual patient correspond to the criteria set by the AAT (minimum improvement). The following critical raw scores or T scores, respectively (one-sided, alpha-level 10%), are given for the AAT: Token Test: 6.5, 4.36; Repetition: 13.61, 3.06; Written Language: 10.58, 3.58; Naming: 14.71, 3.82; and Language Comprehension: 21.04, 8.09.

TABLE 9.5
Number of Patients with Significant Subtest Improvement as a
Function of Syndrome for Computer and Control Groups

Subtest	Syndrome				
	Global[a]	Wernicke[b]	Broca[c]	Amnesic[d]	Others[e]
Token Test					
Computer	1	5	10	4	0
Control	1	3	5	3	1
Repetition					
Computer	4	1	6	1	0
Control	2	2	2	0	2
Written Language					
Computer	3	7	10	2	1
Control	2	1	4	2	1
Naming					
Computer	3	4	4	1	0
Control	0	2	2	1	0
Language Comprehension					
Computer	0	2	0	0	0
Control	1	0	1	1	0

[a]Computer group, $n = 13$; control group, $n = 13$.
[b]Computer group, $n = 13$; control group, $n = 12$.
[c]Computer group, $n = 20$; control group, $n = 29$.
[d]Computer group, $n = 13$; control group, $n = 9$.
[e]Computer group, $n = 5$; control group, $n = 6$.

Table 9.5 shows the number of patients, classified according to syndrome, from each group who showed significant improvement in the subtests. For instance, the table shows that 10 of 20 patients with Broca's aphasia in the computer group and only 5 of 29 patients in the control group demonstrated significant improvements.

With regard to Repetition, one can see that patients with Broca's aphasia benefited the most from the supplementary computer-based training. The computer-assisted training had the most effects on Written Language; 7 of 13 patients with Wernicke's aphasia and 10 of 20 patients with Broca's aphasia improved significantly in the computer group compared with 1 of 12 and 4 of 29 in the control group, respectively. A focal point of the program was the simultaneous presentation of graphics, written texts, and audio recordings. Several tasks required the patients to type in a letter or a word. Thus, the results clearly reflect the focus of the program's contents. On the other hand, we were astonished at the low proportion of patients in the control group who showed significant improvements. This shows that only intensive therapy is successful. The supplementary training, which of course could even be intensified, points to the right direction.

With regard to Naming and Language Comprehension, Table 9.5 shows that, seen as a whole, only a few patients (with the computer group having a slight edge) showed significant improvements in these two subtests. Our data, which needs to be more exactly analyzed, appear to suggest less improvement with relatively high baseline results (with the exception of Repetition). Thus, the computer group and the control group achieved the following respective percentages of correct responses in the initial AAT: Token Test: 44.6% versus 41.6%; Repetition: 67.8% versus 66.5%; Written Language: 48.3% versus 44.3%; Naming: 54.5% versus 55.8%; and Language Comprehension: 68% versus 67.4%. Classification according to severity (based on the initial test) showed different rates of improvement for the groups of mildly, moderately, and severely impaired patients. In Naming, improvement for the two groups was, respectively, only significant for 7.7% versus 5.6% of the patients with mild impairments, 28.6% versus 14.3% for patients with moderate impairments, and 20% versus 16% for patients with severe impairments. With regard to the results from Language Comprehension, it remains to be seen whether the 20 multiple-choice tasks for testing reading comprehension produced different results than the 20 used to test oral comprehension. Unfortunately, these are not treated separately in the AAT.

The influence of age, gender, and duration of illness can only briefly be touched on here. In general, age did not seem to be a decisive factor in the success of therapy. There were some gender differences, but these appeared to be associated with locations of lesion. Duration of illness had a clear influence on the success of therapy. In the computer group as well as the control group, therapy was less effective the longer the duration of illness. Nevertheless, the intensity of treatment seemed to affect this. Up to 20% of the patients in the computer group ill for longer than 2 years showed significant improvement (Written Language), whereas the corresponding percentage in the control group was only 4%. Thus, it is possible that even chronic aphasias can be treated with some success if treatment is intensive enough. Computers seem to be a suitable medium for this. With respect to the long life expectancy following brain injury, further studies must examine whether computer-based home training is a valid option to aid brain-damaged persons who, due to the high costs, are not given inpatient treatment.

Discussion

If one looks at the results in detail, many of the improvement rates do not seem to be particularly high in comparison with the significant improvement rates established by Poeck et al. (1989): for 78% of the patients in early phase (1–4 months), for 46% of the patients in the middle phase (4–12 months), and for 68% of the patients in the chronic phase (more than 12 months). However, it must be remembered that the sums given in their study are a total of all patients showing an improvement in at least one of the five subtests. This is valid because the aphasias often have language modality-specific deficits. It is important to report if the patient has improved even if improvement is restricted to the modality primarily affected (e.g., Naming). Unfortunately, the Aachen study, which is based only on data collected at the clinic there, lacks information about the detailed effects of therapy probably due to the relatively small number of patients. Our analysis attempts to make evident the detailed structure of the improvements. For instance, if we were to add all the patients with Wernicke's aphasia who showed significant improvement in at least one of the subtests of the AAT, the number would be similarly high.

In summary, the majority of the aphasic patients who participated in our study showed improvements in performance, as measured by the AAT, following a 6-week therapy of at least 1 hour of individual speech therapy daily. In the cases where conventional speech therapy was supplemented by an hour of computer-based speech therapy, more patients showed significant improvements, and the level of performance was also raised considerably. On the one hand, this shows that the intensity of therapy is a decisive factor in the rehabilitation of aphasic patients. On the other hand, it shows that the computer is an effective means to intensify therapy when a linguistically and therapeutically founded program is used that is tailored to the patient's needs.

CONCLUSIONS AND FUTURE DIRECTIONS

The foremost goal in the treatment of language-impaired persons is oriented toward the general goal set for every type of rehabilitation of patients with neurological disorders, namely reducing the handicap caused by brain damage. To this end, there are two groups of specific objectives. On the one hand, there is the reduction of the language deficit (i.e., the restitution of language competence or the language system in its linguistic components) or the promotion of the use of remaining linguistic abilities, respectively, to achieve optimal results with limited capabilities. On the other hand, there is the psychosocial rehabilitation of the patient, which should aid him or her to use language means to communicate in daily situations with family, friends, the authorities, while shopping, and so on so that he or she can fulfill needs as independently as possible.

These two objectives tend to lead toward two approaches: a symptom-specific approach concerned with the details of the language deficit, and a "holistic" approach emphasizing the general setting of the patient's life. We promote an integrative therapy that combines the most important aspects of the two approaches (Schädler, Seggewies, Willeke, Stachowiak, & Grassau, 1992). In most German clinical facilities, aphasic patients receive language therapy as well as coordinated neuropsychological and cognitive therapy, ergotherapy, psychotherapy, physiotherapy, and work with social workers who assist them with lodging, social security, and occupational questions.

To assess the efficacy of aphasia therapy, we are thinking of using evaluation sheets as well as scales like those used to measure self-reliance and psychosocial situations of patients with brain trauma (Truelle & Brooks, chapter 19, this volume) in addition to the specific language structural and modality related aphasia tests like the AAT. One focus will be on showing that computer-based techniques can be integrated as a supplementary form of therapy, and that they will in the long run offer good possibilities for long-term improvement for aphasic patients, especially in home training. In the meantime, we are working on interactive multimedia therapy programs containing videos with prototypical situations taken from daily life to promote the bond between computer-assisted training and daily living.

REFERENCES

Basso, A. (1987). Approaches to neuropsychological rehabilitation: Language disorders. In M. J. Meier, A. L. Benton, & L. Diller (Eds.), *Neuropsychological rehabilitation* (pp. 294–314). Edinburgh: Churchill Livingstone.

Basso, A., Capitani, E., & Zanobio, M. E. (1982). Pattern of recovery of oral and written expression and comprehension in aphasic patients. *Behavioural Brain Research, 6*, 115–128.

Enderby, P., & Petheram, B. (1992). Self administered therapy at home for aphasic patients. *Aphasiology, 6*(3), 321–324.

Griessl, W., Stachowiak, F. J., & Burbulla, U. (1992). Computer-assisted speech therapy. In W. Zagler (Ed.), *Proceedings of the 3rd International Conference "Computers for Handicapped Persons"* (pp. 194–202). Vienna: R. Oldenburg Verlag.

Katz, R. C., & Wertz, R. T. (1992). Computerized hierarchical reading treatment in aphasia. *Aphasiology, 6*(2), 165–177.

Kotten, A., Stachowiak, F. J., & Willeke, A. (1985, November). *Veranschaulichung als methodisches Prinzip der Sprachtherapie.* Paper presented at the annual meeting of the "Arbeitsgemeinschaft für Aphasieforschung and Behandlung," Rotterdam, the Netherlands.

Lincoln, N. B., Mulley, G. P., Jones, A. C. et al. (1984). Effectiveness of speech therapy of aphasic stroke patients. *Lancet 1*, 1197–1200.

Loverso, F. L., Prescott, T. E., & Selinger, M. (1992). Microcomputer treatment applications in aphasiology. *Aphasiology, 6*(2), 155–163.

Petheram, B. L. (1992). *The use of microcomputers in non-professionally supervised dysphasia remediation for stroke affected patients*. Unpublished doctoral dissertation, University of West England, Bristol.

Poeck, K., Huber, W., & Willmes, K. (1989). Outcome of intensive language treatment of aphasia. *Journal of Speech and Hearing Disorders, 54*, 471–479.

Schädler, U., Seggewies, G., Willeke, A., Stachowiak, F. J., & Grassau, R. (1993). Methodological aspects of comprehensive speech therapy. In F. J. Stachowiak, R. De Bleser, G. Deloche, R. Kaschel, P. North, L. Pizzamiglio, I. Robertson, & B. Wilson (Eds.), *Developments in the assessment and rehabilitation of brain-damaged patients—Perspectives from a European concerted action*. Tübingen: Narr Verlag.

Schuell, H. (1974). Aphasia theory and therapy. In L. F. Sies (Ed.), *Selected lectures and papers of Hildred Schuell*. Baltimore: University Park Press.

Seron, X., Deloche, G., Moulard, G., & Rouselle, M. (1980). A computer-based therapy for the treatment of aphasic subjects with writing disorders. *Journal of Speech and Hearing Disorders, 45*, 45–58.

Shewan, M. S., & Kertesz, A. (1984). *Effects of speech and language treatment on recovery from aphasia*. Brain and Language, 23, 272–299.

Stachowiak, F. J. (1989). *Entwicklung, Konstruktion und Erprobung eines mikroelektronischen Therapiesystems zur Behandlung hirnorganisch bedingter Sprachstörungen* [Development, construction and trial of a micro-computer-based therapy system for the treatment of patients with language disorders caused by brain damage]. Bonn: MS Rheinische Landesklinik Bonn und BMFT.

Stachowiak, F. J. (1993). Computer-based aphasia therapy with the Lingware/STACH system. In F. J. Stachowiak, R. De Bleser, G. Deloche, R. Kaschel, P. North, L. Pizzamiglio, I. Robertson, & B. Wilson (Eds.), *Developments in the assessment and rehabilitation of brain-damaged patients—Perspectives from a European concerted action*. Tübingen: Narr Verlag.

Stachowiak, F. J., Willeke, A., Grassau, R., Schädler, U., & Rivetto, N. (1991). *Report: European concerted action on "The Evaluation of the Efficacy of Technology in the Assessment and Rehabilitation of Brain-Damaged Patients."* Paris: Inserm.

Wepman, J. (1972). Aphasia therapy: A new look. *Journal of Speech and Hearing Disorders, 37*, 203–226.

Willmes, K., & Poeck, K. (1984). Ergebnisse einer multizentrischen Untersuchung über die Spontanprognose von Aphasien vaskulärer Ätiologie [Results of a multicentric study on the spontaneous prognosis of aphasias with vascular etiology]. *Nervenarzt, 55*, 67–71.

CHAPTER TEN

A New Approach to Physical Rehabilitation

Gitte Rasmussen

ABSTRACT

Most brain-injury patients are usually offered physical therapy where the treatment principles follow the Proprioceptive Neuromuscular Facilitation (PNF) theories by Bobath (1970). However, the Bobath concept appears to be insufficient in meeting the special cognitive, social, and emotional problems and integrating these variables into patient examination and physical rehabilitation of stroke or cranial trauma after 2 years or more. If the physical treatment and education in an intensive neuropsychological rehabilitation program takes place in "normal" surroundings, the results tend to demonstrate a greater "transfer effect" than it has been possible to achieve in an institutional environment.

Improvement of both upper and lower extremity function is one of the major objectives of stroke and cranial trauma rehabilitation because extremity function greatly affects the overall outcome in the acute and subacute states. Traditionally, physical and occupational therapists provide the retraining of ambulation and activities of daily living, respectively, sometimes so strictly defined that the physical therapists train the legs and the occupational therapists train the arms. In the hospital setting, they supervise the nursing staff in handling the patients according to the treatment principles of Bobath (1970).

At the time when the Bobath concept was introduced, other physical therapists developed a similar concept in which Proprioceptive Neuromuscular Facilitation (PNF) techniques inhibit the abnormal spastic motor pattern in order to develop and restore motor function within a 24-hour treatment regime. Knott and Voss (1968), Brunnstrom (1970), and Johnstone (1978) have different ways of approaching the PNF techniques, but nevertheless the Bobath concept is still the predominant approach to rehabilitation among physical therapists, as it has been for at least 30 years, and it has been the most well-known principle among other professionals during the last 10 years.

The aim of the 24-hour Bobath techniques is restoration of normal motor function and to dispense with walking aids. It is true that walking with one cane increases spasticity and spoils the intention of relearning a normal gait and balance. However, it can be very frustrating to the physical therapists to abandon this aim from time to time. If the options are (a) no ability to walk independently without a cane or (b) to walk with a cane but with increased tone in the paretic limb as a consequence, the therapist and patient may often choose the option with the greatest functional potential.

TIME SPAN AND TREATMENT ONSET
AND LENGTH

It is a common view among physical and occupational therapists that no further spontaneous motor recovery from a brain injury can be expected more than 2 years postinjury. However, Danish neurologist Tom Skyhøj Olsen published a paper (1990) with quite different results. His investigation of 75 stroke patients predicts that the majority of functional recovery occurs within the first 3 months. In each patient, extremity paresis was quantified according to the 5-point scoring system recommended by the Medical Research Council, upper extremity function was quantified using the Barthel Index score for dressing the upper body and feeding, and lower extremity function was quantified according to a 5-point scoring of the ability to walk. Improvement was recorded for upper extremity function in 52% of the patients and for lower extremity function in 89%. Best extremity function was reached at a mean of 9 weeks (*SEM* +/− 3) and 10 weeks (*SEM* +/ −4) after stroke for the upper and lower extremities, respectively.

In 135 stroke patients studied by Andrew, Brocklehurst, Richards, and Laycock (1981), maximum improvement in walking distance was reached with 8 weeks after stroke in 88% of the patients. Best upper and lower extremity function was obtained between 9 and 10 weeks, respectively, after stroke, and 95% of the patients had reached their best upper and lower extremity function with 13 and 14 weeks, respectively.

It is a special challenge to predict leg and arm improvement in comatose patients where the only physical rehabilitation that can be offered during coma is contracture profylaxis and positioning in antispastic patterns. There are numerous reports of patients who regained a functional gait several years postinjury. Outcome improvement indices can never be anything but guidelines. In fact, how far the individual comatose patient comes in his or her rehabilitation goals is uncertain.

Several years postinjury abnormal muscle tone and spasticity may still be a remaining physical problem. The question is whether this phenomenon is at all tractable. Strengthening the muscles may reduce spasticity for some time, but the spasticity returns instantly with a yawn or a cough, or may be provoked by a sudden loud noise like the slamming of a door, thus spoiling a permanent decrease in muscle tone. Spasticity can perhaps be treated medically, but side effects such as tiredness, dizziness, and nausea outweigh the benefits derived from a decrease in paretic muscle tone. The nonparetic muscles are also affected because it is difficult to administer spasmolitic drugs locally.

However, the worst consequence of spasticity is social isolation. Anxiety and worrying also increase muscle tone in paretic muscles. Consequently, patients grow increasingly unwilling to engage in social interaction due to repeated experiences of difficulties in controlling gait and arm movements. Moreover, crowds and noise tend to increase spasticity further. Psychological intervention and education in the physiological aspects of spasticity are necessary to reduce the problem and to relax the patients. When the patients know what spasticity is, how it is likely to increase, and how they can control it (instead of being afraid of it), they will no longer let the spasticity control their lives.

METHODOLOGY

The Bobath concept will always be an important tool in the restoration of motor function, but in the long run it will not meet the patients' special cognitive, social, and emotional problems. The 24-hour Bobath treatment regime cannot prevent spasticity from developing if the damaged area is so extensive that abnormal tone persists half a year postinjury. Another question is whether the brain is able to absorb all new information and put it to use in the acute and subacute phases.

The merits of the Bobath concept are mainly founded on two areas. First and foremost, it constitutes a tool for guiding the recovery of motor function into a more functional movement pattern during the first 3 months. In describing the plasticity of the working brain, neuroscience has proved that the compensatory mechanisms in restoration of brain damage often take place in arbitrary ways. It seems likely that intervention by guiding at an early stage in which the therapist tries to inhibit abnormal movement patterns can reduce abnormal tone so that it will not affect the final state of recovery so much. It is to be expected that patients who do not receive specific physical treatment and who try to get back into normal movement patterns without guidance will develop a higher degree of nonfunctional motor patterns.

Another area where the Bobath concept has had and still has a great influence is on managing patients and teaching the nursing staff to pay proper attention to the paretic side. Thus, correct handling of patients has resulted in a marked drop in the number of shoulder problems of the hemiparetic patients during the last decade.

INTRODUCTION OF NEW METHODOLOGY

Some years ago, the Danish Physical Therapy Association distributed a colorful poster in order to make the profession more well known. The poster had a jumping jack with strings to pull. Unfortunately, one very important body part was missing—the head. This poster illustrates perfectly well what physical therapy to brain-injured persons should not be in future. First, one has to integrate the patients' head and possible cognitive deficits into the physical therapy treatment program. Second, brain-injured persons need to take responsibility for their own rehabilitation in order to become less dependent and have less of a need for a physical therapist to "pull the strings."

When it comes to functional physical retraining, Brodal (1973) contributed an important viewpoint on motor restoration. His written self-observations on recovery after his own stroke are very interesting. He used to be an eager cross-country skier. His highest wish was to be able to ski again. Being a physician, he was aware of the importance of physical training, and consequently spent much time engaged in the physical therapy. However, the first time he tried skiing was a complete failure—he could not move the skis. His conclusion was that specific training must go hand in hand with functional training.

Luria (1948/1968) not only provided the fundamental principles of the cognitive and psychological training at the Center for Rehabilitation of Brain Injury, but also inspired the physical retraining principles of the program. His views on motor recovery in *Restoration of Function after Brain Injury* are as realistic as the results published by Olsen (1990) and Andrews et al. (1981). In the chapter "Restoration of Motor Function after Brain Injury" Luria suggested early implementation of compensatory strategies for motor deficits following injuries at lower cortical levels of integration such as pareses and disorders of tone and coordination. As opposed to lesions at lower cortical levels of integration, lesions at higher cortical levels permit reorganization strategies. The examiner should first try to establish the psychological nature of the apraxia, and then find the defective link primarily responsible for disintegration of the motor act. Only then should the examiner try to correct this deficit by introducing the disturbed function into a new and intact system. This method of intersystemic reorganization is the main method of correction of the deficits in these cases. Luria also stated that it is more important to find out and analyze the intact functional systems than to list the deficits.

DEVELOPMENT IN THE PHYSICAL TRAINING AND EDUCATION AT THE CENTER

Since the start of the Center for Rehabilitation of Brain Injury in 1985, the physical rehabilitation in the program has developed from a more traditional neurological treatment approach. The term *physical therapy* has changed into *physical training and education* in the program. Education about their own dysfunctions and deficits affords the patients an opportunity to improve their physical condition. The integration of awareness of cognitive deficits into the physical therapy has produced treatment principles called *cognitive physical* therapy.

Apart from the previously mentioned considerations, two other areas have been essential for the development of new treatment principles. The first area is the nature of the persistent physical deficits most commonly seen in patients referred to the Center. Second, the fact that the Center is located in a university environment rather than a hospital setting has turned out to be important.

PHYSICAL DEFICITS

About one-third of patients have a hemiparesis, most commonly of the right side, and over 20% have fine motor defects. The overriding physical problem of the patients is, however, a very poor physical condition. Most patients have received strengthening exercises and antispastic and contracture profylaxis treatment, but the majority have no postinjury experience of physical exercise with a markedly increased pulse rate for a prolonged period of time. Consequently, they tend to be more fatigable than the average healthy individual.

About 20%–30% of a group experiences other physical problems at the beginning of a program. These typically include: (a) seizures, (b) headaches, (c) sleep disturbances, (d) disturbed appetite regulation, (e) neglect/inattention, (f) apraxias, (g) hemianopsia, and (h) sensation deficits. Impaired balance and ambulation were found in 30%–40%. Most patients had respiratory and voice problems.

TRAINING FACILITIES

The Center for Rehabilitation of Brain Injury is located at a university, which means that the patients use the same public transportation, buy lunch in the same canteen, and sometimes even buy sweatshirts with the insignia of the "University of Copenhagen" just as any other student attending the university might do. These all increase their self-confidence. The patients start and end their training program following the semesters of the university. Patients in the program at the Center are also called *students*, never *patients*. This attitude supports the brain-injured persons to leave the patient role and take the responsibility for their own education and training. The wide open area in which the university is located also lends itself to the possibility for jogging.

Some of the physical conditioning takes place in a fitness center at a nearby hotel. The students use the facilities together with the hotel guests and other users of the center. Here students also meet former students who have continued their physical training after their program ended.

A nearby sailing club located at a lake has two, one-man sailing boats designed mainly for physically disabled persons. They are mini 12-meter sailing boats—miniature versions of the America's Cup 12-meter class. This type of boat has also proved to be suitable for brain-injured persons.

PHYSICAL EXAMINATION

In the early days of physical rehabilitation at the Center, all patients were subjected to a neurological examination to map all physical and neurological data. This was not very motivating to the patients because the end of the program saw a reiteration of the same deficits. The data were more diagnostic than a measure of improvement.

At present, the most important tool in the physical therapy examination is a so-called fitness index, which contains three different tests that have been applied to American soldiers and to a control group consisting of a standard population. Namely, the Åstrand Biking Test (Åstrand & Rodahl, 1970), the Harvard Step-Test (Åstrand & Rodahl, 1970), and the Cooper Walking and Running Distance Test (Åstrand & Rodahl, 1970). The advantages of these tests are that they are easy and quick to perform in a modified form. Moreover, the patients become motivated to continue physical training. It is easy to measure an improvement within a short time (i.e., over a period of 3–4 weeks). Because the students are in such a poor condition at the start, a moderate investment in physical training quickly shows results, which also promotes increased self-confidence.

The Åstrand Biking Test equipment is a Swedish ergometer bike (Monark), a pulse rater around the chest of the type "Respiratory" (VAS, Visual Analogue Scale), Borg's Subjective Evaluation Scale, and the scoring system recommended by the Danish Heart Association. By means of these systems, it is possible to calculate the average fitness level of the student and to show it in a figure. The test takes about 6 minutes—the time it takes for the pulse to reach a steady state at a certain resistance.

For the Harvard Step-Test, you have to step up onto a 50-cm-high footstool at a rate of 30 times per minute for 5 consecutive minutes. Thereafter, over a period of 5 consecutive minutes, measurements are taken of the pulse rate decline. The findings are inserted in a formula, and the resulting figure is yet another indication of physical fitness.

The Cooper Walking and Running Distance Test is carried out in two versions. The first task is to perform a 1,200-m outdoor running or walking distance as quickly as possible. The second version is performed on a treadmill. The students are asked to run and/or walk as many meters as they can in 12 minutes. From these results, an index is obtained that shows the level of physical condition.

THE PHYSICAL TRAINING PROGRAM

Most of the physical training (Table 10.1) is performed in groups, with due consideration given to the students' various cognitive deficits.

However, individual physical training does take place. Typically, this can be supervising the student in his or her home, exercise program, applying for and employing personal aids, education and

TABLE 10.1
Samples of Physical Activities

Activities
Morning gymnastic exercises
Fitness center
Running group
Ball games (volleyball, badminton, table tennis, billiards)
Aerobics
Dancing (Les Lanciers, dance movement therapy)
Transportation program (at the Center and on location)
ADL training (at the Center and at home)
Leisure activities (sailing, bowling, darts, stamps, chess, etc.)
Follow-up activities (fitness center, sailing course)

support in diet maintenance, or teaching the patients to ride a bike or drive a car again. But treatments like manipulation, ultrasound, shortwave, laser or manual active/passive resistance, and physical strengthening exercises are no longer applied. Relaxation therapy and massage have been attempted but with little or no success. This type of therapy tends to lower the general level of concentration and alertness to the detriment of the cognitive training. What most patients need is stimulation and support to minimize the initiation difficulties and the general psychomotor slowing that often are seen as sequelae of brain injury.

After a fortnight of instruction by the therapists, the students take turns in leading the exercises at the morning meetings. The overall aim of the meeting every morning is to increase awareness, alertness, and concentration. Sometimes music is used to support the students' recollection of rhythm and sequence of the morning exercises. However, music is not always a support, and some brain-injured patients describe it as a source of distraction. Problems with divided attention are also seen when the students train at the fitness center where noise from the workout apparatus and background music disturb concentration. Nevertheless, this is also a way to train continuity without becoming distracted during the normal daily stream of unsorted information.

Twice a week there are sometimes two types of physical activity included in the program. One type is usually a ball game (e.g., volleyball). Another type of physical activity is dancing, such as a French minuet-like dance called Les Lanciers, which consists of five sequences with eight participants. The sequences grow increasingly complex. Thus, memory techniques, visuospatial positioning, and polite greetings are required.

At the fitness center one or two times a week, the students have their own chart to fill out during their training. Here, the aim of the physical training is not only improvement of strength and fitness but also body awareness, social behavior, memory, concentration, and general awareness. After the bicycle warm-up, the students measure their own pulse, calory output, resistance, rounds per minute, and duration of the warm-up. The students have to remember four figures on a display before they stop pedaling because the display disappears as soon as they stop. To start and read the display of the treadmill is another cognitive challenge. Besides improving physical condition, the treadmill is also suitable for training balance and stride. In the swimming pool, 2 or 3 persons of a group of 10 learn to swim again. Other physical activities are badminton, table tennis, billiards, jogging, and sailing. The mini 12-meter boat is a suitable type of boat class not only for physically disabled persons, but also brain-injured persons (see Fig. 10.1).

A sailing course is one of the latest physical activities at the Center. The Center has purchased five membership cards in a sailing club to try out sailing as a possible future activity or to rekindle an old interest. If the students want to learn to sail, they can attend a sailing course within the framework of the established evening classes at night school open to the public and pay the ordinary price for such a course.

Often it is difficult to find a relevant sporting activity for brain-injured persons in the Handicap Sport Association in Denmark. There are lots of activities for the disabled and psychiatric patients, but none for brain-injured persons. At first, members of the sailing club expressed a rather negative attitude toward having brain-injured persons frequent their club. However, when they met them they were very relieved to discover that brain-injured persons are no more difficult to get along with than anyone else. Often the effects of the brain injury are not immediately apparent, and that in itself may be a problem as well.

The sailing course is composed of a winter program with theory and physical training once a week, a summer program with sailing in practice twice a week, and visits to different clubs and harbors to integrate the participants in their local harbor environments. This boat type is primarily designed for disabled persons, therefore the students may participate in racing with other nondisabled persons. In the World Championship in Norway last year, 50% of the 100 participants were nondisabled persons. To develop the course further, the plan is to issue a special certificate and examination as is the case in any ordinary sailing course.

Two or three students per group require transportation training. They are often afraid to travel by bus, train, car, or bike because of (a) a

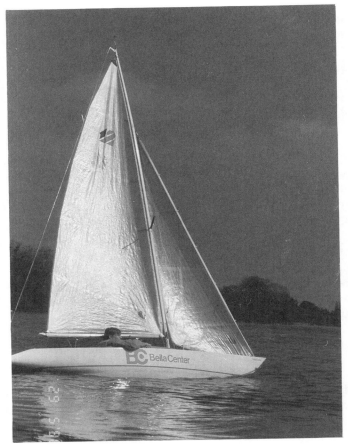

FIG. 10.1. A brain-injured patient at the helm of a mini 12-meter sailing boat.

tendency to seizure, (b) sudden increases of spasticity, (c) orientation and memory problems, or (d) a sense of uneasiness in public places.

PHYSICAL FOLLOW-UP ACTIVITIES

An important element in the Center's program is to try out different sport and leisure activities while the students are still in the program. Such activities may be bowling, playing the guitar, sailing, rowing, flamenco dancing, collecting stamps, chess, or going to the theater. Many sport and leisure activities provide a setting where movement patterns are enhanced far more functionally than is possible in a traditional physical training program. Thus, balance can be trained while sailing, and arm movements can be trained during flamenco dancing.

Quality of life is not always a question of getting a job or being able to study again, but also having sport and/or leisure activities. Former students are offered continued use of the facilities of the fitness center. Typically 10% of each group continues.

CONCLUSION

Most brain-injury patients receive physical therapy treatment together with occupational therapy as inpatients. A majority of the brain-injury patients also continue as outpatients in a hospital setting or private clinic. The treatment principles mostly follow the PNF theories of Bobath (1954).

One year after a stroke or cranial trauma, the Bobath concept is insufficient to meet the patients' special cognitive, social, and emotional problems, and to integrate them in the physical rehabilitation. Spasticity may be a great physical problem, but it is also a psychological one.

During the last 7 years, the physical therapeutic treatment at the Center for Rehabilitation of Brain Injury has changed from being traditionally Bobath oriented to being more functional and pedagogically cognitive. It has been inspired by Luria, whose ideas constitute the basis of the retraining principles used by all the members of the interdisciplinary team.

The physical therapists do not "treat" but offer physical training, consultation, and education. The physical training takes place in normal surroundings, and has demonstrated a greater degree of transfer effect than has been possible to achieve in an institutional environment.

In conclusion, in the future physical therapists will need to integrate the cognitive, psychological, and social deficits into the physical rehabilitation, and not simply focus on arms and legs rehabilitation. This approach will avoid the frustration of failing to make spasticity permanently disappear. Additionally, a physical therapist has more challenge and satisfaction when a greater repertoire is offered rather than a single system.

REFERENCES

Åstrand, P.-O., & Rodahl, K. (1970). *Textbook of physiology.* New York: McGraw-Hill.
Andrews, K., Brocklehurst, J. C., Richards, B., & Laycock, P. J. (1981). The rate of recovery from stroke—and its measurement. *International Journal of Rehabilitation Medicine, 3,* 155–161.

Bobath, B. (1954). A study of abnormal postural reflex activity in patients with lesions of the central nervous system. Parts 1–4. *Physiotherapy, 40,* 259, 295, 326, 368.

Bobath, B. (1970). *Adult hemiplegia: Evaluation and treatment.* London: William Heinemann.

Brodal, A. (1973). Self-observations and neuroanatomical considerations after a stroke. *Brain, 96,* 675–694.

Brunnström, S. (1970). *Movement therapy in hemiplegia.* New York: Harper & Row.

Johnstone, M. (1978). *Restoration of motor function in the stroke patient.* Edinburgh: Churchill Livingstone.

Knott, M., & Voss, D. E. (1968). *Proprioceptive neuromuscular facilitation.* New York: Harper & Row.

Luria, A. R. (1968). *Restoration of function after brain injury.* New York: Pergamon. (Original work published 1948)

Olsen, T. S. (1990). Arm and leg paresis as outcome predictors in stroke rehabilitation. *Stroke, 21,* 247–251.

CHAPTER ELEVEN

Individuality, Lesion Location, and Psychotherapy After Brain Injury

George P. Prigatano

ABSTRACT

An attempt is made to address Christensen and Rosenberg's (1991) critique of a previous article on psychotherapy of brain-dysfunctional patients (Prigatano, 1991a). Specifically, three questions are addressed: (a) How does psychotherapy of the brain-injured person attend to individual needs and characteristics? (b) Is there anything about the nature of the brain injury that influences the psychotherapeutic approach? (c) Is the psychotherapeutic approach in (my) neuropsychological rehabilitation program essentially a form of Freudian psychoanalytic supportive psychotherapy?

In their critique of the role of psychotherapy in brain-injury rehabilitation, Christensen and Rosenberg (1991) reviewed, among others, a recent article that expressed some of my ideas concerning psychotherapy with brain-dysfunctional patients (Prigatano, 1991a).

The purpose of this chapter is to address these comments and clarify my position on the points they raised. However, before doing so a few comments concerning psychotherapy within the context of neuropsychological rehabilitation are needed.

NEUROPSYCHOLOGICAL REHABILITATION
AND PSYCHOTHERAPY

Neuropsychological rehabilitation consists, at a minimum, of the following activities:

1. Cognitive rehabilitation

2. Psychotherapy

3. Milieu (therapeutic) environment

4. Protected work trial

5. Family involvement

Within the context of this model, the patient's higher cerebral dysfunctions are explored, and the patient is helped to compensate for those impairments and, in some instances, find alternative ways to solve various cognitive tasks. Second, individuals are helped to deal with their emotional reactions to their brain injury and establish or reestablish a sense of purpose or meaning in the face of the tragedy of brain injury. Neuropsychological rehabilitation often requires the development of a therapeutic milieu to help patients adequately participate in cognitive retraining and psychotherapy efforts. This therapeutic milieu frequently involves working with patients in small groups to facilitate the adaptation to brain injury in the context of interpersonal exchange. In addition, the rehabilitation staff must deal with their own affective reactions toward brain-dysfunctional patients in order to be of maximum service to them (Ben-Yishay & Prigatano, 1990; Prigatano, 1989a; Prigatano, Fordyce, Zeiner, Roueche, Pepping, & Wood, 1986).

Finally, to help patients become productive, it is necessary to develop a working alliance with both them and their families (Prigatano et al., in press). Family involvement and the development of a protected work trial complement and extend traditional forms of neuropsychologically oriented rehabilitation. Because of the scope of this chapter, the various therapies are not discussed. Such a discussion can be found elsewhere (Ben-Yishay & Prigatano, 1990; Prigatano, 1991a, 1991b; Prigatano et al., 1986).

However, it is appropriate to ask why psychotherapy should be considered in the context of neuropsychologically oriented rehabilitation. The answer is that, in working with brain-dysfunctional patients, one repeatedly encounters them asking three questions:

1. Why did this happen to me?

2. Will I be normal again?

3. Is life worth living after brain injury?

These questions are highly personal and require more than a scientific approach to address them. The canons of science require dispassionate, controlled observations and repeatable measures (Meadows, 1987). However, one cannot be dispassionate when faced with personal tragedy. Patients with brain dysfunction need a forum to explore these questions even though they may not be asked early or directly. That forum is typically psychotherapy. Therefore, it is important that neuro- psychologically oriented rehabilitation incorporate psychotherapeutic interventions to address these important phenomenological issues.

It is necessary to ask the question of whether psychotherapeutic interventions can be demonstrated to improve the patient's adaptation and quality of life following brain injury. Because no two patients are alike, it is impossible to scientifically assess the efficacy of psychotherapeutic work with a given patient. However, the effectiveness of psychotherapy can be indirectly assessed when comparing programs of neuropsychological rehabilitation. Those programs that differ in their use of psychotherapeutic intervention with similar brain-dysfunctional patients can be compared using various outcome measures. I predict that programs that actively utilize psychotherapeutic interventions will show the greatest rate of sustained employment several years after brain injury. This is based on the notion that those individuals who have truly come to grips with the consequences of their brain injury will make greater commitments to life—and one of those commitments is, of course, being productive (Prigatano, 1989b; Prigatano et al., 1986).

A recent outcome article on the efficacy of the present neuropsychological rehabilitation program documented that the quality of the therapeutic alliance was positively related to the productivity status of brain-dysfunctional patients following discharge (Prigatano et al., in press). These data indirectly support the important role of psychotherapy for some patients.

INDIVIDUATION AND PSYCHOTHERAPY
AFTER BRAIN INJURY

From the Jungian perspective, the process of psychotherapy can be compared to the hero's journey that is described in literature (Campbell, 1989). This is primarily a journey in which the individual leaves the security of a certain psychological position and ventures out to face his or her destiny. Within the course of this journey, the individual often becomes challenged by some threatening or negative force. It is not uncommon for the individual to feel perplexed over how to handle the threat. In the face of that perplexity, he or she must use whatever ingenuity he or she has to solve the problem. Thus, it involves more than bravery. It requires cunningness as well as bravery to be a hero. Once what is feared is faced, the patient returns "home" as a more "integrated" or mature person. In his introduction to *The Man with a Shattered World*, Luria (1972) referred to his patient Zazetsby as a hero. That patient had spent 25 years attempting to improve his higher cerebral functioning, and eventually came to grips with the long-term consequences of his devastating brain injury. Thus, the general process of psychotherapy, as a personal journey, is a unique venture, and Jung (1957) described this process as individuation.

In discussing his "Principles of Practical Psychotherapy," Jung defines *individuation* as the process by which a person (patient) "becomes what he really is" (p. 10). In another chapter, Jung stated that "Individuation has two principal aspects: In the first place it is an internal and subjective process of integration, and in the second it is an equally indispensable process of objective relationship" (p. 234).

It would again be beyond the scope of this chapter to discuss in detail precisely what is "integrated" when one speaks of individuation or achieving a sense of individuality. However, at its most basic level, integration refers to helping patients with the problem of opposites in their lives. They want this, which is in conflict with that. They do this, but later feel angry, guilty, or depressed over what they have done. There is a struggle over what direction to take in life to make "sense" of the living experience and to enjoy the process of living, which means eventually preparing for tragedy and ultimately the end of one's biological/psychological existence as we know it (i.e., the problem of death).

Many brain-injured patients, whether they are young, middle aged, or older, were progressing along some course or direction in life when an unexpected insult to their brain occurred. Many want to continue along the same road, but now have altered higher cerebral functions. For some it is still possible to continue along that road, but for most it is not. Curiously, some patients appear to be painfully aware of impaired motor and speech functions, whereas others are not. Some recognize a memory disorder but think it is of no practical significance to them in their day-to-day activities. Still others, when confronted about changes in their personality, feel that these are greatly exaggerated by others and see no true alteration in their basic personality structure or characteristics. This can exist despite painful and obvious complaints from their relatives.

Does the dialogue of psychotherapy have anything to offer these individuals? You can answer this question for yourself by imagining the following scenario. Suppose that you suffered a stroke involving the lenticulostriate artery in your left hemisphere, and you observed a loss of function in your right arm and leg without any substantial loss of consciousness. Would you eventually need help in dealing with your emotional reactions to these motor deficits and associated subcortical language-based impairments? How would you face the consequences of the cerebrovascular accident (CVA) as it relates to work and family life? Would you feel it would be better to leave emotional things alone, or possibly work on them simply by yourself? Would you wish to focus solely on obtaining another line of work? Would you require help in dealing with a loved one who now may become frustrated and angry with you because he or she notices personality changes that you are not aware of?

The answers are likely to be highly individual. Some might ask for help and others would not want help, at least at certain points in the recovery course. A wide variety of conditions can exist. Being attentive to these phenomena and recognizing the legitimate individual needs of each patient is a cornerstone to the Jungian approach to psychotherapy, which I embrace along with other theoretical models.

It is against this background of observations that the three questions or observations raised by Christensen and Rosenberg (1991) are addressed.

How Does Psychotherapy of Brain-Injured Persons Attend to Their Individual Characteristics?

Christensen and Rosenberg (1991) raised the question: How does psychotherapy of brain-injured persons attend to their individual characteristics? The answer is by attempting to enter their phenomenological experience of being brain injured, and helping them reconstruct a sense of direction or purpose in life given their unique premorbid personality characteristics. Elsewhere, I tried to provide clinical vignettes of how individual differences dictate how the psychotherapeutic process unfolds (Prigatano, 1991a, 1991b). Before giving a few examples taken from those articles, it is important to focus on the neglected problem of premorbid personality characteristics in neuropsychological research.

A central problem in describing how psychotherapy should progress with a brain-dysfunctional person relates directly to the fact that individuals vary greatly in terms of their premorbid dynamics and personality characteristics. Thus, how they are approached within the context of a psychotherapeutic intervention is heavily dependent on the kind of person they were prior to the injury, as well as the kind of person they are following the injury.

It has long been known that premorbid variables influence the neuropsychological picture. For example, the most obvious moderator variables in neuropsychological assessment are age and education. Typically, older individuals do worse on certain tests of memory and speed of information processing compared with younger individuals. These two dimensions are commonly affected following brain injury. Conversely, more educated individuals often do better on certain neuropsychological measures (see Parsons & Prigatano, 1978). Recently, my colleagues and I demonstrated significant negative correlation between age and performance on a new screening test referred to as the Barrow Neurological Institute (BNI) Screen for Higher Cerebral Functions. Likewise, a high positive correlation was obtained between educational level and the total score obtained from this screening measure. Brain injury reduced the magnitude of these correlations, but the relationships were nevertheless maintained (Prigatano, Amin, & Rosenstein, 1991). This type of observation has been reported in many studies throughout the world, and presents a convenient example of how premorbid characteristics interact with brain injury to produce the symptom picture.

However, when faced with a given individual who has had a certain social history, cultural background, and preexisting pattern of intellectual and personality strengths and weaknesses, it is impossible to provide a simple directory of how the individual should be approached within the context of neuropsychological rehabilitation. Only by extensive history taking and interacting with the patient daily over various therapeutic activities does one begin to develop a collective view or picture of how this individual experiences his or her brain injury and how he or she might best be approached when working with emotional reactions to the consequences of the brain injury.

As noted elsewhere (Prigatano, 1991a, 1991b), the symbolic expressions of patients can provide valuable clues as to how to approach them psychotherapeutically. Their artistic expressions give useful information about the central issue or issues that they are experiencing at a given time (Kalff, 1984). Recently, I reported on a young woman who had suffered a left temporal parietal brain injury following a shotgun wound to the left side of the cranium. Although she was engaged in most of her rehabilitation activities, at one point she became unexpectedly defiant and was unwilling to participate in a certain therapeutic activity. In the course of her psychotherapy, she agreed to "draw anger." Her artistic representation of feeling angry clarified that she was feeling not only angry, but very sad if not depressed. Moreover, her drawing identified a basic existential issue she was facing. That is, she no longer could be "perfect" for others, which included the therapists. This was a major change from her premorbid stance in which she was often judged as "perfect." Entering this patient's phenomenological field via her artistic expressions proved to be valuable in helping her and the rehabilitation staff manage her reaction. She subsequently remained in rehabilitation. Ultimately, she showed an excellent adjustment to residual language and memory impairments (Prigatano, 1991a, 1991b).

A second patient also drew a picture that compared himself before and after brain injury. Although the picture clarified his feeling useless after brain injury (Prigatano & Klonoff, 1988), the psychotherapist was not able to utilize this information to help the patient relate to symbols that would help foster a feeling of personal value. The patient deteriorated in his emotional reactions and eventually alienated his wife and children. By not being able to adequately enter the patient's phenomenological field, the therapist was unable to help the patient identify with symbols that might have helped restore a sense of direction or meaning in life (Jaffe, 1984). Unfortunately, this failure is all too common in rehabilitation programs throughout the world.

A third example highlights the fact that not all patients need psychotherapy. Some are able to deal with their existential dilemmas given their own unique personal and cultural backgrounds. As described by Prigatano (1991a), a Vietnamese pilot who had suffered a brain injury in the United States was extremely well adjusted to the consequences of the injury. He showed none of the anxiety and anger that is typically seen following such injuries, even when a change in work status became inevitable. Why? The patient related a childhood story that had greatly influenced his life. The story made the point that you do not know the impact of an apparent negative event on your life until very late in life. This helped sustain his positive view toward life, and was a tremendous aid in coping with his brain injury. Also, this patient's ability to rely on religious values helped guide him through difficult times. A brief description of this case and the story he told can be found in Prigatano (1991a).

Although I did not go into details of each of these three clinical vignettes, they provide examples of how entering the patient's phenomenological field helps the psychotherapist better understand what the patient is experiencing. The patient's spontaneous symbols, as reflected by music, drawings, fairy tales, and stories, often provide valuable insights. In some instances, one is able to use the information to help the patient. In other instances, one is not able to help them. Still in other situations, the patient is able to use symbols independently, and does not need psychotherapeutic intervention per se.

Is There Anything About the Nature of the Brain Injury That Influences the Psychotherapeutic Approach?

Christensen and Rosenberg (1991) raised the question of whether there is anything about the nature of brain injury that dictates what is actually done within the course of psychotherapy. The answer is "yes," but we are only at the beginning of an understanding of how lesion location relates to psychotherapeutic efforts. To answer this rather difficult question, consider research on altered self-awareness associated with brain injury.

Early clinical observations (Prigatano, 1991c, 1991d) emphasized the close connection between the patient's awareness of the effects of brain injury on their day-to-day functioning and their actual ability to become productive following a rehabilitation program. Later findings (Prigatano & Altman, 1990; Prigatano, Altman, & O'Brien, 1990) demonstrated that there was a relationship between lesion location and the lack of insight patients have about their disabilities. Moreover, the nature of the lack of insight seems related to lesion location (Prigatano, 1991c).

A recent study emanating from Japan (Mizuno, 1991) showed that patients who suffer right-cerebral dysfunction tend to repeatedly overestimate their behavioral capacities even in the face of repeated feedback about their actual performance. In contrast, patients with left-hemisphere dysfunction often repeatedly underestimate their capacities.

In addition, there has been a body of literature that emphasizes that bilateral frontal injuries, particularly involving the orbital frontal cortex, frequently result in impulsive, childlike behavior (Prigatano, 1992; Stuss, Gow, & Hetherington, 1992). Finally, temporal lobe lesions have long been implicated in the development of psychotic reactions, particularly paranoid ideation (Cummings, 1985; Lishman, 1978; Prigatano, O'Brien, & Klonoff, 1988).

I have retrospectively attempted to classify how different types of brain injury have guided the psychotherapeutic process of patients involved in neuropsychologically oriented rehabilitation. The following observations are offered as hypotheses based on clinical experience.

Typically, patients with left-hemisphere damage, particularly involving the more posterior regions of the brain, require guidance and support when overcoming their overly cautious and self-doubting attitude. These individuals are often easily discouraged and frightened by their disabilities. Consequently, to help them adjust, encouragement and support are frequently given. In contrast, right-hemisphere patients involving both anterior and posterior lesions frequently appear less cautious and less doubting over their actual abilities. As noted earlier, they often overestimate their capacities, and consequently they need help to inhibit inappropriate responding. These individuals are often asked to go "slowly" before making decisions. They are given guidance to help them obtain a more global view of how their brain injury affects their behavior and impact on others. Thus, the lateralization of the cerebral lesion influences the psychotherapeutic process by considering differences of "cognitive style" seen after right- versus left-hemisphere brain injury.

Also, patients who have frontal-lobe lesions are approached differently than patients who have temporal-lobe lesions (see Prigatano, 1988). Obviously, in traumatic brain injury, lesions can occur in both regions. However, in those patients who show primarily frontal- versus temporal-lobe damage, different behavioral patterns emerge. Bilaterally frontal-injured patients, particularly involving orbital frontal cortex, often are impulsive, volatile, and less likely to plan a strategy. Frequently, they are described as childish. These patients often need structure, and are worked with to develop a more "mature" stance to the world. It is not uncommon for the psychotherapist to behave more like a "parent" toward this type of patient.

In contrast, patients with temporal-lobe injury often tend to misperceive the environment or misremember what was said or done. Consequently, they tend to develop a distrustful attitude, and in some instances they can develop frank paranoid ideations. These patients need to be encouraged to write down what is said in a psychotherapeutic session, and specific agreed on plans of action are undertaken with them to improve the therapeutic alliance. Frequently the therapist is very task oriented and attempts to clarify intentions so as to undercut the development of a misperception of the environment (Prigatano et al., 1988).

Thus, lesion location does influence the psychotherapeutic approach to the patient. However, it is the brain-behavior disturbance, coupled with the premorbid personality characteristics of the individual, that ultimately determine how the psychotherapist approaches the patient. Therefore, it is clear that the psychotherapist does have something to say to the neuroscientist and vice versa.

However, to imply that the lesion location and neuropsychological deficits are the sole determinants of what the psychotherapist does of course misses the major point of my approach to psychotherapy. One must take into consideration the richness of the individual's background, how he or she may perceive the deficits, as well as the actual deficits themselves on planning a course of rehabilitation that includes psychotherapy.

Is the Psychotherapeutic Approach in (My) Neuropsychological Rehabilitation Program Essentially a Supportive Form of Psychoanalytic Psychotherapy That Is Influenced Primarily by Freudian Concepts and Ideas?

This last question raised by Christensen and Rosenberg (1991) may have already been answered in light of what has been discussed. There is no question that my approach to psychotherapy is heavily influenced by psychodynamic theories. Clearly Freud's appreciation of the role of the unconscious and the role of what he broadly described as libidinal and death wish instincts can clearly be seen in the behavior of patients that I work with, as well as a wide variety of psychiatric patients. I believe the Freudian approach provides one basis for interventions, and for some of the therapists who work within my program that particular model still is the primary model (Klonoff & Lage, 1991). However, from my own perspective, I see a combination of both Freud's and Jung's ideas as the cornerstone of what I attempt to do in psychotherapy. As the issue of meaning in life after brain injury is dealt with, Jung's ideas are more useful.

From the Freudian perspective, the primary goal of psychotherapy is to help the patient deal with unconscious conflicts in such a manner as to free up psychic energy and thereby make greater commitments to life. The emphasis is often on helping the patient become more productive in his or her work and more competent in interpersonal or love relationships. Within the context of this model, the symbols of work and love are clearly deemed important for psychological health. To this degree, Freud's theories have clearly influenced my approach to psychotherapy. However, Jung has pointed in the direction of a third dimension that is equally important. Besides the capacity to work and love, Jung emphasized the need for people to develop along their own personal course. There is no doubt that Jung's concept of *individuation* developed in reaction to his professional and personal separation from Freud. Yet Jung's appreciation of this dimension is especially relevant to work with brain-dysfunctional patients.

Brain-dysfunctional individuals have to develop a renewed sense of individuality. They must face the tragedy in their life even though it frightens them, and they have perhaps less cognitive capacities for dealing with it than they did in the past. Nevertheless, individuals can use whatever cunning they have in conjunction with the guidance of an experienced psychotherapist knowledgeable about brain-behavioral relationships to face the thing that frightens them the most following their brain injury. The symbol of play can be used to reflect not only recreation but the playful attitude. It is the symbol of the individual doing what he or she enjoys the most. Consequently, the symbol of play should be placed next to the symbols of work and love as the primary goals of psychotherapy (Prigatano, 1989b; Prigatano, 1991a, 1991b). These observations hopefully clarify the fact that both Freudian and Jungian ideas form the basis of my psychotherapeutic approach, with Jung clearly having the primary influence as it related to meaning in life after brain injury.

Some may argue that these ideas are rather abstract and difficult to apply to brain-dysfunctional individuals. In reality, I believe this language is easily understood by brain-dysfunctional patients, even severely brain-injured individuals. When I talk about how brain injury affects one's capacity to work, it makes sense to the brain-dysfunctional person. When I talk to them about how brain injury influences their capacity to love someone else or maintain intimate interpersonal relationships, it also makes sense to them. Finally, when I talk to a brain-dysfunctional person about their ability to follow whatever course in life they felt was going to be most fulfilling to them, it also makes sense to them. Consequently, these ideas can be applied as "living symbols" in a manner that has intuitive appeal to brain-dysfunctional patients and the psychotherapist. However, besides the intuitive appeal, these symbols allow one to guide one's objective assessment of rehabilitation outcome. Elsewhere I have argued for the importance of using work as a major outcome variable (Prigatano et al., 1986). Although not all patients have to "work" per se, almost everyone needs to be productive in the course of their daily existence. Thus, brain-dysfunctional patients also need to experience a sense of productivity, therefore this is an important outcome measure.

Although my model is heavily influenced by Freudian and Jungian perspectives, these are not the only theoretical systems that I find useful. There are other models that can be quite helpful. For example, the concept of learned helplessness, which has emanated from learning theory and behavior research (Seligman, 1975), can be applied to some brain-dysfunctional patients' behavior as well as their families' behavior and the treatment staff's behavior. In the context of my daily staff meeting, I work with my own emotional reactions to brain-dysfunctional patients and how the patient's inability to show major changes despite my therapeutic efforts at times leads to a sense of depression in the treatment team (Prigatano, 1989a).

Thus, as any experienced psychotherapist knows, one has to take information from various theoretical models in order to deal with a given patient. A given patient might best respond to a certain theoretical perspective, but not all patients will respond to a single perspective. Recognizing this and adjusting to it is the hallmark of effective psychotherapy. In so doing, the psychotherapist appreciates the importance of the scientific approach to working with individuals while still insisting on the importance of entering the patient's phenomenological experience through applying artistic efforts to the psychotherapeutic process when needed.

CONCLUSION

This chapter attempted to emphasize the potential role of psychotherapy within the context of neuropsychologically oriented rehabilitation after brain injury. It described some of the concepts involved in working with brain-dysfunctional patients, particularly those borrowed from the work of Jung and Freud. In responding to Christensen and Rosenberg's (1991) useful critique, an attempt was made to demonstrate that the idiosyncratic differences of each patient are incorporated in the psychotherapeutic process. This means attending to their premorbid personality characteristics, as well as the neuropsychological characteristics they show following focal or diffuse brain dysfunction. Although briefly considered, a series of hypotheses were offered as to how lesion location may influence the "cognitive style" of patients and thereby dictate in part how the patients are approached within the context of rehabilitation and psychotherapy in particular.

It is extremely important that neurorehabilitationists develop (a) methods for assessing the efficacy of their work, and (b) clear guidelines for which types of patients they can successfully help. This is also true of the psychotherapists working with brain-dysfunctional patients. Greater efforts need to be made in evaluating how one might best deal with the emotional and motivational disturbances of a given brain-dysfunctional patient, and to clarify which patient seems to benefit most from what types of psychotherapeutic interventions. However, psychotherapy remains an individualistic process, and a pure technique-oriented approach will never be sufficient.

Although psychotherapy cannot be expected to move the patient into a state of "false happiness" following the tragedy of his or her brain injury, it can be used to help them face the realities of life in a more productive manner, as the following quote from Jung's early work clearly demonstrated: ". . . the principal aim of psychotherapy is not to transport the patient to an impossible state of happiness, but to help him acquire steadfastness and philosophic patience in the face of suffering" (Jung, 1957, p. 81).

REFERENCES

Ben-Yishay, Y., & Prigatano, G. P. (1990). Cognitive remediation. In M. Rosenthal, E. R. Griffith, M. R. Bond, & J. D. Miller (Eds.), *Rehabilitation of the adult and child with traumatic brain injury* (pp. 393–409). Philadelphia: F. A. Davis.

Campbell, J. (1989). *The hero with a thousand faces.* Princeton, NJ: Princeton University Press.

Cummings, J. (1985). Organic delusions: Phenomenology, anatomical correlations, and review. *British Journal of Psychiatry, 146,* 184–197.

Christensen, A.-L., & Rosenberg, N. K. (1991). A critique of the role of psychotherapy in brain injury rehabilitation. *Journal of Head Trauma Rehabilitation, 6*(4), 56–61.

Jaffe, A. (1984). *The myth of meaning in the work of C. G. Jung.* Zurich, Switzerland: Daimon Verlag.

Jung, C. G. (1957). *The practice of psychotherapy. Bollinger Series XX* (Vol. 16). Princeton, NJ: Princeton University Press.

Kalff, D. M. (1984). *Sandplay: A psychotherapeutic approach to the psyche.* Boston, MA: Sigo Press.

Klonoff, P. S., & Lage, G. (1991). Narcissistic injury in patients with traumatic brain injury. *Journal of Head Trauma Rehabilitation, 6*(4), 11–21.

Lishman, W. A. (1978). *Organic psychiatry.* Oxford, England: Blackwell Scientific Publications.

Luria, A. R. (1972). *The man with a shattered world.* (L. Solotaroff, Trans.). New York: Basic Books.

Meadows, J. (1987). *This history of scientific discovery.* Oxford, England: Pharden Press.

Mizuno, M. (1991). Neuropsychological characteristics of right hemisphere damage: Investigation by attention tests, concept formation and change test, and self-evaluation task. *Keio Journal of Medicine, 40*(4), 221–234.

Parsons, O. A., & Prigatano, G. P. (1978). Methodological considerations in clinical neuropsychological research. *Journal of Consulting and Clinical Psychology, 46,* 608–619.

Prigatano, G. P. (1988). Emotion and motivation in recovery and adaptation to brain damage. In S. Finger, T. LeVere, C. Almli, & D. Stein (Eds.), *Brain injury and recovery: Theoretical and controversial issues* (pp. 335–350). New York: Plenum.

Prigatano, G. P. (1989a). Bring it up in milieu: Toward effective traumatic brain injury rehabilitation interaction. *Rehabilitation Psychology, 34*(2), 135–144.

Prigatano, G. P. (1989b). Work, love, and play after brain injury. *Bulletin of the Menninger Clinic, 53*(5), 414–431.

Prigatano, G. P. (1991a). Disordered mind, wounded soul: The emerging role of psychotherapy in rehabilitation. *Journal of Head Trauma Rehabilitation, 6*(4), 1–10.

Prigatano, G. P. (1991b, November). *Science and symbolism in neuropsychological rehabilitation after brain injury.* Paper presented at the 10th annual James C. Hemphill lecture, Rehabilitation Institute of Chicago, IL.

Prigatano, G. P. (1991c). Disturbances of self-awareness of deficit after traumatic brain injury. In G. P. Prigatano & D. L. Schacter (Eds.), *Awareness of deficit after brain injury: Clinical and theoretical issues* (pp. 111–126). New York: Oxford University Press.

Prigatano, G. P. (1991d). The relationship of frontal lobe damage to diminished awareness: Studies in rehabilitation. In H. S. Levin, H. M. Eisenberg, & A. L. Benton (Eds.), *Frontal lobe function and dysfunction* (pp. 381–397). New York: Oxford University Press.

Prigatano, G. P. (1992). Personality disturbances associated with traumatic brain injury. *Journal of Consulting and Clinical Psychology, 60*(3), 44–55.

Prigatano, G. P., & Altman, I. M. (1990). Impaired awareness of behavioral limitations after traumatic brain injury. *Archives of Physical Medicine and Rehabilitation, 71,* 1058–1064.

Prigatano, G. P., Altman, I. M., & O'Brien, K. P. (1990). Behavioral limitations that brain injured patients tend to underestimate. *Clinical Neuropsychologist,4*(2), 163–176.

Prigatano, G. P., Amin, K., & Rosenstein, L. D. (1991). *Manual for the BNI screen for higher cerebral functions.* Unpublished manual.

Prigatano, G. P., & Klonoff, P. S. (1988). Psychotherapy and neuropsychological assessment after brain injury. *Journal of Head Trauma Rehabilitation, 3*(1), 45–56.

Prigatano, G. P., O'Brien, K., & Klonoff, P. S. (1988). The clinical management of paranoid delusions in postacute traumatic brain-injured patients. *Journal of Head Trauma Rehabilitation, 3*(3), 23–32.

Prigatano, G. P., Fordyce, D. J., Zeiner, H. K., Roueche, J. R., Pepping, M., & Wood, B. C. (1986). *Neuropsychological rehabilitation after brain injury.* Baltimore, MD: Johns Hopkins University Press.

Prigatano, G. P., Klonoff, P. S., O'Brien, K. P., Altman, I., Amin, K., Chiapello, D. A., Shepherd, J., Cunningham, M., & Mora, M. (in press). Returning TBI patients back to work and school using a neuropsychologically oriented, milieu rehabilitation program. *Journal of Head Trauma Rehabilitation.*

Seligman, M. E. P. (1975). *Helplessness.* New York: W. H. Freeman.

Stuss, D. T., Gow, C. A., & Hetherington, C. R. (1992). "No longer Gage": Frontal lobe dysfunction and emotional changes. *Journal of Consulting and Clinical Psychology, 60*(3), 349–359.

CHAPTER TWELVE

Rehabilitating Psychosocial Functioning

Zeev Groswasser

ABSTRACT

The rehabilitation of patients sustaining traumatic brain injury is aimed at restoring proper psychosocial functioning. The latter is variously defined, depending on national and cultural backgrounds. I have found that, in Western countries, the return of the patient to work at a job commensurate with his or her residual capacity constitutes an objective, integrative, and measurable index of outcome that is well correlated with the patient's subjective evaluation of the quality of life as determined by the Rehabilitation Need and Status Scale (RNSS). I have used this criterion in outcome studies of traumatic brain-injured patients at the Loewenstein Rehabilitation Hospital since 1974. In the last few years, it has gained a central place in the planning of the rehabilitation program.

Traumatic brain injury (TBI) has been recognized by the National Institutes of Health as a major problem of modern society. Among others, Goldstein (1990) described TBI as the "silent epidemic." Most TBI patients in developed countries are victims of road accidents. In the United States, road accidents take the lives of almost 100,000 people annually, and reduce an additional 70,000–90,000 people to a life-long debilitating loss of function. The estimated yearly cost to society is $25 billion (Goldstein, 1990).

Israel is no exception. From 1964 to 1974, the death toll from automobile accidents in this country almost doubled, from 325 to 716 persons annually without significant changes in population. In

1985, 387 persons were reported killed (lowest incidence over years—8.3/100,000).

It is important to keep in mind when comparing national statistics that definitions vary from country to country. In some cases, overall incidence is recorded; in others, accidents per kilometers driven or accidents per number of vehicles is recorded (Table 12.1). Death by accident is defined in accordance with the length of time after the event that death occurred. This criterion also may vary (the World Health Organization [WHO] definition is death within 30 days of accident; Table 12.2). The same is true with regard to severity of the injury resulting from the accident (Table 12.2).

A common language for describing the initial state of the central nervous system (CNS) after trauma became available with the introduction of the Glasgow Coma Score (GCS) by Teasdale and Jennett (1974). Ill-defined terms such as *stupor* and *delirium* were eliminated, and a basis was established for evaluating the treatment provided TBI patients at different centers in different countries. In addition, the GCS served the clinician as a prognostic measure for TBI patients. However, it has been shown that victims of road accidents often suffer not only CNS damage, but polytrauma. According to Groswasser, Cohen, and Blankstein (1990), 58% of TBI patients show additional injuries, and psychosocial outcome is usually worse in TBI patients with multiple trauma than in those with CNS damage only. Therefore, perhaps the GCS should be combined and weighed with results of other scales that measure trauma, such as the Injury Severity Score introduced by Baker,

TABLE 12.1
Comparison of Different Accident Rates in Various Countries

Country	Accidents/10^5 vehicles	Accidents/100 million km driving	Death toll/10^5 people
Israel	1,626	97	11
Holland	652	46	9
Japan	866	112	8
Jordan	2,501	445*	14*
Spain	680	115	16
France	580	44	19
United States	1,184	78	19*
United Kingdom	1,050	86	9
Switzerland	592	—	14

Note. From *Injuries from Road Accidents—Circumstances of Accident, Evacuation and Outcome* (p. 5) by M. Avizur, 1992, Jerusalem: Hebrew University and Hadassa Medical Organization. Copyright © 1992 by Hebrew University and Hadassa Medical Organization. Reprinted by permission.
*Figures for 1987.

TABLE 12.2
Death and Severity of Injury: Definitions
of Different European Countries

Country	Death	Very Severe Injury	Severe Injury
Israel	Within 30 days		24 hours in hospital
Germany (FRG)		Within 30 days	24 hours in hospital
Czechoslovakia		Within 30 days	At least 42 days in hospital
France	Within 6 days		6 days in hospital
Italy	Within 7 days		
Greece	Within 3 days		
Austria	Within 3 days	At least 21 days in hospital	Sick leave > 24 hours in hospital
Spain	Within 24 hours		
Portugal	Prehospital		
Norway		Life threatening	Not life-threatening invalidity

Note. From *Injuries from Road Accidents—Circumstances of Accident, Evacuation and Outcome* (p. 5) by M. Avizur, 1992, Jerusalem: Hebrew University and Hadassa Medical Organization. Copyright © 1992 by Hebrew University and Hadassa Medical Organization. Reprinted by permission.

O'Neill, Haddon, and Long (1974), to obtain better prognostic information during the acute phase.

The Loewenstein Rehabilitation Hospital (LRH) had been dealing with TBI patients since 1965. At that time, most physicians believed that little could be done for TBI patients surviving the acute phase. However, after the Six Day War in June 1967, many war veterans with TBI were referred to the LRH, together with an increasing number of civilians with accident-related injuries. This concentration of a large number of TBI patients in one institution provided a tremendous amount of experience in the management and study of the multiple aspects of brain damage. In 1973, the Ministries of Health and Defense declared the LRH the national center for the rehabilitation of TBI patients in Israel. Since then, it has expanded its services to include an Intensive Care Unit for unconscious patients, an Inpatient Rehabilitation Department, a Day Center, and a follow-up Outpatient Clinic. A Vocational Rehabilitation Center was added in 1982, and the pediatric TBI patients got a separate unit in 1988. The basic advantage of having a TBI rehabilitation center as part of a rehabilitation hospital was the change in emphasis, right at the outset, away from minimizing specific neurological and neurobehavioral deficits, to the achievement of normal daily functioning, including psychosocial reintegration.

Approximately 160 new TBI patients are admitted each year to the LRH. This figure represents those with very severe diseases, suffering from polytrauma, usually after a period of unconsciousness of varying length. Although most patients are referred for rehabilitation, those without overt motor deficits are often sent home directly after receiving treatment in a general hospital. Some of the latter are seen in the Outpatient Clinic at a much later phase, usually because of a failure to resume their previous position within the family, inability to return to work, or psychosocial dysfunctioning. A number adopt abnormal behavior patterns when their immediate environment is unguided, and these are very difficult to change after a long term. Moreover, as a result of vast experience, I believe that the true incidence of patients with severe TBI injury is higher than reported, and that patients who suffer from the neurobehavioral sequelae of traumatic insult to the CNS often continue to be misdiagnosed as neurotic. It is important that the general medical community be made aware of the possibility of such problems and refer affected patients as soon as possible. I believe that early intervention and guidance for both patient and family may avoid late behavioral problems and can improve the overall psychosocial adaptability of the TBI patient.

ASSESSMENT OF CNS DAMAGE
AND PSYCHOSOCIAL OUTCOME

Traumatic injury to the CNS may affect any or all of the four main domains of human functioning: (a) motor control, (b) communication, (c) cognition, and (d) behavior. The precise assessment of each of these domains is necessary for obtaining prognostic information, evaluating the efficacy of treatment, and epidemiologically studying head injury as a public health problem.

The prognostic information is very important because it also affects the relatives of TBI patients. These relatives need to know what lies ahead of them, and they must handle the enforced change in lifestyle and family relationships. In 1975, Jennett and Bond introduced the Glasgow Outcome Scale (GOS), which gained popularity because of its practicality and ease of use. However, a closer look at its subscales reveals that it is a measure of dependence and independence, rather than a measure of psychosocial functioning. Therefore, it is not precise enough for the rehabilitation setting (Rao et al., 1990). Jennett and Bond regarded the patient's return to work as "an unrealistic index of recovery." However, it should be remembered that patients at the late phase of disease in need of comprehensive rehabilitation programs were not treated at that time by them.

Today, the main concern of the rehabilitation process is attainment of the best possible quality of life for the patient in accordance with his or her optimal residual capacity. Strictly medical definitions are too narrow, and broader measurements of psychosocial functioning are necessary. I believe that the time to assess outcome is not at discharge from the rehabilitation program, but at a later phase when the patient has had time to experience the realities of life within family and society. Evidence for this was provided by Najenson, Groswasser, Mendelson, and Hackett (1980), who showed that there was a contrast between the relatively good outcome predicted at time of discharge from an inpatient rehabilitation program and the poor actual state of the patient half a year or more after discharge.

The manner of assessment of psychosocial functioning is a key problem in measuring outcome. It is especially complicated by the lack of a "golden standard" and by the range of preceptions of good psychosocial functioning by different cultures and different societies. Because TBI rehabilitation is practiced mostly in Western countries, "back to work" is its goal and *raison d'etre* (Livneh, 1988). It is believed that patient's return to work at a job commensurate with his or her residual capacity can be used as an integrative, objective, and measurable criterion of outcome providing a good indication of the psychosocial functioning of TBI patients. In Israel, Najenson et al. (1974) successfully used this criterion to measure the rehabilitation outcome of TBI patients. Lezak (1986) considered employment important because it helps structure lifestyle, provides stability and purpose, and creates independent lifestyle. Stanbrook, Moore, Deviane, and Hawryluk (1990) concluded that vocational programs and planning are essential targets in holistic rehabilitation. This goal is realistic. Rao et al. (1990) showed that 66% of consecutive patients who were admitted to an intensive rehabilitation program returned to work. A British committee established in 1987 to assess the after care of brain-injured patients concluded that "returning to work is regarded as a major aim for brain damaged patients . . . however, the transition between medical and vocational rehabilitation is difficult and is poorly catered for" (Conference, 1987). At the LRH, the vocational rehabilitation program is part and parcel of the comprehensive rehabilitation program of the TBI patient. Thus, there is no need to transition from the inpatient rehabilitation program to an outside vocational rehabilitation center.

TABLE 12.3
Age Groups and Predicted Vocational Outcome at Discharge
from a Comprehensive Inpatient TBI Rehabilitation Program
at the LRH

	Percentages of patients within each age group				
Outcome	5–15	16–29	30–44	45–59	60–65
Good recovery	71.0	76.7	73.0	73.0	75.0
Poor recovery	29.0	23.3	24.1	27.0	25.0

Age, Brain Damage, and Vocational Outcome

I have found that the patient's capacity to resume a self-supporting work position is highly correlated with the type and amount of brain damage affecting the four main domains of life (i.e., motor control, communication, cognition, and behavior). During the years 1981–1985, 328 TBI patients ages 5–65 years were discharged from the LRH. This group was studied with regard to the influence of age and of deficits in the four domains on expected vocational outcome at the time of discharge. *Good recovery* was defined as employment on the open job market; *poor recovery* was defined as working in a shelter or unemployed. Patients who returned to a regular school were considered with those who returned to work.

The male/female ratio of the group was 3.63, with no significant age differences between the genders. Outcome was found to be unrelated to age, as shown in Table 12.3. This finding is of interest because it is commonly believed that increased age is negatively correlated with outcome following TBI. In a study of the relationship between patient age and clinical outcome following closed-head injury, Vollmer et al. (1991) could not identify any factor that accounted for the adverse effects of age on outcome. Multivariate analysis of their data failed to eliminate age as an independent variable. They suggested that the effect of age on outcome is dependent on an alteration in the pathophysiological response of the aging CNS. It is suggested here that, in the case of severe TBI, these alterations are common in all age groups. Therefore, the effect of age alone is negligible.

With regard to CNS damage, motor control, as evaluated by the presence of hemiparesis, was found to be significantly related to vocational outcome, as shown in Table 12.4. Language and speech disturbances were each seen in one fifth of the TBI patients and were significantly related to poor recovery. Similarly, cognitive and behavioral disturbances were adversely linked to vocational outcome (Tables 12.5

TABLE 12.4
Hemiparesis and Predicted Vocational Outcome at Discharge
from a Comprehensive Inpatient TBI Rehabilitation Program
at the LRH

Outcome	Good Recovery (open market)		Poor Recovery (sheltered work and unemployed)	
	N	%	N	%
Hemiparesis N = 166 (50.6%)	102	61.4	64	38.6
No overt motor deficit N = 162 (49.4%)	144	88.9	18	11.1
Total	246	75.0	82	25.0

$p < .001$, χ^2.

and 12.6). Cognitive disturbances were the most common deficit (almost 71% of patients).

Subjective Rehabilitation Outcome

A basic question that remains to be answered is: What do patients think of the rehabilitation goals set by their therapists? Do these goals represent what they believe is a good quality of life?

I used the Rehabilitation Need and Status Scale (RNSS), introduced by Kravetz (1973) for patients with physical disabilities, to learn how TBI patients subjectively perceive their quality of life and the relationship of this perception to work placement. The RNSS was found suitable for use with TBI patients because the alpha coefficients

TABLE 12.5
Cognitive Disturbances and Predicted Vocational Outcome at
Discharge from a Comprehensive Inpatient TBI Rehabilitation
Program at the LRH

Outcome	Good Recovery (open market)		Poor Recovery (sheltered work and unemployed)	
	N	%	N	%
Cognitive disturbances N = 232 (70.7%)	160	69.0	72	31.0
No overt cognitive disturbances N = 96 (29.3%)	86	89.6	10	10.4
Total	246	75.0	82	25.0

$p < .001$, χ^2.

TABLE 12.6
Behavior Disturbances and Predicted Vocational Outcome at
Discharge from a Comprehensive Inpatient TBI Rehabilitation
Program at the LRH

Outcome	Good Recovery (open market)		Poor Recovery (sheltered work and unemployed)	
	N	%	N	%
Behavioral disturbances N = 135 (41.2%)	81	60.0	54	40.0
No overt behavioral disturbances N = 193 (58.8%)	165	85.5	28	14.5
Total	246	75.0	82	25.0

$p < .001$, χ^2.

for TBI patients for each subscale resembled those obtained by Kravetz for physically disabled patients (Melamed, Groswasser, & Stern, 1992).

The RNSS is composed of 80 items distributed among seven subscales. Scores for each item, which range from one to five, are weighed to gain greater homogeneity. The subscales are as follows:

1. Physiological need satisfaction subscale—measures the frequency with which a person experiences physical symptoms, such as headache, palpitations, dizziness.

2. Emotional security need satisfaction subscale—measures the frequency of feelings of unhappiness, depression, worry about becoming old, uncertainty with regard to solving personal problems, and so on.

3. Family need satisfaction subscale—measures satisfaction gained from various family activities and the ability to communicate feelings among family members.

4. Social need satisfaction subscale—measures the frequency of participation in social activities, maintenance of social contacts, number of new social contacts made over a certain period, and number of friends.

5. Economic self-esteem subscale—measures auto assessment of the degree to which the patient's present job is better or worse than those he or she held in the past, whether he or she is self-supporting, and the number of jobs held over the past 6 months.

6. Economic security need satisfaction subscale—measures the frequency with which the patient feels secure with regard to his or her economic situation.

7. Vocational self-actualization need satisfaction subscale—measures the frequency with which the patient experiences feelings of satisfaction about his vocational activity. The items refer to utilization of capabilities, opportunity to try own ideas, appreciation received at work, and relationship with employers.

Melamed et al. (1992) studied 84% of the total number of consecutive TBI patients ages 18–59 years who were discharged from the inpatient TBI rehabilitation program at the LRH. Evaluation was conducted 1–2 years after discharge. The authors hypothesized that employed TBI patients would have higher RNSS scores than unemployed patients. Results support this hypothesis, which links objective and subjective rehabilitation goals as defined by the test subscales.

Melamed et al. (1992) found that acceptance of disability (Linkowski, 1971) was significantly associated with work status in TBI patients. Those working at jobs obtained on the open market had the highest RNSS scores. Significantly, high correlations were found between acceptance of disability and six of the subscales. However, it is difficult to know which comes first: Does the return to work precede acceptance of disability, or vice versa? In either case, these findings stress the importance of acceptance of disability as a factor to be addressed during the rehabilitation process.

Johnson (1987) found time to be a crucial factor in the return to work for TBI patients. That is, those who will resume regular work will do so within 2 years following trauma; after 2 years, the chances of the patient returning to work are much lower. Successful return to work depends on the (a) opportunity to work at the previous job, (b) opportunity for a work trial period, (c) opportunity for employment at a job commensurate with capability, and (d) strong and long-term support by family and friends. Johnson could not predict which specific factors preclude a return to work, but he did show that variables such as the initial GCS bore little relationship to final cognitive outcome, and that the length of posttraumatic amnesia (PTA) was also not a key factor (60% of patients who returned to work had PTA for more than 3 weeks). He recommended that educational programs and information on TBI be made available to potential employers of these patients.

PSYCHOSOCIAL FUNCTIONING OF THE FAMILIES
OF TBI PATIENTS

The majority of TBI patients are males in their second or third decade. Normally, these are the years in which people complete their education, take on a profession or vocation, and establish new family relationships or reestablish old ones—in short, they arrange their lives with an eye toward the future. Thus, a brain injury at this time of life is extremely hard on the patient and his or her family.

During the acute phase, the immediate concern of the family is the survival of the patient. Usually, however, physicians are unable to predict with certainty even short-term outcome. This state of suspense, coupled with the fear of imminent disaster and grief while the patient may still be unconscious, may lead to mistrust of the medical staff by the family, who cannot understand the physician's hesitation in this age of advanced technology. These feelings are exacerbated when they discover that in most cases of blunt brain injury, no surgery is needed, and treatment is for the great part supportive only. If the patient remains in a state of prolonged postcomatose unawareness (Sazbon & Groswasser, 1991), there may even be open aggression toward the medical personnel (Stern, Sazbon, Becker, & Costeff, 1988). To help family members overcome these feelings and enable them to function well and relate with care and understanding toward each other and the patient, a meaningful dialogue must be established between the caretaker personnel and the family as early as possible after the trauma. In addition, families must receive emotional and informational support, either on an individual basis or via support groups.

These problems do not disappear when the patient recovers consciousness. It soon becomes very evident that he or she will require a long period of rehabilitation and that he or she has undergone profound changes in every aspect of life. Families must now deal with the problem of how to live with a brain-injured member. There may be children or elderly parents who also need care and attention. Often the necessary information and resources are not provided to them by the medical world (McMordie, Rogers, & Barker, 1991). Livingstone, Brooks, and Bond (1985) found that female relatives of TBI patients show significant psychiatric morbidity at about 3 months following the trauma, with the severity of symptoms proportional to the severity of the patient's injury. Their social functioning at home becomes poor and may not show improvement with time. Brooks, Campsie, Symington, Beattie, and McKinlay (1986) showed that psychiatric symptoms of family members were more severe after 5 years of injury than after 1 year, and that relatives were under great strain and exhibited constant anxiety.

McMordie et al. (1991) observed that families of TBI patients had questions about prognosis, care, and referral resources after initial hospitalization. Their main concerns were focused on expectation and outcome. The authors concluded that educational programs should be implemented for families of TBI patients.

Experience tells us that it is almost impossible to rehabilitate a TBI patient without the family. It is the family that provides physical and moral support, cares for the patient in the long run, and facilitates his or her reintegration into society. Therefore, it is mandatory that families be involved in the rehabilitation process from the very beginning, that any and all available information be shared with them, and that they be aided in adjusting their expectations on a realistic level. Only in this manner can the best possible psychosocial outcome of patients be achieved.

CONCLUSIONS

To help the TBI patient achieve optimal psychosocial functioning through the rehabilitation process, objective, integrative, and measurable criteria for success must be established. I chose the patient's ultimate return to employment on the open market or his or her return to school as my index for successful outcome. My choice was supported by results of the RNSS, which revealed that the patient's subjective evaluation of the quality of his or her life is highly correlated with his or her vocational status. I concluded that the psychosocial functioning of TBI patients can be determined on the basis of their employment status in a real-life situation after discharge from the rehabilitation program.

I suggest that age alone is not an independent factor in determining the psychosocial outcome of TBI patients, and that outcome is influenced by the presence and severity of deficits in motor control, communication, cognition, and behavior.

Family involvement in the rehabilitation process is crucial, and family members must be given emotional support and information starting from the very early phases after trauma. This eases anxiety, decreases uncertainty, and provides them with resources for the care and support of patients within the family and for facilitating their reintegration into society.

REFERENCES

Avizur, M. (1992). *Injuries from road accidents—circumstances of accident, evacuation and Outcome.* Jerusalem: Hebrew University and Hadassa Medical Organization.

Baker, S. P., O'Neill, B., Jr., Haddon, W., & Long, W. B. (1974). The injury severity score: A method for describing patients with multiple injuries and evaluating emergency care. *The Journal of Trauma, 14,* 187–196.

Brooks, N., Campsie, L., Symington, C., Beattie, A., & McKinlay, W. (1986). The five year outcome of blunt head injury: A relative's view. *Journal of Neurology, Neurosurgery and Psychiatry, 49,* 764–770.

Goldstein, M. (1990). Traumatic brain injury: A silent epidemic. *Annals of Neurology, 27,* 327.

Conference (1987, November). *The aftercare of brain injury on inter-professional co-operation and guidelines for the future.* Paper presented at the conference of the Royal College of Physicians, London.

Groswasser, Z., Cohen, M., & Blankstein, E. (1990). Polytrauma associated with traumatic brain injury: Incidence, nature and impact on rehabilitation outcome. *Brain Injury, 4,* 161–166.

Jennett, B., & Bond, M. (1975). Assessment of outcome after severe brain damage. A practical scale. *Lancet, 1,* 480–484.

Johnson, R. (1987). Return to work after severe head injury. *International Rehabilitation Studies, 9,* 44–49.

Kravetz, S. (1973). *Rehabilitation need and status: Substance, structure and process.* Unpublished doctoral dissertation, University of Wisconsin, Madison.

Lezak, M. D. (1986). Psychological implications of traumatic brain damage of the patient's family. *Rehabilitation Psychology, 31,* 241–250.

Linkowski, D. C. (1971). A scale to measure acceptance of disability. *Rehabilitation Counseling Bulletin, 14,* 236–244.

Livingstone, M. G., Brooks, N. D., & Bond, M. (1985). Three months after head injury: Psychiatric and social impacts on relatives. *Journal of Neurology, Neurosurgery and Psychiatry, 48,* 870–875.

Livneh, H. (1988). Assessing outcome criteria in rehabilitation: A multicomponent approach. *Rehabilitation Counseling Bulletin, 32,* 72–94.

McMordie, W. R., Rogers, K. F., & Barker, S. L. (1991). Consumer satisfaction with services to head-injured patients and their families. *Brain Injury, 5,* 43–51.

Melamed, S., Groswasser, Z., & Stern, M. J. (1992). Acceptance of disability, work involvement and subjective rehabilitation status of traumatic brain-injured (TBI) patients. *Brain Injury, 6,* 233–243.

Najenson, T., Groswasser, Z., Mendelson, L., & Hackett, P. (1989). Rehabilitation outcome of brain damaged patients after severe head injury. *International Rehabilitation Medicine, 2,* 17–22.

Najenson, T., Mendelson, L., Schechter, I., David, C., Mintz, N., & Groswasser, Z. (1974). Rehabilitation after severe head injury. *Scandinavian Journal of Rehabilitation Medicine, 6,* 5–122.

Rao, N., Rosenthal, M., Cronin-Stubb, D., Lambert, R., Barnes, P., & Swanson, B. (1990). Return to work after rehabilitation following traumatic brain injury. *Brain Injury, 4,* 49–56.

Sazbon, L., & Groswasser, Z. (1991). Editorial. Prolonged coma, vegetative state, postcomatose unawareness—semantics or better understanding? *Brain Injury, 5,* 3–8.

Stanbrook, M., Moore, A. D., Deviane, C., & Hawryluk, G. A. (1990). Effects of mild, moderate and severe head injury on long-term vocational status. *Brain Injury, 4,* 183–190.

Stern, M. J., Sazbon, K., Becker, E., & Costeff, H. (1988). Severe behavioral disturbances in families of patients with prolonged coma. *Brain Injury, 2,* 259–262.

Teasdale, G., & Jennett, B. (1974). Assessment of coma and impaired consciousness: A practical scale. *Lancet, 2,* 81–84.

Vollmer, D. G., Torner, J. C., Jane, J. A., Sadovnic, B., Charlebois, D., Eisenberg, H. M., Foulkes, M. A., Marmarou, A., & Marshall, L. F. (1991). Age and outcome following traumatic coma: Why do older patients fare worse? *Journal of Neurosurgery, 75,* 37–49.

CHAPTER THIRTEEN

Traumatic Brain-Injury Rehabilitation Outcome Studies in the United States

D. Nathan Cope

ABSTRACT

Tremendous expansion of rehabilitation services for survivors of traumatic brain injury (TBI) has occurred in the United States. The expansion is both vertical (through the course of the patients' continuum of recovery) as well as horizontal (geographically more complete). Until recently, data supporting the efficacy of such a continuum of rehabilitation interventions have been lacking. Over the past 5–10 years, such studies have appeared with increasing frequency, and they do support the efficacy of these treatments. The most salient of these studies are reviewed here. Although no blinded, prospective, random-assignment study has been done, the accumulation of other studies with "quasi-experimental" designs now makes it difficult to argue against a true and clinically important treatment effect.

Outcome studies in relation to traumatic brain injury (TBI) tend to follow a few general patterns. The goal of describing a "natural history" of such injuries, with current techniques of medical and surgical acute care, is evident in most early and many current studies. These naturalistic studies have tended to utilize more gross measures of outcome ranging from simple assessment of survival and mortality, to only somewhat more finely delineated measures of outcome such as the Glasgow Outcome Scale (GOS). Much of the recent outcome data of this sort may be considered refinement of, or addition to, previous studies of TBI dating back at least 70–80 years. These outcome studies typically have involved the efforts of clinicians located in trauma centers. More recently, formal trauma registries have been established that have also added refinement to our knowledge of the epidemiology, demographics, and general outcomes of this condition. In large part, through these efforts, it is now reasonable to say the magnitude and significance of the problem of TBI is appreciated by health-care professionals. Among these professionals, at least, it is probably no longer precise to refer to TBI as "the silent epidemic" (as it has been characterized in the United States).

It also seems to have been demonstrated that aggressive surgical and medical management of the emergency and early acute care periods following TBI have produced pronounced beneficial effects on the outcomes in this condition (Becker et al., 1977; Langfitt, 1978; Nordstrom, Sundbarg, Messeter, & Schalen, 1989). Clearly, there is increased survival over earlier periods. It appears that this increased survival is also accompanied by decreased morbidity in terms of rates of long-standing disability.

A more recent type of TBI outcome study has to do with the results of rehabilitation interventions. The bulk of these interventions take place in later phases of TBI care outside of acute medical/surgical hospital settings. These rehabilitation outcome studies tend to utilize more detailed outcome measures. Outcome of rehabilitation of TBI can be described at many possible levels. It has become customary to utilize the World Health Organization (WHO) schema on these matters (Frey, 1984). With this perspective, one may look at outcomes in terms of alteration in the fundamental impairment or deficit, the disability, or the handicap. For example, it is of great interest to understand whether cognitive retraining programs alter the underlying impairment (of memory, attention, etc.) itself. It is another important question to ask whether such intervention alters the patients' disability or competence in simple isolated tasks or everyday activities. Finally, however, the outcome question must be asked in terms of rehabilitation's ability to affect the patients' ultimate handicap or ability to fulfill various social role requirements (irrespective of effect on underlying deficit and disability). There are multiple unresolved theoretical and practical difficulties in pursuing outcome studies in the area of TBI at all of these levels. Brooks (1989) and Diller and Ben-Yishay (1987) recently reviewed these issues in depth.

THE STUDIES

Acute Rehabilitation

Heinemann et al. (1990) reported on a comprehensive analysis of TBI patients discharged from their inpatient rehabilitation program between January 1, 1985, and May 31, 1987. Follow-up was performed by assessment at discharge and by means of formal telephone interviews at 3 months postdischarge. Sixty-six such patients were interviewed for this study. Patients younger than 18 months and in the program for less than 1 week were excluded. Activity of daily living scores were determined on a modified Barthel index, possible range 0–100. The measure of severity utilized was the Glasgow Coma Score (GCS). The onset to admission interval was also reported for this sample. Results of this analysis are given in Table 13.1.

Although primarily descriptive, it looks at longer term (3 month postdischarge) outcomes and demonstrates that functional gains in Activity Daily Living (ADL) scores are achieved from admission to discharge and are maintained for this postdischarge interval. There is difficulty in this study in determining the specific contribution of rehabilitation to the improved function because the average length of time from injury to admission was only 146.7 days. However, the authors stated that statistical analysis revealed that the extent of recovery in their series was unrelated to the length of time from injury to admission to program.

To discuss the next major study, I must first review a study by Cope and Hall (1982). In 1981, they reported an analysis of 34 brain-injured

TABLE 13.1
Data on Heinemann et al. (1990)

Measure	Admission	Discharge	Follow-up	Significance
Age	32.7			
	(13.0)			
Length of Stay		65.8		
		(35.3)		
Glasgow Coma	14.1			
Score (3–15)	(SD: 2.1)		80.3	
Activity Daily	49.9	78.9	(30.0)	$p < .0001$
Living (0–100)	(SD: 30.5)	(28.9)		adm–disch
Onset-admission	146.7 days*			
interval	(SD: 531.0)			

*Time injury to admission was unrelated to extent of recovery.

patients based on prospectively gathered data. They showed that TBI patients, equally matched on severity of injury, demographics, and comorbidity measures, but varying only on whether they had been referred early or late to a comprehensive inpatient rehabilitation program, had a greater than 50% reduction in total hospital treatment days required. The late and early rehabilitated groups both experienced reductions in days: Acute hospital days went from 55.8 to 20.9, and inpatient rehabilitation days went from 88.8 to 43.5. This amounted to a total savings of 80 hospital days per patient. The patients were found to reach equivalent degrees of functional recovery at discharge from rehabilitation and of social status (living situation and productivity) at 2 years postinjury. This was a dramatic finding and, if true, has great implications for the manner in which the care of these patients should be managed. However, this provocative study had, until recently, remained unreplicated.

Hall and Wright (1991) recently carried out an independent replication of this earlier study based on an analysis of a separate cohort of patients. The authors analyzed data gathered prospectively from 68 brain-injured patients, in 1990–1991, from the same acute inpatient brain-injury rehabilitation program. The median time from injury to admission to the program for this group of sequential admissions was 22 days. The patients were matched for severity of injury on a variety of measures (including demographics, GCS, length of coma, length of time from injury to admission, CT scan abnormalities, etc.) similar to the previous study. No significant differences were found between groups except for incidence of general surgeries. The length of inpatient rehabilitation stay was an average of 28 days for early admissions and 60 days for late admissions. Dependent variables were length of rehabilitation and functional return as assessed by the Rappaport Disability Rating Scale (DRS; Rappaport, Hall, Hopkins, Belleza, & Cope, 1982; Hall, Cope, & Rappaport, 1985; range 0 = minimal impairment; 30 = death) and the Social Status Outcome Scale (SSO; Berrol, Rappaport, Cope et al., 1982; range 0 = maximal independence and productivity; 3 = maximal handicap), a measure of productivity and living status. Upon long-term follow-up (30 months postinjury), the early admitted patients were found to be mildly disabled, with an average DRS of 1.79, and the later admitted patients were moderately disabled, with an average DRS of 4.07.[1] In terms of actual social functioning, assessed by the SSO, the early rehabilitation group had a score of 0.52, and the late rehabilitation group had a score of 2.30.

---

[1]A difference significant at the $p < .008$ level.

Thus, the findings have strongly confirmed the conclusions of the previous study. Two benefits from early intervention are suggested by these two studies. First, total medical care resources are saved, both in the acute and in the rehabilitation phases of care, by rapid aggressive rehabilitation. Second, ultimate functional outcomes are also, in high likelihood, improved by such early rehabilitation interventions. Theoretical reasons for explaining such results have been detailed by Cope and Hall (1982) and include both the prevention of unnecessary secondary complications and deterioration, as well as possible better absolute neurologic recovery.

It is worth noting at this point as well that the median delay in referral from acute trauma care to rehabilitation, from the first to the second study, approximately a decade later, fell from 35 to 22 days. The reasons for this significantly shorter referral time may include more general awareness and acceptance of the need for early and aggressive rehabilitation in these cases, as well as changed economic incentives.[2] These issues are considered more fully later.

Finally, Aronow (1987) reported on essentially the only quasi-experimental, case-controlled study available to date regarding the effectiveness of comprehensive inpatient rehabilitation of TBI. She matched patients from an inpatient TBI program, from 1977 to 1979, with similar patients derived from an acute neurotrauma program who received no formal rehabilitation, on measures likely to influence outcome, including age, gender, race, severity, and time postonset. She also controlled for severity by measures of posttraumatic amnesia (PTA) obtained at follow-up. Outcomes were assessed utilizing formal scales of (a) living arrangement, (b) functional status, (c) daily care requirement, (d) vocational status, (e) and others. The patients receiving rehabilitation had a significantly better outcome on these scales than similarly injured TBI patients who received (excellent) neurotrauma care only. Aronow also did a cost-outcome analysis. Costs of care and opportunity between rehabilitation and nonrehabilitation cases varied by degree of severity of injury. For patients with up to 1 month PTA, savings achieved by the rehabilitation group averaged \$11,949[3]; for the group with 2–3 months of PTA, the savings

---

[2]Shorter retention time in acute hospital settings may be in part an artifact of the institution of diagnosis-related group (DRG) reimbursement policies by the U.S. government as well, which financially rewards hospitals for early discharges to rehabilitation. If so, it is an artifact with apparent beneficial consequences for the patient.

[3]1979 dollars.

were $3,102. Aronow did not calculate an average savings for the 4-month and higher PTA group because there was only one such case in the nonrehabilitation group. However, the annual cost of that one unrehabilitated case was calculated at $16,388, compared with the average cost of $7,117 for the equivalently severely injured rehabilitated group. It was further reported that the cost for rehabilitating the 60 cases in the rehabilitation group was approximately $1 million; the annual savings in cost of care for these patients was calculated to be $335,842, a rate estimated to allow recouping of treatment cost within 3 years.

At this point in considering the sum of these studies, it becomes increasingly difficult to argue against the clinical value of acute inpatient rehabilitation for TBI patients, and that it should be provided as early as feasible after their injury.

Postacute Rehabilitation

As would be expected for a treatment approach with such a brief history as postacute TBI rehabilitation, only limited studies addressing the results of these programs have been available to date. These have included: reports on the results of behavioral (Eames & Wood, 1985a), vocational (Ben-Yishay, Silver, Piasetsky, & Rattik, 1987; Burke, Wesolowski, & Guth, 1988; Prigatano et al., 1984), cognitive retraining (Scherzer, 1986), and general (Fryer & Haffey, 1987) measures of outcome. These early reports addressed only specific elements of a comprehensive system, and also have had a number of methodological shortcomings discussed by Cope, Cole, Hall, and Barkan (1991). However, several recent reports looked at the effect of such comprehensive systems of postacute care in a methodologically more sophisticated manner. The design of all these studies is to rely on the quasi-experimental strategy of utilizing the patients studied as their own control (i.e., treatment interventions at sufficient time postinjury to largely remove spontaneous recovery as a confounder of change).

Mills, Nesbeda, Katz, and Alexander (1992) reported on 42 TBI patients who were evaluated during and following treatment in a structured outpatient, postacute rehabilitation program. Mean length of time postinjury was reported as 50.3 months (all patients were at least 6 months postinjury; only 9 of the 42 were less than 1 year postinjury). The authors found no relationship between time postinjury and amount of improvement achieved. All traditional outpatient treatments (i.e., physical, occupational, speech therapies, etc.) had been completed. Outcomes were determined utilizing both pre- and posttreatment functional scales (5-point scale: 5 = independent, 1 =

dependent/total care or supervision) and formal cognitive assessments. Follow-up was done at 6, 12, and 18 months after treatment. Significant improvement in the 5-point functional level ($p < .05$) was found.[4] They failed to show change in cognitive measures, although a trend toward improvement was noted. Follow-up data at 6, 12, and 18 months showed essentially all gains being maintained or continuing to demonstrate improvement.

Johnston (1991) reported on 82 patients discharged in the first quarter of 1988 from a group of nine postacute programs within one such system of care. Outcomes were assessed at 1 year after discharge via a structured telephone interview. Only 2.4% of cases were lost to follow-up. A 5-point hierarchical global rating was done of need for supervision and care. Independent living outcomes were similarly assessed. Appropriate regressive statistical analysis was done to adjust for the effect of patient chronicity at time of admission on relative degrees of improvement. The mean interval from injury to admission was 812 days or 2.2 years (median 451 days). Johnston reported highly significant decreases in need for supervision or care. These findings were true even for a subgroup of more chronic patients (more than 1 year postinjury to treatment). Outcomes were (M. V. Johnston, personal communication, 1992) statistically analyzed by both simple pre- and post- 1-year chronicity, as well as by a curvilinear regression analysis. In both analyses, more improvement was seen in more acute cases, as would be expected because higher degrees of spontaneous improvement would occur in these. However, significant clinical improvement in outcomes was present in excess of what would be predicted by variance in chronicity alone. Roughly 50% of the degree of improvement was beyond that expected based on chronicity (Johnston, 1991). In terms of productive activity, 81% were improved, 16.5% were unchanged, and 2.5% were found worse at follow-up than at entry to the program.[5] This study clearly provides evidence that significant patient improvement in independence and productivity was achieved during treatment in these programs. The finding of significant improvement in the more chronic cases supports the conclusion that this improvement was not simply the result of spontaneous improvement.

A companion analysis by Johnston (1991) of the same population reported the mean length of stay in the postacute programs as 267.0 days (8.8 months) and the median length as 230 days. Based on the

---

[4]Although statistically significant functional improvement is reported, the magnitude of such change is not apparent from the data presented.

[5]All these positive results are reported to have had statistical significance.

average cost per day of such programs, he estimated that the average cost of delivering this postacute care was $106,000. Johnston's analysis also found a correlation between the severity of a case and postacute rehabilitation expenditures, as would be expected. However, no correlation was found between cost and any measure of improvement, nor did the analysis reveal the usual relationship between effort and outcome seen in other similar data (i.e., one finds such statistical relationships for reported outcome analyses of hospital-based acute rehabilitation). In the postacute system under analysis, those patients who stayed a lesser number of months improved as much as those who stayed several years. The long-stay cases (greater than 1–2 years) tended to be discharged into institutional settings and were found in higher numbers residing within institutional settings at long-term follow-up significantly more than the shorter stay cases. Analysis of measures of severity between the two groups did not reveal any statistical difference (i.e., the long-stay cases that tended to end in institutional settings were not shown to be more severely impaired at admission than the shorter stay cases). Also, those long-term cases that came out of community settings into the postacute settings (i.e., from home settings) tended to go into institutions at discharge and follow-up. In attempting to explain these findings, it is possible that entry into postacute residential settings, by relieving families of ongoing burden of care, allowed them to develop resistance to resuming obligation of care following treatment. One can argue whether this is beneficial for the families, and institutionalization may be a justified outcome in certain cases.

My organization (Cope et al., 1991) recently reported on an analysis of our total experience in providing comprehensive rehabilitation to brain-injured patients in a coordinated system of postacute programs. Changes in function and social integration from admission to discharge and at 6, 12, and 24 months follow-up from discharge were reported. The population reported on was 192 patients. Patients seen only for evaluation were excluded from analysis (19 cases), leaving a study population of 173; 145 patients were found for follow-up, resulting in a follow-up rate of 83.8%. The patient populations were prospectively characterized by chronicity (time from injury to program admission), severity at time of admission to program, and other independent variables of significance in projecting care need and outcome. Outcome was assessed utilizing a single-blind interview methodology. Rated on formal hierarchical scales, measures of outcome included residential status and productivity status, and a measure of dependency (number of hours per day of care or supervision) of patients at these various points postdischarge. Analysis of the whole group and a subgroup (greater than 1 year from time of

TABLE 13.2
Residential Status, Total Sample

Location	Admission		Follow-up	
	N	%	N	%
Home or apartment	65	44.8	101	69.7
Board and care	2	1.4	12	8.3
Skilled nursing facility	1	0.7	6	4.1
Chronic institution	6	4.1	4	2.8
Treatment facility	71	49	22	15.2
Total	145	100	145	101.1

Note. From "Brain Injury: Analysis of Outcomes in a Post-Acute Rehabilitation System: Part 1. General Analysis" by D. N. Cope, J. R. Cole, K. M. Hall, and H. Barkan, 1991, *Brain Injury, 5,* p. 119. Copyright © 1991 by Taylor & Francis Ltd. Reprinted by permission.

TABLE 13.3
Productive Activity, Total Sample

Type of Activity	Admission		Follow-up	
	N	%	N	%
Competitive employment or academic	8	5.6	50	34.5
Vocational training	0	0	5	3.5
Noncompetitive employment or academic	2	1.4	16	11
Volunteer activity	0	0	6	3.4
Recreational or day activity	0	0	11	7.6
No productive activity	132	92.3	40	27.6
Homemaker or retired	1	0.7	12	8.3
Other	0	0	6	4.1
Total	143	100	145	99.9

Note. From "Brain Injury: Analysis of Outcomes in a Post-Acute Rehabilitation System: Part 1. General Analysis" by D. N. Cope, J. R. Cole, K. M. Hall, and H. Barkan, 1991, *Brain Injury, 5,* p. 119. Copyright © 1991 by Taylor & Francis Ltd. Reprinted by permission.

injury and time of admission and not admitted out of another treatment facility) was done. Tables 13.2, 13.3, and 13.4 present results in terms of percentage change from admission to follow-up for the whole population.[6]

Clear improvement on the three measures, residential status, productivity, and dependency, is seen. Tables 13.5, 13.6, and 13.7 present results for a subgroup of patients composed of only those who were

---

[6]Results significant at $p < .001$ or more.

TABLE 13.4
Hours of Attendant Care or Supervision Per Day, Total Sample

Hours/Day	Admission		Follow-up	
	N	%	N	%
0	36	25	114	78.6
1–4	36	25	5	3.5
5–8	19	13.2	3	1.4
9–12	6	4.2	4	2.8
13–16	0	0	0	0
17–20	0	0	0	0
21–24	47	32.6	20	13.8
Total	144	100	145	100.1

Note. From "Brain Injury: Analysis of Outcomes in a Post-Acute Rehabilitation System: Part 1. General Analysis" by D. N. Cope, J. R. Cole, K. M. Hall, and H. Barkan, 1991, *Brain Injury, 5*, p. 120. Copyright © 1991 by Taylor & Francis Ltd. Reprinted by permission.

TABLE 13.5
Residential Status*

Location	Admission		Follow-up	
	N	%	N	%
Home or apartment	32	91.4	24	68.6
Board and care	1	2.9	2	5.7
Skilled nursing facility	0	0	2	5.7
Chronic institution	2	5.7	1	2.9
Treatment facility	0	0	6	17.1
Total	35	100	35	100

Note. From "Brain Injury: Analysis of Outcomes in a Post-Acute Rehabilitation System: Part 1. General Analysis" by D. N. Cope, J. R. Cole, K. M. Hall, and H. Barkan, 1991, *Brain Injury, 5*, p. 121. Copyright © 1991 by Taylor & Francis Ltd. Reprinted by permission.
*Residential status at > 1 year, not from treatment facility.

more than 1 year from time of injury at entrance into treatment (average 2.2 years) and who were also not being referred from an active treatment facility (i.e., who had previously "finished" their rehabilitation).[7]

The most significant results found from admission to follow-up for the total population included: (a) an increase in residence at home from 44.8% to 69.7%, (b) an increase in competitive activity from 5.6% to 34.5%, (c) a decrease in "no productive activity" from 92.3% to 27.6%,

[7]Residential status nonsignificant; productive activity and reduction in attendant care significant at the *p* < .005 or greater.

TABLE 13.6
Productive Activity*

Type of Activity	Admission		Follow-up	
	N	%	N	%
Competitive employment or academic	2	6.1	8	22.9
Vocational training	0	0	0	0
Noncompetitive employment or academic	1	3.0	7	20.0
Volunteer activity	0	0	3	8.6
Recreational or day activity	0	0	1	2.9
No productive activity	30	91.0	13	37.1
Homemaker or retired	0	0	2	5.7
Other	0	0	1	2.9
Total	33	100	35	100

Note. From "Brain Injury: Analysis of Outcomes in a Post-Acute Rehabilitation System: Part 1. General Analysis" by D. N. Cope, J. R. Cole, K. M. Hall, and H. Barkan, 1991, *Brain Injury, 5,* p. 121. Copyright © 1991 by Taylor & Francis Ltd. Reprinted by permission.

*Productive activity at > 1 year, not from treatment facility.

TABLE 13.7
Hours of Attendant Care Per Day*

Hours/Day	Admission		Follow-up	
	N	%	N	%
0	8	23.5	27	77.1
1–4	11	32.3	1	2.9
5–8	6	17.6	1	2.9
9–12	1	2.9	1	2.9
13–16	0	0	0	0
17–20	0	0	0	0
21–24	8	23.5	5	14.3
Total	34	99.8	35	100.1

Note. From "Brain Injury: Analysis of Outcomes in a Post-Acute Rehabilitation System: Part 1. General Analysis" by D. N. Cope, J. R. Cole, K. M. Hall, and H. Barkan, 1991, *Brain Injury, 5,* p. 122. Copyright © 1991 by Taylor & Francis Ltd. Reprinted by permission.

*1 year from treatment, N = 35.

(d) an increase in patients independent for an entire 24-hour period from 25% to 78.6%, (e) a decrease in patients requiring 24-hour care from 32.6% to 13.8%, and (f) an average reduction in hours per day care required from 10.2 hours to 3.8 hours. For the most part, these findings were confirmed in the "chronic" subgroup, greater than 1 year from

TABLE 13.8
Residence, Admission to Follow-up at 6 Months, 1 Year,
and 2 Years*

	Follow-up (%)		
Location	6 Months	1 Year	2 Years
Home or apartment	66.7	71.8	75.0
Board and care	7.0	9.4	8.3
Nursing facility	7.0	3.1	0
Hospital or institution	3.5	3.1	0
Treatment facility	15.8	12.5	16.7

Note. From "Brain Injury: Analysis of Outcomes in a Post-Acute Rehabilitation System: Part 1. General Analysis" by D. N. Cope, J. R. Cole, K. M. Hall, and H. Barkan, 1991, *Brain Injury, 5*, p. 136. Copyright © 1991 by Taylor & Francis Ltd. Reprinted by permission.
*χ^2 = no significant difference.

TABLE 13.9
Productive Activity, Admission to Follow-up at 6 Months, 1 Year,
and 2 Years*

	Follow-up (%)		
Type of Activity	6 Months	1 Year	2 Years
Competitive employment or academic	38.6	43.6	54.2
Voctional training	5.3	4.7	0
Noncompetitive employment or academic	1.6	1.6	0
Volunteer activity	3.5	3.1	4.2
Recreational or day activity	8.8	7.8	4.2
No productive activity	29.8	26.6	25.0
Homemaker or retired	7.0	9.4	8.3
Other	5.3	3.1	4.2

Note. From "Brain Injury: Analysis of Outcomes in a Post-Acute Rehabilitation System: Part 1. General Analysis" by D. N. Cope, J. R. Cole, K. M. Hall, and H. Barkan, 1991, *Brain Injury, 5*, p. 136. Copyright © 1991 by Taylor & Francis Ltd. Reprinted by permission.
*χ^2 = no significant difference.

injury and not from treatment facility: (a) an increase in competitive activity from 6.1% to 22.9%, (b) a decrease in "no productive activity" from 91.0% to 37.1%, (c) an increase in patients independent for an entire 24-hour period from 23.5% to 77.1%, and (d) a decrease in patients requiring 24-hour care from 23.5% to 14.3%. Tables 13.8, 13.9, and 13.10 show that for the three follow-up intervals, there was no significant drop-off in percentages of patients in any outcome category (i.e., there is no apparent drop-off in therapeutic gains achieved at 6, 12, or 24 months after discharge from the programs).

TABLE 13.10
Attendant Care, Admission to Follow-up at 6 Months, 1 Year,
and 2 Years*

Hours/Day	Follow-up (%)		
	6 Months	1 Year	2 Years
0	77.2	79.7	79.2
1–4	3.5	3.1	4.2
5–8	1.8	0	4.2
9–12	3.5	3.1	0
13–16	0	0	0
17–20	0	0	0
21–24	14.0	14.1	12.5

Note. From "Brain Injury: Analysis of Outcomes in a Post-Acute Rehabilitation System: Part 1. General Analysis" by D. N. Cope, J. R. Cole, K. M. Hall, and H. Barkan, 1991, *Brain Injury,* 5, p. 137. Copyright © 1991 by Taylor & Francis Ltd. Reprinted by permission.
*Analysis of variance = no significant difference.

In relation to treatment duration and cost of the programs analyzed, the authors reported lengths of stay and average costs by breaking down the 145 cases into three subgroups based on severity of disability at admission to program: (a) mild (DRS 1–3), (b) moderate (DRS 4–7), and (c) severe (DRS 7–20). These were 140 days and $22,449, 173 days and $50,670, and 212 days and $68,333, respectively. They also calculated annual "savings" based on reduction in attendant care requirement alone for the three subgroups: (a) mild = $2,696, (b) moderate = $14,365, and (c) severe = $41,288 (see Tables 13.11 and 13.12).

Taken as a whole, these studies provide good, if not irrefutable, evidence that the sum effect of postacute rehabilitation is significantly reduced disability and social handicap. It is also evident that these programs can produce, in theory, sufficient societal savings to justify their support on a cost/benefit basis.

Behavioral Programs

In somewhat of a landmark study, Eames and Wood (1985b) described the efficacy of an intensive inpatient behavioral and rehabilitation intervention in 24 severely brain-damaged, behaviorally disordered patients with mean coma duration of 7–8 weeks (range 0–20). This was the first study to document the efficacy of interventions in the "late" period after brain injury; the mean chronicity of their 24 patients from time of injury to initiation of the treatment program was 44.7 months (range 10–126). Therefore, patients were justifiably used as their own controls in a pre- and posttreatment comparison design. Follow-up was

TABLE 13.11
Length of Stay and Cost by Diagnosis-Related Group (DRG)

DRG	Average Time in Program (days)	Range in Program (days)	Average Cost	Range of Cost	Average Cost/Day
Mild[a]	140	46–281	$22,449	$2,880–$87,285	$160
Moderate[b]					
	173	51–417	$50,670	$1,915–$120,670	$293
Severe[c]	212	122–485	$68,333	$5,980–$159,369	$322

Note. From "Brain Injury: Analysis of Outcomes in a Post-Acute Rehabilitation System: Part 1. General Analysis" by D. N. Cope, J. R. Cole, K. M. Hall, and H. Barkan, 1991, *Brain Injury, 5*, p. 137. Copyright © 1991 by Taylor & Francis Ltd. Reprinted by permission.
[a]DRG = 1–3, *N* = 39. [b]DRG = 4–6, *N* = 52. [c]DRG = 7–20, *N* = 54.

TABLE 13.12
Projected Savings Due to Reduced Attendant Care

DRG	Average Hours per Day per Case of Reduced Attendant Care (range)	Projected Annual Savings (per case)
Mild[a]	0.82 (0.87–0.05)	$2,926
Moderate[b]	4.37 (6.60–2.23)	$14,365
Severe[c]	12.56 (20.85–8.29)	$41,288

Note. From "Brain Injury: Analysis of Outcomes in a Post-Acute Rehabilitation System: Part 1. General Analysis" by D. N. Cope, J. R. Cole, K. M. Hall, and H. Barkan, 1991, *Brain Injury, 5*, p. 137. Copyright © 1991 by Taylor & Francis Ltd. Reprinted by permission.
[a]DRG = 1–3, *N* = 39. [b]DRG = 4–6, *N* = 52. [c]DRG = 7–20, *N* = 54.

at a mean of 18.8 months posttreatment. At follow-up, utilizing a hierarchical scale, more than two thirds of the patients had shown substantial improvement in residential or "placement" options after treatment. They also reported that "the outlook for a good response to treatment was not affected by the length of time since injury" (p. 615); those who received their treatment many years after injury had equivalent changes in their outcomes as those treated in the more acute period. However, the reported length of time spent in program by their patients is a mean of 12.2 months for all patients and a mean of 15.6 months for responders with full treatment programs. They reported that "length of stay in the program was determined . . . by achievement and tempo of improvement. As long as measurable improvements were appearing at a rate which suggested that further achievements could be made cost-effectively, treatment was continued" (p. 618).

This study has been followed by other reports of general benefit from programs that treat head-injured populations with a significant component of behavioral disturbances. Ashley, Krych, and Lehr (1990) reported on 218 patients assessed on admission and discharge by the DRS and the Living Status Scale ([roughly] range: 1 = living independently; 9 = locked facility). The analysis showed significant benefits to the postacute intervention. Depending on the degree of dependence at admission and discharge, they calculated a range of annualized cost savings produced by the program for each patient. The amounts of savings on reducing dependency are obviously quite large. There are some methodological problems in interpreting their findings. Principally, these are the (a) nonblinded nature of the outcome assessments, (b) lack of any long-term follow-up to assess durability of change, and, most significantly, (c) lack of notation about the chronicity of the population, thus making spontaneous improvement a serious confounding concern.

Sundance, Jolander, Bryant, Cope, and Rozance (1992) recently submitted data suggesting that a much reduced interval of formal inprogram treatment is necessary to successfully integrate severely behaviorally disturbed patients into their communities than these previous reports imply. Twenty-five brain-injured patients, a mean of 361 days from injury, with "maladaptive behaviors restricting community placement" admitted to a residential neurobehavioral program for behavioral analysis and establishment of behavioral strategies were reported on. Families were behaviorally analyzed and educated. Transition into the community environment was affected by teams providing care within the discharge setting (i.e., in the home and community). Inpatient treatment averaged 49 days. Outcome improvements included: (a) Rancho Los Amigos scores improved from 5.4 admission to 6.7 discharge, and (b) the DRS score improved from 9.0 admission to 4.8 discharge. Discharge disposition included: (a) 84% home, (b) 8% community reentry programs, and (c) 8% group home. Durability of discharge at both 6 and 12 months was: (a) 88% home, and (b) 12% group home. A further analysis of follow-up information on relative outcomes compared three groups of patients: (a) those who received normal (long-term) inpatient behavioral treatment, (b) all patients who received abbreviated inpatient behavioral treatment coupled with aggressive in-home behavioral interventions, and (c) those patients who received abbreviated inpatient and in-home behavioral interventions based on limited funding only.[8] This follow-up revealed no significant

---

[8]The separate analysis of patients treated in the abbreviated inpatient program because of funding limitations only was to discount any bias toward less severely involved patients naturally falling into the general abbreviated treatment inpatient program group.

differences in outcome among the three groups (i.e., the shortened length of stay in inpatient behavioral programs was not associated with any discernable decrement in clinical outcome).

DISCUSSION

Strong evidence for the overall effectiveness of rehabilitation on general measures of handicap has emerged in the past 5 years. In general, there is a distinct trend away from discrete measures of deficit or disability, and toward more global measures of general handicap. These are becoming accepted as the measures of most significance for policy and reimbursement questions regarding rehabilitation in any case.

There remain important methodological problems with these studies as a group. They all fall short of achieving true experimental design in which a randomly assigned control group is prospectively compared to rehabilitation interventions. Aronow's (1987), Cope and Hall's (1982), and Hall and Wright's (1991) studies rely on matching to create controls and come closest to this ideal. But even with the careful matching of these studies, the authors cannot entirely rule out an unknown bias influencing selection of those patients who do or do not receive rehabilitation and prejudicing relative outcomes. The remaining studies essentially rely on utilizing patients largely as their own control. The problems that spontaneous recovery creates for this design are easily appreciated. However, when sufficient time has elapsed from injury to allow some stability in the recovery process, the design can be very persuasive. There are some suggestions in the literature of meaningful ongoing recovery beyond 1–2 years postinjury (e.g., Thomsen, 1984, reported on late improvement in function found at 10–15 years after injury, and extended periods of recovery have been reported by Dikmen, Reitan, & Temkin, 1983). However, for the studies reported here, with subanalyses of cohorts composed of patients generally greater than 1 year postinjury (and in most cases with average chronicity of several years), results showing significant improvement may be given a great deal of weight. It seems unlikely that spontaneous improvement is a reasonable explanation for the magnitude of reported changes in outcome reported in these groups of chronic patients.

It is becoming increasingly difficult to carry out a true random assignment research project in this area of rehabilitation. It has become difficult to hold the view that such rehabilitation of neurologically damaged patients may be ineffective or reflect only placebo action. With the accumulation of evidence of efficacy, ethical considerations have now become fairly prohibitive of denying rehabilitation to any control group for research purposes.

A further point of interest is evident from recent research and reflects a commonly appreciated clinical fact. In general, there has been a substantial decrease in average lengths of time in all phases of TBI rehabilitation over earlier reports. The average length of stay in a model hospital TBI rehabilitation program was 93 days in the late 1970s (Berrol et al., 1982). In 1990, this same facility had an overall average length of stay of 50–55 days (K. M. Hall, personal communication, 1990). The Heinemann et al. (1990) report listed an average length of stay of 65.8 days. TBI patients are now shown by U.S. national model TBI system data to have an average length of stay in the acute medical-surgical phase of care of 27 days, and in the rehabilitation phase for 49 days (Shilling, 1992). The most comprehensive reflection of current inpatient stays for TBI is reflected by the report of the Uniform Data System Annual Report, which gives brain dysfunction a national average length of stay of 42 days (Granger & Hamilton, 1992). It is clear that impressive gains have been made in efficiency in delivering acute rehabilitation care.

Other barriers emerging to carrying out outcome research bear comment. Our study (Cope et al., 1991) had originally been designed to have a control group from a TBI population with similar demographic and acute health-care service characteristics. This population was to be drawn from a large regional health maintenance organization (HMO) in the same area of service as the postacute program system. The suitability of these patients as controls derived from their demographic and economic similarities to the rehabilitation patients in the study who had funding to receive postacute rehabilitation (i.e., both groups were insured patients). At that time, this HMO was not providing rehabilitation to TBI patients other than traditional inpatient and hospital-based, general outpatient services. However, due to concerns by the legal department of the HMO regarding potential liability should a differential in outcome be found, which favored the formal postacute rehabilitation system (the experimental group), the HMO declined at the last moment to participate in the study.

It is clear that, to some extent, the studies fail to reflect the most current clinical practice. To the experienced clinical eye, it is evident that the reports reviewed reflect a more lavish approach to rehabilitation than that which is actually being practiced in a number of areas. In my organization, which 5 years ago had a nearly total focus on residential, facility-based delivery of care, a major change in perspective has taken place based on clinical experience. We now believe that optimum treatment is usually delivered within the patient's own home and community, rather than in residential, facility-based settings. This is clinically so for reasons of minimizing problems of generalizability, as well as increased patient and family motivation and acceptance. It is also considerably less costly. Only those few patients who require complete 24-hour structure, or who have limited family/home resources, are usually appropriate for residential programs. Thus, the outcomes reported on by Cope et al. (1991) reflect practices of several years ago. Our distinct clinical impression is that home- and community-based rehabilitation is both less costly and more effective than our previous residential model. Further research will be necessary to confirm this clinical belief.

There is no question that the comprehensive rehabilitation represented in the discussed studies is an extremely expensive undertaking. The point that such expenditures may ultimately decrease the cost of care for these patients is strongly supported by the emerging data. This is a finding of great magnitude. A sophisticated analysis of the cost of head injuries in the United States for 1988 has been given by Max, MacKenzie, and Rice (1991). When one takes into account minor, moderate, and severe injuries and includes direct medical costs, indirect societal support, and the cost of premature death, the total calculated annual cost is $44 billion. Interestingly, the proportion of cost due to increased social dependency represents 54% of the total ($20.6 billion). It is in this area that rehabilitation has the greatest potential to affect savings.

Although none of the outcome research provides definitive proof of rehabilitation efficacy, the sum of many studies, some reviewed herein, provides reasonably convincing evidence that comprehensive rehabilitation does make a substantial difference in outcome of handicap for TBI patients. If possible, a prospective matched study would be ideal, but practically speaking future research more properly should focus on comparative designs for delivering rehabilitation services. Studies should now be designed to discriminate the active or effective elements of treatment from that which is inactive, nonessential, or simply inefficient. We have already seen some vision of the future of rehabilitation in the reports reviewed here; it will be characterized by decreased length of stays in all phases of treatment. Perhaps it will also involve movement of treatment out of facilities and into the home and community, a decreased ratio of professional to lay and family treaters, and so on. Research will be necessary to help us understand the benefits and dangers of these new models of rehabilitation. However, based on these early reports, it is evident that TBI rehabilitation is efficacious. It can also possibly be done more efficiently than at present, and hence can be more affordable and accessible than traditional models suggest.

REFERENCES

Aronow, H. U. (1987). Rehabilitation effectiveness with severe brain injury: Translating research into policy. *Journal of Head Trauma Rehabilitation, 2,* 24–36.

Ashley, M. J., Krych, D. K., & Lehr, R. P. (1990). Cost/benefit analysis for post-acute rehabilitation of the traumatically brain-injured patient. *Journal of Insurance Medicine, 22,* 156–161.

Becker, D. P., Miller, J. D., Ward, J. D., Greenberg, R. P., Young, H. F., Sakalas, R. (1977). The outcome from severe head injury with early diagnosis and intensive management. *Journal of Neurosurgery, 47,* 491–502.

Ben-Yishay, Y., Silver, S., Piasetsky, E., & Rattik, J. (1987). Relationship between employability and vocational outcome after intensive holistic cognitive rehabilitation. *Journal of Head Trauma Rehabilitation, 2,* 35–49.

Berrol, S. M., Rappaport, M., Cope, D. N., Cervelli, L., Hall, K., Mackworth, N., et al. (1982). *Severe head trauma: A comprehensive medical approach* (Project 13-P-59158/9, Vol. 1). National Institute for Handicapped Research. San Jose, CA: Santa Clara Valley Medical Center.

Brooks, N. (1989). Defining outcome. *Brain Injury, 3,* 325–329.

Burke, W. H., Wesolowski, M. D., & Guth, M. L. (1988). Comprehensive head injury rehabilitation: An outcome evaluation. *Brain Injury, 2,* 313–322.

Cope, D. N., Cole, J. R., Hall, K. M., & Barkan, H. (1991). Brain injury: Analysis of outcomes in a post-acute rehabilitation system: Part 1. General Analysis. *Brain Injury, 5,* 111–125.

Cope, D. N., & Hall, K. (1982). Head injury rehabilitation: Benefit of early intervention. *Archives of Physical Medicine and Rehabilitation, 63,* 433–437.

Dikmen, S., Reitan, R., & Temkin, N. (1983). Neuropsychological recovery in head injury. *Archives of Neurology, 40,* 333–338.

Diller, L., & Ben-Yishay, Y. (1987). Outcomes and evidence in neuropsychological rehabilitation in closed head injury. In H. S. Levin, J. Grafman, & H. M. Eisenberg (Eds.), *Neurobehavioral recovery from head injury* (pp. 146–165). New York: Oxford University Press.

Eames, P., & Wood, R. (1985a). Rehabilitation after severe brain injury: A special-unit approach to behavior disorder. *International Rehabilitation Medicine, 7,* 130–133.

Eames, P., & Wood, R. (1985b). Rehabilitation after severe brain injury: A follow-up study of a behavior modification approach. *Journal of Neurology, Neurosurgery, and Psychiatry, 48,* 613–619.

Frey, W. D. (1984). Functional assessment in the 80's: A conceptual enigma, a technological challenge. In A. S. Halpern & M. J. Fuhrer (Eds.), *Functional assessment in rehabilitation* (pp. 11–45). Baltimore: Paul H. Brookes.

Fryer, J., & Haffey, W. (1987). Cognitive rehabilitation and community readaptation: Outcomes from two program models. *Journal of Head Trauma Rehabilitation, 2,* 51–63.

Hall, K., Cope, N., & Rappaport, M. (1985). Glasgow Outcome Scale and Disability Rating Scale: Comparative usefulness in following recovery on traumatic head injury. *Archives of Physical Medicine and Rehabilitation, 66,* 35–37.

Hall, K., & Wright, J. (1994). Benefit of early rehabilitation in traumatic brain injury: A replication study. Manuscript submitted for publication.

Heinemann, A. W., Saghal, V., Cichowski, K., Ginsburg, K., Tuel, S. M., & Betts, H. B. (1990). Functional outcome following traumatic brain injury rehabilitation. *Journal of Neurological Rehabilitation, 4,* 27–37.

Johnston, M. V. (1991). Outcomes of community re-entry programmes for brain injury survivors: Part 2. Further investigations. *Brain Injury, 5,* 155–168.

Langfitt, T. W. (1978). Measuring the outcome from head injuries. *Journal of Neurosurgery, 48,* 673–678.

Max, W., MacKenzie, E. J., & Rice, D. P. (1991). Head injuries: Costs and consequences. *Journal of Head Trauma Rehabilitation, 6,* 76–91.

Mills, V. M., Nesbeda, T., Katz, D. I., & Alexander, M. P. (1992). Outcomes for traumatically brain-injured patients following post-acute rehabilitation programmes. *Brain Injury, 6,* 219–228.

Nordstrom, C. H., Sundbarg, G., Messeter, K., & Schalen, W. (1989). Severe traumatic brain lesions in Sweden: Part 2. Impact of aggressive neurosurgical intensive care. *Brain Injury, 3,* 267–281.

Prigatano, G. P., Fordyce, D. J., Zeiner, H. K., Roueche, J. R., Pepping, M., Wood, B. C., et al. (1984). Neuropsychological rehabilitation after closed head injury in young adults. *Journal of Neurology, Neurosurgery and Psychiatry, 47,* 505–513.

Rappaport, M., Hall, K., Hopkins, H. K., Belleza, T., & Cope, N. (1982). Disability rating scale for severe head trauma patients: Coma to community. *Archives of Physical Medicine and Rehabilitation, 63,* 118–123.

Scherzer, B. P. (1986). Rehabilitation following severe head trauma: Results of a three year program. *Archives of Physical Medicine and Rehabilitation, 67,* 366–374.

Shilling, M. (1992). Brain injury model systems. *Update, II*(2), 5.

Sundance, P. L., Jolander, D. K., Bryant, E. T., Cope, D. N., & Rozance, J. E. (1992). *Short-term neurobehavioral program for achievement of stable community placement.* Presented at the annual meeting of American Academy of Physical Medicine and Rehabilitation (AAPM & R), San Francisco, CA.

Thomsen, I. V. (1984). Late outcome of very severe blunt head trauma: A 10–15 year follow-up. *Journal of Neurology, Neurosurgery and Psychiatry, 47,* 260–268.

CHAPTER FOURTEEN

Rehabilitation Treatment Variables that Affect Outcome After Brain Injury

David W. Ellis
George Spivack
Claire M. Spettell

ABSTRACT

Two studies were performed to examine the effects of temporal factors in rehabilitation and the effects of intensity of rehabilitation treatment on outcomes following traumatic brain injury. First, the effects of length of acute hospitalization on social disability and length of rehabilitation stay (LOS) were examined. Although severity of brain injury had the greatest effect on the patient's outcome, length of acute hospitalization also had a significant effect on social disability and length of rehabilitation. The second study examined the effects of length and intensity of rehabilitation on cognitive and physical outcomes. There was a significant interaction between length of stay and treatment outcome, with the long LOS group starting out more disabled at admission but improving to the same level as the short LOS group at discharge. A similar pattern of results was found for the effects of intensity of rehabilitation on physical outcomes. However, when cognitive outcomes were studied, a different pattern emerged. For short LOS patients, high- and low-intensity treatment groups improved equally, but for the long LOS patients those treated more intensely made significantly more progress. The theoretical and clinical significance of these results is discussed.

This chapter discusses various factors that may affect treatment outcomes after traumatic brain injury (TBI). The conclusions are based on a review of the literature as well as two studies that we have done at Mediplex Rehab-Camden in Camden, New Jersey (Spettell et al., 1991; Spivack, Spettell, Ellis, & Ross, 1992).

A review of a number of recent studies has shown that a variety of nontreatment factors may have predictive significance for outcome. These factors include (a) severity of injury (Braakman, Gelpke, Habhema, Maas, & Minderhoud, 1980; Gelpke, Braakman, Habhema, & Hilden, 1983; Williams, Gomes, Drudge, & Kessler, 1984), (b) increased age of the patient (Braakman et al., 1980; Giannotta, Weiner, & Karnaze, 1987), and (c) the presence of multiple injuries (Bowers & Marshall, 1980; Klauber et al., 1989; Mayer, Walker, Shasha, Matlak, & Johnson, 1981).

When we look further at the effects of severity of brain injury on outcome, we find that the following indicators of severity appear to affect outcome: (a) depth and duration of coma (Alexandre, Colombo, Nertempi, & Benedetti, 1983; Bergman, Rockswold, Haines, & Ford, 1987; Braakman et al., 1980; Overgaard et al., 1973; Young et al., 1981), (b) pupillary response (Choi, Narayan, Anderson, & Ward, 1988; Overgaard et al., 1973), (c) the presence of intracranial mass lesions (Bowers & Marshall, 1980; Overgaard et al., 1973), (d) elevated intracranial pressure (Becker et al., 1977; Miller et al., 1977), and (e) blood and cerebrospinal fluid factors (Woolf, Hamill, Lee, Cox, & McDonald, 1987).

Treatment factors that have been studied in relation to outcome include (a) expeditious entry into intensive rehabilitation (Cope & Hall, 1982), (b) intensive sensory stimulation (Kater, 1989; LeWinn & Dimancescu, 1978; Mitchell, Bradley, Welch, & Britton, 1990; Pierce et al., 1990), and (c) intensity of rehabilitation treatment (Blackerby, 1990).

A variety of outcome measures were employed in these studies. Thus, the meaning of *outcome* depends on what measure was used. For example, the Glasgow Outcome Scale (GOS) has been used as a measure of overall social disability (Jennett & Bond, 1975), whereas the Disability Rating Scale (DRS) has been used to assess a patient's functional status (Rappaport, Hall, Hopkins, Bellzella, & Cope, 1982). Measures of outcome have also assessed the patient's residential status (i.e., whether the patient is in a rehabilitation facility, nursing home, or independent living situation; Burke, Wesolowski, & Guth, 1988; Cope, Cole, Hall, & Barkan, 1991a, 1991b), capacity for productive activity (Brooks, McKinlay, Sumington, Beattie, & Campsie, 1987; Burke et al., 1988; Cope et al., 1991a, 1991b), and level of psychosocial functioning (Bond, 1975).

Because of methodological differences among these outcome studies, it is difficult to identify the most salient features in a given group of variables. For example, in some studies using nontreatment variables as predictors, the bivariate analyses have not controlled for possible confounding variables. Although appropriate bivariate analyses have been used in many studies investigating effects of treatment factors on outcome, the findings have nevertheless been inconsistent. Additionally, controls over nontreatment variables have been generally inconsistent. Finally, there has often been no partialling out of the effects of the different treatment variables, so it is not clear what treatment factor is at work.

In an attempt to resolve some of these difficulties, we conducted two studies that looked at how these diverse measures correlated with two factors that we suspected were also important in determining eventual outcome: the timing of the patient's entrance into rehabilitation after acute hospitalization, and the length and intensity of treatment given the patient while in the rehabilitation facility. The methodology also controlled for the potential confounding effects of these correlated measures.

TIMING OF REHABILITATION SERVICES

In our first study, we examined the effect of the timing of entrance into rehabilitation services on patients' outcomes (as measured by the GOS). We examined 59 subjects (40 males, 19 females) who were admitted for intensive rehabilitation between January 1987 and December 1988. The patients' mean age was 31 (range 15–67 years); their mean educational level was 11.6 years. Measures of severity of brain injury indicated that most of this group had sustained severe brain injuries. Seventy-three percent of subjects were in coma at the time of admission to the acute-care hospital.

Table 14.1 shows the correlation coefficients among all independent and dependent variables. Our goal was to control for the effects of severity of injury, as well as other variables that were correlated with our dependent variables, in order to more clearly examine the independent effects of timing of rehabilitation services on outcome. Table 14.1 informed us that gender, duration of coma, head AIS-85 (Abbreviated Injury Scale [AIS]-85 score reflects the severity of head injury, measured by the AIS score head), motor score, and acute hospitalization length of stay would need to be partialled out in the subsequent multiple regression analyses (American Association of Automotive Medicine, 1985).

In the first analysis (see Table 14.2), we examined predictors of disability outcome, as measured by the GOS. Insofar as age,

TABLE 14.1
Correlation Coefficients Among All Independent and Dependent Variables

Variables	Education	Gender	Motor Score	Duration of Coma	Head AIS	Extracranial Injury	Acute LOS	Rehab LOS	Glasgow Outcome
Subject									
Age	-.15	-.02	+.24	-.20	-.10	+.12	+.32[a]	+.03	+.02
Education		+.01	+.01	+.08	+.14	-.19	-.06	+.12	-.06
Gender*			+.08	-.28[a]	-.18	-.15	-.01	-.28[a]	+.23
Brain Injury									
Motor score				-.49[b]	-.41[b]	+.15	-.11	-.31[a]	+.38[b]
Duration of coma					+.41[b]	-.07	+.46[b]	+.39[b]	-.60[b]
Head AIS						-.21	+.17	+.23	-.37[b]
Other									
Extracranial injury							+.35[a]	+.20	-.05
Acute length of stay								+.46[b]	-.46[b]
Rehab. length of stay									-.74[b]

[a]$p < .05$. [b]$p < .01$.
*0 = female, 1 = male.

TABLE 14.2
Stepwise Multiple Regression Analysis on GOS Scores

Variables Entered	Unstandardized Coefficient	t value[a]
Step 1*		
Constant	4.962	7.151
Motor Score	0.021	0.215
Duration of coma	−0.063	−4.841[c]
Head AIS	−0.111	−1.135
Step 2**		
Constant	5.111	7.507
Motor Score	0.041	0.435
Duration of coma	−0.051	−3.652[c]
Head AIS	−0.096	−1.011
Acute length of stay	−0.011	−1.952[b]

[a]One-tailed test of significance used to evaluate t value. [b]$p < .05$. [c]$p < .01$.
*$N = 58$, multiple $R = .652$, squared multiple $R = .428$, and $F(3, 54) = 13.446$, $p < .001$.
**$N = 58$, multiple $R = 683$, squared multiple $R = 466$, and $F(4, 53) = 11.561$, $p < .001$.

education, and gender were not correlated with GOS, these variables were not included in this analysis. When the severity of brain injury measures (i.e., Motor Score of the Glasgow Coma Scale [GCS; Teasdale & Jennett, 1974], duration of coma, and head AIS-85) were entered into the analysis, duration of coma was the variable that was demonstrated to have a significant effect on GOS. When length of acute hospitalization was added to the set of predictor variables, it was found that both duration of coma and length of acute hospitalization had significant effects on GOS. Thus, length of acute hospitalization increased our ability to predict disability outcome above and beyond our ability using duration of coma alone.

We repeated our analyses using rehabilitation LOS as the dependent variable to test the hypothesis that moving people out of acute-care settings quickly makes the rehabilitation process more efficient, resulting in shorter stays in rehabilitation (see Table 14.3). In addition, the ability to predict rehabilitation LOS at the beginning of the course of treatment has practical value for rehabilitation professionals.

The gender of the patient was a significant predictor for rehabilitation LOS. Female patients tended to have longer rehabilitation LOS. Severity of brain injury (as measured by the Motor Score) was also a significant predictor. As in the previous analysis, length of acute hospitalization added independent predictive power to the model over and above that

TABLE 14.3
Stepwise Multiple Regression Analysis on Rehabilitation LOS

Variables Entered	Unstandardized Coefficient	t value[a]
Step 1*		
Constant	22.445	6.781
Sex	−64.723	−2.365[c]
Step 2**		
Constant	185.581	3.008
Sex	−43.556	−1.626
Motor Score	−13.660	−1.309
Duration of Coma	2.564	1.768[b]
Step 3***		
Constant	161.098	2.802
Sex	−55.028	−2.201[b]
Motor Score	−17.538	−1.806
Duration of Coma	0.193	0.126
Acute Length of Stay	1.983	3.189[c]

[a]One-tailed test of significance used to evaluate *t* value. [b]$p < .05.$ [c]$p < .01.$
*$N = 58$, $F(1, 56) = 5.591$, $p < .05.$ **$N = 57$, $F(3, 53) = 4.59$, $p < .01.$ ***$N = 57$, $F(4, 52) = 6.480$, $p < .001.$

accounted for by gender and severity of brain injury. Together, these variables explained 34% of the variability in rehabilitation LOS.

TREATMENT INTENSITY DURING REHABILITATION, AND LENGTH OF STAY IN REHABILITATION SERVICES

We conducted a second study to learn what effects intensity of treatment and LOS in rehabilitation might have on outcomes at discharge from rehabilitation. The subjects in the study were 95 adults (61 men, 34 women) who had sustained traumatic brain injuries. The median age of the subjects was 35. Subjects were admitted to rehabilitation between December 1988 and June 1990. Their Rancho levels on admission ranged from IV to VII (Hagen, Malkmus, & Durham, 1979; the Rancho scale is used for classifying the cognitive status of patients with brain injuries).

The independent variables in the study were intensity of rehabilitation treatment and LOS in rehabilitation. Two sets of 2×2 analyses were performed: (a) using average daily intensity of treatment during the first month of rehabilitation and LOS as independent variables; and (b) using average daily intensity of treatment over the entire course of rehabilitation and LOS as independent variables.

The levels of the independent variables were determined based on median splits of each variable. Thus, because the median daily number of treatment hours during the first month of rehabilitation was 3.8 hours, subjects in the high-intensity group received treatment for 3.8 hours or more per day; those in the low-intensity group received less than 3.8 hours of treatment per day.

Similarly, when average daily intensity of treatment over the entire course of rehabilitation was used as the independent variable, subjects who received, on average, 4 or more hours of treatment per day were grouped into the high-intensity group, whereas subjects who received less than 4 hours per day were assigned to the low-intensity group.

The median length of rehabilitation hospitalization was 58 days. Thus, subjects who stayed 58 days or more were classified into the Long LOS group; those who stayed less than 58 days were classified into the Short LOS group.

Dependent variables were rated by the clinical team at admission and discharge. Dependent variables included Rancho level scores as well as ratings of: (a) physical functioning (motor control, strength of extremities, bladder control, physical ability, capacity for feeding oneself); (b) higher cognitive function (problem solving, functional memory, awareness of potential for injury, auditory comprehension); and (c) cognitively mediated physical functioning/skills (nutritional status, ability to swallow, visual-perceptual functioning, leisure skills).

To specifically examine the effects of intensity and length of rehabilitation on outcomes, without contamination from other factors that correlate with outcome, we used analyses of covariance techniques to control for the effects of potential moderator variables. These moderator variables were (a) depth of coma as measured by the GCS, (b) duration of coma, (c) extent of extracranial injury, (d) severity of the head injury as measured by the head AIS-85, and (e) the length of acute hospitalization.

Table 14.4 shows the correlation coefficients between the moderator variables and the dependent variables. Moderator variables that were correlated with dependent variables were entered as covariates in the analyses of covariance. Analyses of variance were conducted for those dependent variables that had no significant correlates among the mod-

TABLE 14.4
Pearson Product-Moment Correlation Coefficients Between
Moderator Variables and Dependent Variables

Variables	Age	Duration of Coma (days)	Time (between injury and admission)	Extracranial Injury	GCS
Physical performance (admissions)	−.07	.02	−.41[a]	−.30	.27
Physical performance (discharge)	−.04	.09	−.66[b]	−.23	.10
Higher level cognitive skills (admissions)	.09	−.01	.04	.08	.02
Higher level cognitive skills (discharge)	−.14	−.43[a]	.12	.17	−.20
Cognitively mediated physical skills (admissions)	−.03	.00	−.36[a]	−.09	−.01
Cognitively mediated physical skills (discharge)	−.12	−.40[a]	−.75[b]	−.04	−.09
Rancho (admissions)	.12	.12	−.05	.17	.12
Rancho (discharge)	−.09	−.17	.05	−.02	−.06

[a]$p < .05.$ [b]$p < .01.$

erator variables. In all analyses, repeated measures designs were used to control for the effects of subjects' starting levels on their outcomes.

These analyses led to the following conclusions:

1. There were significant treatment effects over all conditions on all four dependent variables (i.e., subjects improved significantly over the course of rehabilitation).

2. There was a significant interaction between treatment effects and LOS on the three functional factor scores. Long LOS patients began treatment at significantly lower functional levels than patients in the Short LOS group, but at discharge they equaled the levels of patients in the Short LOS group. In other words, Long LOS patients started out more disabled than the Short LOS patients, but at discharge they were equal in functioning to the Short LOS patients.

3. Intensity of treatment during the first month of rehabilitation bore no significant relationship to outcome.

4. When we looked at cognitive factors, we found a significant interaction between treatment effects and intensity of treatment over the entire course of rehabilitation. In other words, the more intensely treated patients started out lower in cognitive skills, yet at discharge

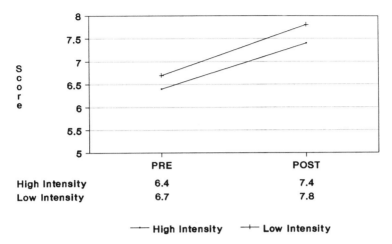

FIG. 14.1. Change in Rancho level from admission to discharge as a function of average intensity of treatment for Short LOS group.

they were functioning on par with less intensely treated cases. This pattern of results was similar to that of LOS effects.

5. However, unlike LOS findings, the intensity findings could not be explained away on the basis of different starting levels on overall functional level. When subjects' scores on all three functional factors were examined, subjects in the Long LOS group were clearly more disabled than subjects in the Short LOS group. Ninety percent of subjects in the Short LOS group had above-median scores on all three factors, whereas only 9% of the Long LOS group did. However, no significant differences in starting levels of functional disability were found between the low-intensity and high-intensity groups.

6. Finally, when Rancho scores were used as the dependent variable, there was a triple interaction among LOS, intensity of treatment, and Rancho scores (see Figs. 14.1 and 14.2). The nature of this triple interaction shows that patients in the Short LOS group improved during the course of rehabilitation, although there was no differential effect of intensity of treatment. There was a differential effect of intensity of treatment on patients in the Long LOS group, however. Patients who received more intense treatment started out somewhat lower on Rancho level than those who received less intense treatment. However, by discharge this group made significantly greater gains than the group that received less intense treatment, achieving at discharge a superior level of functioning.

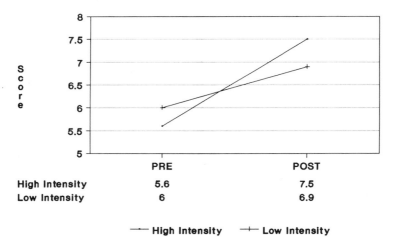

	PRE	POST
High Intensity	5.6	7.5
Low Intensity	6	6.9

FIG. 14.2. Change in Rancho level from admission to discharge as a function of average intensity of treatment for Long LOS group.

CONCLUSIONS

The following conclusions can be drawn from the two studies we conducted at Mediplex Rehab-Camden:

1. The shorter the acute-hospital LOS, the shorter the subsequent intensive rehabilitation LOS. Therefore, it is important for patients to move into intensive rehabilitation as soon as it is medically feasible.
2. Long (e.g., 4–5 months) rehabilitation LOS may be justified by patient needs, as reflected in low admission functional levels.
3. Intensity of treatment plays a role in enhancing patients' cognitive capacities, above and beyond LOS.
4. For intensity of care to "pay off," it must be maintained for a sufficient length of time.

In addition, these studies and others suggest the following:

1. Short LOS in acute hospitalization increases the chances of decreased cost of intensive rehabilitation (Cope & Hall, 1982; Spettell et al., 1991) and better outcomes (Rappaport, Herrero-Backe, Rappaport, & Winterfeld, 1989.)
2. Although the efficacy of structured sensory stimulation with patients in coma is still an open issue, once patients are out of coma, a high intensity of rehabilitation treatment may shorten

LOS (Blackerby, 1990) and enhance positive cognitive outcomes (Spivack et al., 1992.)

3. Intensity of rehabilitation treatment of at least 5–6 hours a day over at least 4 months yields clinically better results than treatment of less than 3 hours a day for less than 2 months (Spivack et al., 1992).

4. Payment systems that arbitrarily restrict rehabilitation LOS without considering patients' admission functional status, or that arbitrarily restrict treatments without requiring a certain minimal level of treatment intensity, may limit patients' eventual functional outcomes.

REFERENCES

Alexandre, A., Colombo, F., Nertempi, P., & Benedetti, A. (1983). Cognitive outcome and early indices of severity of head injury. *Journal of Neurosurgery, 59,* 751–761.

American Association for Automotive Medicine (1985). *The Abbreviated Injury Scale—1985 revision.* Arlington Heights, IL: Author.

Becker, D. P., Miller, J. D., Ward, J. D., Greenberg, R. P., Young, H. F., & Sakalas, R. (1977). The outcome from severe head injury with early diagnosis and intensive management. *Journal of Neurosurgery, 47,* 491–502.

Bergman, T. A., Rockswold, G. L., Haines, S. J., & Ford, S. E. (1987). Outcome of severe closed head injury in the Midwest. *Minnesota Medicine, 70,* 397–401.

Blackerby, W. F. (1990). Intensity of rehabilitation and length of stay. *Brain Injury, 4*(2), 167–173.

Bond, M. R. (1975). Assessment of the psychosocial outcome after severe head injury. *CIBA Foundation Symposium, 34,* 141–157.

Bowers, S., & Marshall, L. (1980). Outcome in 200 consecutive cases of severe head injury treated in San Diego County: A prospective analysis. *Neurosurgery, 6,* 237–242.

Braakman, R., Gelpke, G., Habhema, J., Maas, A., & Minderhoud, J. (1980). Systematic selection of prognostic features in patients with severe head injury. *Neurosurgery, 6,* 362–369.

Brooks, N., McKinlay, W., Sumington, C., Beattie, A., & Campsie, L. (1987). Return to work within the first seven years of severe head injury. *Brain Injury, 1,* 5–19.

Burke, W. H., Wesolowski, M. D., & Guth, M. L. (1988). Comprehensive head injury rehabilitation: An outcome evaluation. *Brain Injury, 2,* 313–322.

Choi, S. C., Narayan, R. K., Anderson, R. L., & Ward, J. D. (1988). Enhanced specificity of prognosis in severe head injury. *Journal of Neurosurgery, 69,* 381–385.

Cope, D. N., Cole, J. R., Hall, K. M., & Barkan, H. (1991a). Brain injury: Analysis of outcome in a post-acute rehabilitation system: Part 1. General analysis. *Brain Injury, 5,* 111–125.

Cope, D. N., Cole, J. R., Hall, K. M., & Barkan, H. (1991b). Brain injury: Analysis of outcome in a post-acute rehabilitation system: Part 2. Subanalyses. *Brain Injury, 5,* 127–139.

Cope, D. N., & Hall, K. (1982). Head injury rehabilitation: Benefit of early intervention. *Archives of Physical Medicine and Rehabilitation, 63,* 433–437.

Gelpke, G. J., Braakman, R., Habhema, J. D., & Hilden, J. (1983). Comparison of outcome in two series of patients with severe head injuries. *Journal of Neurosurgery, 59,* 745–750.

Giannotta, S. L., Weiner, J. M., & Karnaze, D. (1987). Prognosis and outcome in severe head injury. In P. R. Cooper (Ed.), *Head injury* (2nd ed., pp. 464–487). Baltimore: Williams & Wilkins.

Hagan, C., Malkmus, D., & Durham, P. (1979). *Levels of cognitive functioning in rehabilitation of the head injured adult: Comprehensive physical management.* Downey, CA: Professional Staff Association of Rancho Los Amigos Hospital, Inc.

Jennett, B., & Bond, M. (1975). An assessment of outcome after severe brain damage: A practical scale. *Lancet, 1,* 480–484.

Kater, K. M. (1989). Response of head-injured patients to sensory stimulation. *Western Journal of Nursing Research, 11,* 20–33.

Klauber, M. R., Marshall, L. F., Luerssen, T. G., Frankowski, R., Tabaddor, K., & Eisenberg, H. M. (1989). Determinants of head injury mortality: Importance of the low risk patient. *Neurosurgery, 24,* 31–36.

LeWinn, E. B., & Dimancescu, M. D. (1978). Environmental deprivation and enrichment in coma. *Lancet, 2,* 156–157.

Mayer, T., Walker, M. L., Shasha, I., Matlak, M., & Johnson, D. G. (1981). Effect of multiple trauma on outcome of pediatric patients with neurologic injuries. *Child's Brain, 8,* 189–197.

Miller, J. D., Becker, D. P., Ward, J. D., Sullivan, H. G., Adams, W. E., & Rosner, M. J. (1977). Significance of intracranial hypertension in severe head injury. *Journal of Neurosurgery, 47,* 503–516.

Mitchell, S., Bradley, V. A., Welch, J. L., & Britton, P. G. (1990). Coma arousal procedure: A therapeutic intervention in the treatment of head injury. *Brain Injury, 4,* 273–279.

Overgaard, J., Hvid-Hansen, O., Land, A., Pedersen, K. K., Christensen, S., Haase, J., Hein, O., & Tweed, W. A. (1973). Prognosis after head injury based on early clinical examination. *Lancet,* 631–635.

Pierce, J. P., Lyle, D. M., Quine, S., Evans, N., Morris, J., & Fearnside, M. (1990). The effectiveness of coma arousal intervention. *Brain Injury, 4,* 191–197.

Rappaport, M., Hall, K., Hopkins, H. K., Bellzella, T., & Cope, N. (1982). Disability Rating Scale for severe head trauma patients: Coma to community. *Archives of Physical Medicine and Rehabilitation, 63,* 118–123.

Rappaport, M., Herrero-Backe, C., Rappaport, M. L., & Winterfeld, K. M. (1989). Head injury outcome up to ten years later. *Archives of Physical Medicine and Rehabilitation, 70,* 885–892.

Spettell, C. M., Ellis, D. W., Ross, S. E., Sandel, M. E., O'Malley, K. F., Stein, S. C., Spivack, G., & Hurley, K. E. (1991). Time of rehabilitation admission and severity of trauma: Effect on brain injury outcome. *Archives of Physical Medicine and Rehabilitation, 72,* 320–325.

Spivack, G., Spettell, C. M., Ellis, D. W., & Ross, S. E. (1992). Effects of intensity of treatment and length of stay on rehabilitation outcomes. *Brain Injury, 6,* 419–439.

Teasdale, G., & Jennett, B. (1974). Assessment of coma and impaired consciousness: A practical scale. *Lancet, 2,* 81–84.

Williams, J. M., Gomes, F., Drudge, O. W., & Kessler, M. (1984). *Journal of Neurosurgery, 61,* 581–585.

Woolf, P. D., Hamill, R. W., Lee, L. A., Cox, C., & McDonald, J. V. (1987). The predictive value of catecholamines in assessing outcome in traumatic brain injury. *Journal of Neurosurgery, 6*, 875–882.

Young, B., Rapp, R. P., Norton, J. A., Haack, D., Tibbs, P. A., & Bean, J. R. (1981). Early prediction of outcome in head-injured patients. *Journal of Neurosurgery, 54*, 300–303.

CHAPTER FIFTEEN

Psychosocial Outcome in Denmark

Tom W. Teasdale and Anne-Lise Christensen

ABSTRACT

Results are presented from a follow-up study of 69 patients who had completed the day program at the Center for Rehabilitation of Brain Injury at the University of Copenhagen. Data from the patients were collected for five time points: (a) preinjury, (b) preprogram, (c) post-program, (d) a 1-year follow-up, and (e) a 3-year follow-up. The results suggest that gains are achieved in the areas of independent living, employment, and leisure activities. These gains appear either immediately following completion of the day program or at the 1-year follow-up, and they are substantially sustained at the 3-year follow-up.

To begin by defining terms of reference, this chapter presents results from one particular center in Denmark, namely the Center for Rehabilitation of Brain Injury (CRBI) at the University of Copenhagen. At the time of writing, there are five centers in Denmark providing rehabilitation programs. But our own center is in fact the oldest, and therefore we are able to present follow-up results for a comparatively large group of patients up to 3 years after completion of the program.

The term *psychosocial* needs to be defined. It here refers to three broad and fundamental aspects of everyday life: first of all, their domestic situation by which we mean whom they live with rather than what kind of physical home people have. Do they live on their own, do they live in a marital or cohabiting relationship, or do they live with parents or guardians? The second aspect is occupation. Do

235

they have a job, or are they perhaps in an educational program? The third aspect is recreation. How do they spend their leisure time, do they have any pastimes or hobbies, and, if so, of what nature?

Table 15.1 lists these three areas of concern: (a) domestic, (b) occupation, and (c) recreation. It also shows the five time points for which we present results. When considering outcome following a rehabilitation program, there are two baselines that are relevant. The first of these is the patient's circumstances before injury. It is necessary to know the patient's level of functioning prior to the brain injury to evaluate the extent to which the patient is brought back to that level of functioning. The second baseline is the level of functioning at the beginning of the program. To evaluate the effectiveness of rehabilitation, one must obviously establish the level of functioning immediately before its commencement. There are three time points of outcome in our study. The first is at the end of the program, the second is a follow-up of the patients 1 year after completion of the program, and the third is a follow-up 3 years after the program.

Table 15.2 shows some details of the admission procedures and general characteristics of our day program. These are described in greater detail elsewhere (Christensen, Pinner, Møller Pedersen, Teasdale, & Trexler, 1992). Here we emphasize that, following completion of the 4-month day program, there is a period of at least 6 months in which active and involved contact is sustained with the patients and, where appropriate, with members of their families, their employers or potential employers, educational establishments, and their social workers. We argue later that this sustained contact following the day program is a major element in the rehabilitation process and contributes greatly to the generally encouraging results that are presented here.

The Copenhagen Center opened with a grant from the Egmont foundation in 1985. It admits patients in groups of about 10–15 twice a year. By 1988, a total of 67 patients had completed the program.

Table 15.3 shows some demographic and medical characteristics of these patients. That there was an excess of males in the sample is of course related to the fact that cranial trauma is the largest single

TABLE 15.1
Psychosocial Outcome

Areas of Concern	Time Points
Domestic situation	Before injury
Occupation	Beginning of program
Recreation	End of program
	1-year follow-up
	3-year follow-up

TABLE 15.2
CRBI Copenhagen—Day Program

Admission	Program Elements
Groups of 10–15	Morning meeting
4–5 months	Cognitive training
4 days per week	Psychotherapy
6 hours per day	Physical training
Thereafter regular contact for minimum of 6 months	Language therapy, etc.

diagnostic group. As can be seen, median age at injury was comparatively young, but there was rather a large variation. A quarter of our patients were 37 years or older at the time of injury. The skewed distribution for age comes about because our Center is restricted to adult patients. We rarely have patients above 50 years of age because the funding agencies, most often the social services department of the local authority where the patient resides, are usually unwilling to pay for the rehabilitation of older patients.

Table 15.3 also shows coma duration for the cranial trauma patients and indicates a typically severe level of head injury. For this sample of patients, the median time interval between the injury and entry into the program was over 2 years. Here, too, there is quite some variation. However, in more recent years, namely since 1988, the interval between injury and entering the program has actually fallen closer to 1 year.

Our data derive from interviews with the patients, reference to medical records, and discussions with relatives and social workers. It needs to be emphasized that our follow-up is not complete. We have

TABLE 15.3
1985–1988 Patient Characteristics

Characteristics		%
Gender		
Male		61
Female		39
Type of injury		
Cranial trauma		53
Stroke		30
Other		17
	Median	25–75 percentile
Age at injury (years)	24	(18.7–36.3)
Coma duration (days)	8	(4–21)
Hospitalization (days)	82	(30–180)
Age at program entry (years)	26.8	(22.0–39.6)
Injury to entry (years)	2.2	(1.5–3.2)

3-year data on 84% of our subjects. Inspection has not shown drop-out to be related to severity of injury or to favorable or unfavorable outcome. In many cases, it is due to the patient in question having moved to some more distant part of Denmark or abroad.

Because of skewed distributions and scaling at the ordinal level only, statistical analyses of the data have been conducted using nonparametric methods. For each variable, comparison has been made between successive time points (i.e., preinjury with preprogram, preprogram with postprogram etc.).

Figure 15.1 shows distributions for domestic situation across the five time points for our patients. As defined here, *domestic situation* can encompass a multitude of complex relationships, but for present purposes we have combined them into three categories. The first of these categories is what we call dependent: living with parents, other responsible relatives, foster parents, and so on. This, of course, is particularly characteristic for the younger patients. The second category is living alone. The third category is living with a spouse or other partner in a stable cohabiting relationship. These three categories can plausibly be regarded as an ordinal scale, therefore comparisons were made using the Wilcoxon matched-pairs test.

Figure 15.1 shows that, prior to injury, over 40% of our patients were living in situations involving dependence. As mentioned before, these comprise the younger patients who, at the time of injury, were still living at home with their parents. Also over 40% of the patients

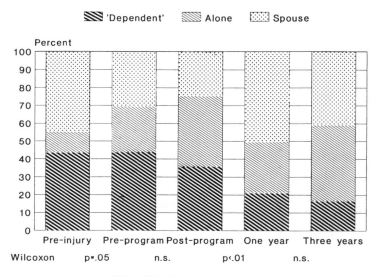

FIG. 15.1 Domestic situation.

were living in partner relationships, and comparatively few were living alone. From preinjury to preprogram, a period of a little over 2 years, the overall pattern changes significantly. The proportion living in dependent situations remains almost exactly the same, but the proportion living alone more than doubles, and there is a corresponding breakup of marital relationships.

Returning to the dependent cases, it needs to be emphasized here that they are the same individuals who comprise the over 40% at both preinjury and preprogram. In other words, individuals who lived at home with their parents at the time of injury tended very strongly to remain in that situation thereafter until they entered the program.

Between entering the program and completing the program, there is no significant change, although a small decline in the proportion number in dependent situations is apparent. In the time from postprogram up to 1 year after the program, a substantial and significant change does occur. The number living in dependent situations declines further to just a little over 20%, namely half of what it was at the time of entering the program. Correspondingly, the numbers living in marital relationships increase to over 50%.

With regard to changes from preinjury to preprogram, one is considering a 2-year time interval—the time interval during which any spontaneous recovery from the effects of injury are most often considered to take place. By contrast, the time from preprogram to 1-year follow-up involves an interval of less than 1½ years—an interval during which substantial changes in psychosocial situation are not to be expected. However, it is the period that commences with the 4-month day program and thereafter proceeds to approximately 6 months of concentrated involvement in the patients' resocialization. The rehabilitation program actively seeks to promote the redevelopment of social skills and to counter tendencies toward social isolation. Were such efforts successful, an increase in partner relationships would not be surprising as a consequence. Correspondingly, the program deliberately fosters skills of independent living, particularly for the younger patients still living with their parents, and indeed often involves direct negotiations with housing authorities to secure independent apartments for them. The conclusion is therefore inviting: The program is directly responsible for the increase in partner relationships and the decline in dependent situations.

Between 1 year and 3 years after completion of the program, there are no significant changes. As can be seen from Fig. 15.1, only a small decline in the proportion of marital relationships appears to occur. This too could be considered to support the previous conclusion. After 1 year following completion of the day program, our contact with the patients is often limited. That there is little apparent improvement in their domestic situation from that time once again suggests that the earlier improvements came about because of the direct involvement of the rehabilitation program. Conversely, it is encouraging that we see no real evidence of any relapse from the degree of restored functioning established at 1 year postprogram. The gains made are evidently sustained.

Figure 15.2 shows the distribution for occupation. Here, too, a simplified picture is presented in which a number of different categories have been grouped. For instance, part-time employment and full-time employment are combined. Furthermore, the employment category includes work for which the wages are in some way subsidized by the state. Those patients who are in education programs are shown separately, although for statistical purposes the categories of education and employment are combined and contrasted with the condition of neither occupation or education by means of the McNemar test. Prior to injury, almost all patients were either employed or in educational programs, the latter being the younger of our patients. Following injury, this pattern was severely disrupted: At entry into the program, almost none of our patients were in employment or educational programs. Some 15% were employed, but these patients were usually under threat of losing their jobs if they were not successfully rehabilitated.

Following completion of the program, there was already an immediate and significant improvement: The numbers in employment and, per-

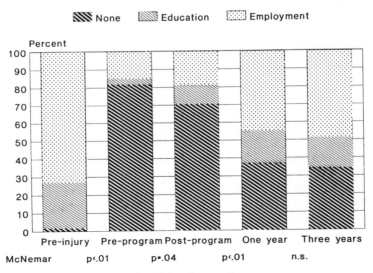

FIG. 15.2. Occupation.

haps even more so, the proportion entering education programs had increased. This again is not surprising because, particularly toward the end of the day program, we concentrate much effort on guiding and steering the patients back into an occupation or educational situation. This process continues after completion of the day program, and its full effects are seen at the 1-year follow-up. By this time, almost 65% of the patients are either in employment or educational programs. At 3 years, the pattern again stabilizes. It very closely resembles, and does not differ significantly from, the 1-year pattern. Thus, the gains achieved during the time of active rehabilitation efforts do not progress further under their own momentum, but neither do they fade when the most direct support is removed.

A return to employment is often rated by brain-injured patients as the highest priority for rehabilitation. In view of this importance, we have looked more closely at the outcome in terms of occupation at 3 years to see whether any of the broad characteristics shown in Table 15.2 had any predictive value regarding those who were able to return to employment or education.

As Table 15.4 shows, we appear to have been somewhat more successful in returning males to employment or education than females, although the gender difference is far from statistically significant. Conversely, comparatively fewer of the cranial trauma patients returned to employment or education than stroke patients, despite the larger proportion of males in the former group.

TABLE 15.4
Prediction of Occupational Status at 3-Year Follow-up

	Employment/Education (%)	Neither (%)
Gender[a]		
Male	71	29
Female	58	42
Type of injury[a]		
Cranial trauma	57	43
Stroke	72	28
	Median	
Age at injury (years)[b]	23.3	25.6
Coma duration (days)[c]	6	14
Hospitalization (days)[d]	70	120
Age at program (years)[b]	25.8	27.7
Injury program (years)	2.2	2.2

[a]$p > .1.$ [b]$p = .17.$ [c]$p = .14.$ [d]$p = .13.$

There were no significant differences in age at injury, coma duration (for those patients who were in coma), hospitalization duration, or in age at entering the program. For all of these variables, there were only marginal tendencies in the direction of those returning to employment or education having been slightly less severely injured. One suspects that it is psychological characteristics, rather than medical or physical, that are decisive for a successful rehabilitation outcome.

It is particularly intriguing that the time interval between injury and program entry was in fact exactly the same for both those patients who were able to return to employment or education and those who were not. This might appear to disconfirm the widely held view that rehabilitation should be implemented comparatively early postinjury. However, it should be recalled, that almost all of our patients entered the program quite late. Table 15.2 shows that only a quarter entered at less than 18 months postinjury. Nonetheless, the present findings suggest that good rehabilitation outcome can still be attained even with patients who are relatively late postinjury.

Figure 15.3 shows the third and final psychosocial variable to be presented here—namely leisure activities. Here again, many different forms can be reported by patients, but for present purposes these have been combined into three broad categories. The first is those patients who report no pastimes or hobbies. The second is those whose leisure activities are either solitary and/or engaged in at home. The reason for this combination is that a tendency to withdraw and become socially isolated is one of the most common characteristics of brain-injury patients. The third category is correspondingly formed by patients reporting leisure activities that take them out of the home and into the company of others. This latter is another major objective of the rehabilitation program. For statistical purposes, these three categories are regarded as forming an ordinal scale, and therefore comparisons are made using the Wilcoxon matched-pairs test.

At preinjury, about 85% of patients had some leisure activities and over 70% included social activities outside the home. There was a significant and dramatic fall in the social activities outside the home following injury, such that on entering the program over 50% of patients reported engaging in no real leisure activities. This development is perhaps all the more striking because they are no longer in employment or in education, hence they really do have rather a lot more spare time. Postprogram there are already some increases in leisure activities, but these become statistically significant at the 1-year follow-up. By that time, the proportion reporting no leisure activities has declined to almost precisely its preinjury level, although

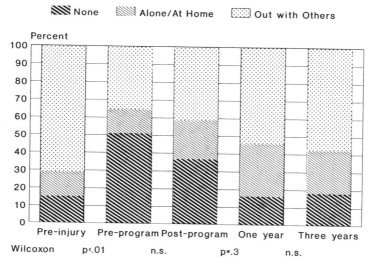

FIG. 15.3 Leisure activities.

social activities outside the home remain lower. At 3 years, the pattern yet again resembles very closely the pattern at 1-year follow-up, with over 50% involved in social activities outside the home and less than 20% reporting no leisure activities at all. In conclusion, we draw these three strands of psychosocial outcome together: domestic situation, occupation, and leisure activities. There are striking parallels. In all three we see a significant decline in level of functioning in the 2-year period between the injury and entering the program; in all three we see substantial improvements in psychosocial functioning in the 1½ years between entering the program and the 1-year follow-up; and in all three we see substantially no change in the situation in the subsequent 2 years.

Although this is not a controlled study, we would nevertheless assert that this pattern of development of psychosocial functioning is atypical when compared with results found from patients not undergoing rehabilitation programs, and they point to two conclusions. There is substantial improvement during the time that we are actively engaged in the patients' lives, and there is little further improvement thereafter. We believe this suggests reasonably strongly that the program has contributed to the improvements seen. As emphasized earlier, the rehabilitation program is quite deliberately geared toward these areas of psychosocial functioning. Although there may be no evidence here of psychosocial gains appearing long after completion of the rehabilitation program, there is conversely evidence that the gains established during the rehabilitation period are robust and enduring.

ACKNOWLEDGMENT

This work was supported, in part, by a grant from the Trock-Jansen Foundation, which is hereby gratefully acknowledged.

REFERENCES

Christensen, A.-L., Pinner, E. M., Møller Pedersen, P., Teasdale, T. W., & Trexler, L. E. (1992). Psychosocial outcome following individualized neuropsychological rehabilitation of brain damage. *Acta Scandinavica Neurologica, 85,* 32–38.

CHAPTER SIXTEEN

Overview of the Economics of Rehabilitation in the United States

Diane V. Bistany

ABSTRACT

This is an overview of private-sector economics of rehabilitation in the United States with emphasis on treatment for persons with head injury and brain damage. Areas to be elaborated on include the (a) limited understanding of rehabilitation, (b) incidence of disability, (c) role of private insurance, and (d) economic consequences. Informed individuals recognize the long-term benefits of rehabilitation and realize the need to control escalating costs. With good rehabilitation, there also exists opportunity for abuse, which requires intervention to reduce and eliminate it. There is a growing awareness among providers, payers, and private citizens to work toward improved services for all disabled in a cost-effective manner.

As we move through the 1990s toward the 21st century, we are embarking on an economic revolution, particularly in health care. However, rehabilitation, which is an aspect of this health-care reform, is often forgotten and remains a "stepchild" of the medical profession.

Although medicine has been a vital part of history for many thousands of years, rehabilitation medicine is barely 50 years old. Specialization in head-injury rehabilitation is even younger, resulting in limited understanding and skepticism for many. The rapid growth of modern research and technology has positively influenced those who survive catastrophic injuries and illnesses. Life expectancy is prolonged and very close to the norm for many. This benefit to humankind also brings

245

with it new and vital issues that have tremendous economic impact. Prolonged life with disability requires additional costs for long-term management with frequent medical intervention to maintain health and quality of life. Brain damage is one of the disabilities requiring acute medical care, extensive rehabilitation, and lifetime management. Because of the advances in treatment and economic factors associated with it, we are faced with a dilemma of (a) how much to treat, (b) for how long, (c) at what expense, and (d) for what outcome.

It is well documented that rehabilitation is a vital specialty. Rehabilitation is expensive to provide, however it can be cost-effective in terms of results with a systematized and comprehensive approach.

This chapter discusses how the United States has dealt with the private-sector economics of rehabilitation, including the (a) evolution of specialized treatment facilities dealing with brain injury, (b) benefit of these programs, (c) present debate of health-care reform, (d) inequities to many, and (e) unanswered questions. Also discussed is the specialization of managing brain injury and how it is not adequately understood, resulting in abuses that are detrimental to those treated and very expensive for the payers.

To confirm the belief among rehabilitation professionals that rehabilitation is indeed a stepchild, a review of a survey conducted by the National Association of Rehabilitation Facilities (NARF) and American Hospital Association (AHA) Section for Rehabilitation Hospitals and Programs (1988) showed the following:

- Most people in the United States do not understand rehabilitation.
- Most doctors are unaware of what goes on in a rehabilitation facility.

INCIDENCE

How extensive is the need for rehabilitation and at what cost? The book *Disability in America* (Pope & Parlor, 1991) and AHA revealed the following statistics:

- 57 million people sustain injuries each year.
- 1.3 million people suffer head injuries each year.
- 70,000–90,000 people sustain moderate to severe traumatic head injuries per year.
- 10,000–20,000 people sustain permanent spinal cord injuries (SCI) each year.

- There are 152 freestanding rehabilitation hospitals in the United States.
- There are approximately 700 specialized brain-injury programs in the United States.

In comparing the two catastrophic injuries cited previously, one notes that the incidence per year of moderate to severe brain injury in relation to permanent SCI is more than 5:1. The average lifetime cost for a SCI person is estimated to be between $210,400 and $751,900. However, many have projected costs exceeding $1 million, particularly those covered by Worker's Compensation benefits, as well as those individuals awarded liability settlements.

Because of the complexity of deficits related to brain damage, acute and rehabilitative treatment is far more extensive than SCI therapy, resulting in costs two to three times greater, particularly for those brain-injured individuals with moderate to severe behavioral and cognitive deficits. Historically, the United States has provided medical coverage from both the public and private sector. In contrast to the private sector, funding for public assistance is through taxation, and individuals qualify only when there is predetermined financial need. There are specific guidelines with rare exceptions, and the services have limitations.

INSURANCE

The major player in private-sector funding is the insurance industry. In researching its roots, it is worthy to note that insurance goes back to ancient times. One of our forefathers, Benjamin Franklin, successfully established the first fire insurance company in the New World in 1752. From that point forward, insurance has expanded to having many facets and providing coverage for risks of all kinds. No attempt is made to enumerate and explain all forms of insurance, but rather attention is given to highlight the specific coverage available that applies to illness and accidents. A definition for this type of insurance would be purchasing protection to fund illness or injuries, should they occur, without depleting individual savings and investments. Types of coverage include:

- Accident and health
- Automobile
- Liability, including medical malpractice
- Worker's Compensation

Accident and health insurance coverage is very specific as to what illness and accidents will be underwritten, for how long, at what type of facility, by which providers, and the dollar amount for allowable charges. This insurance has become somewhat more liberal in recent years, although limitations and restrictions still exist.

Liability insurance, which includes automobile as well as other forms of liability, is protection in the event that an accident occurs that is not work related and it is determined that an individual or individuals cause the specific injury. A drawback here is that it may take months or years before resolution with a final settlement and payout is reached. In these situations, individuals must fund health care and rehabilitation through other resources including private funds.

The literature is unclear as to when insurance coverage for accident and health, automobile, and liability were established. The system of protection for work-related injuries began in New York State in 1910. This offers the most liberal of medical and rehabilitation benefits, particularly since the late 1960s and early 1970s when regulations became more encompassing through state legislation that mandated an increased scope of coverage. This insurance is written by individual insurance companies that also manage the claims and approve any needed medical treatment and rehabilitation. However, these companies have regulations imposed by governing boards in each state.

CONTROLLING ESCALATING COSTS

With each new year, all insurance companies see an increase in charges for health care and rehabilitation. The advances in the medical technology arena have contributed substantially to the increased cost to consumers and taxpayers. For many years, the annual inflation rate has been in the double digits, as calculated by the Consumer Price Index (an organization that calculates the inflation rate each year for the United States). The Index shows that health-care costs increased 700% between 1976 and 1989. As a result, both the government and the private insurance industry have begun to focus on methods to provide needed services at lower or controlled costs.

In *Social Insurance and Economic Security*, Rejda (1989) estimated $425 billion was spent in health care in the United States in 1985, or 10.7% of the Gross National Product. Approximately $158 billion is spent annually for rehabilitation.

In an effort to address increasing health-care costs, the insurance industry has been examining and implementing cost-effective management methods. For over 20 years, the casualty insurance carriers, either with their own staff or by contract with rehabilitation professionals, have provided individual case management. In addition to facilitating quality care, a positive outcome has been the enhanced education of insurance companies in the need for and benefits of rehabilitation. Recently, there have been increased efforts in cost-effective management methods by both casualty and health companies. Some of the methods that have been implemented with success are:

- Using medical health-care professionals to develop rehabilitation plans.
- Consulting with treating medical providers regarding the medical and rehabilitation needs, particularly in catastrophic claims.
- Using health-care professionals to consult with providers.
- Auditing hospital bills to determine if services were actually provided and accurately billed.
- Reviewing medical records to determine if medical services were appropriate.
- Providing options to the injured and their families regarding the facilities and physicians who provide high-quality and cost-conscious treatment.

As complete as these efforts and methods sound, there remains a shortfall because cost awareness may compromise quality and positive outcome. Rehabilitation treatment, standards, and outcome include complex and intertwined variables affecting cost-effective management and long-term maintenance.

The positive effects have included more interaction and dialogue among insurers, treatment facilities, and physicians. This results in each realizing a clearer understanding of the other so that motivation and goals will mesh, achieving quality care, cost-effectively, with optimal outcome for the people treated. Even with these controls and efforts, the major problem of high cost remains.

PROBLEMS FACED IN REHABILITATION

Throughout the United States, businesses (small and large), insurance companies, and the federal government are placing significant emphasis on health-care reform to slow the outpouring of monies in escalating medical costs. Once again, we are seeing politicians and various interest groups advocating a national health-care system. The insurance industry is instituting tighter controls and increasing the amount of money individuals and corporations will pay for health-care coverage. There is a growing concern about health-care costs, which is the largest expense for taxpayers today.

Unfortunately, the emphasis is focused on acute medical needs, with rehabilitation playing a minor role. In 1988, NARF and the AHA Section for Rehabilitation Hospitals and Programs cosponsored a survey that showed that 66% of the then 43 million Americans with disabilities "are not receiving the potential benefits to be realized from rehabilitation services" (pp. 1–3). Twenty-eight million Americans are not receiving the benefits of medical rehabilitation. In addition, administrators of rehabilitation facilities across the United States are sensitive to the lack of understanding about rehabilitation. This signifies the need for the rehabilitation industry to protect its interest by furthering an awareness with patients, physicians, and payers.

In the private sector, most individuals who have work-related injuries are eligible for Workers' Compensation benefits, and are provided with comprehensive medical and rehabilitation opportunities. Insurance companies that have rehabilitation professionals on their staff or contract with independent professionals take a more active role in the entire medical management process. Cases are followed closely, authorization is given for needed care, and, in many instances, referral is facilitated to appropriate rehabilitation programs. In addition, an active role in long-term planning and maintenance is a crucial aspect of the entire process. Unless this phase is properly managed, the benefits of rehabilitation can be compromised. This, in turn, affects quality of life and results in increased costs. In terms of numbers, those eligible for Workers' Compensation benefits are only a small percentage of the people requiring acute medical and rehabilitation treatment. When there is limited knowledge of rehabilitation by the vast majority of lay people and professionals, there are opportunities for abuses to occur. This is particularly true in the care and treatment of brain-damaged people.

Within the last 15–20 years, there emerged a recognition that many individuals with residual deficits resulting from head injury or brain damage can improve beyond what was previously believed, with more structured and comprehensive programming. The treatment-program model became more educational than medical.

Many brain-injured individuals are able to return to their own homes, communities, and, in some instances, work environments. Those who experience behavioral problems are improving sufficiently to avoid placement in institutions and locked psychiatric wards. A significant number return to structured environments with support services provided by families or communities.

All of this has become possible by the formation of specialized programs dealing exclusively with the issues of brain damage. Traditional therapies changed to become more focused and refined. A new method of team approach was developed with clinicians overlapping their skills to provide this "new" approach to rehabilitation. This new comprehensive method has been, and is, very costly with length of stay for this treatment often extended for many months.

ABUSES IN HEAD-INJURY AND BRAIN-DAMAGE REHABILITATION

As with any new method, the process has had a period of trial and error, particularly in the first several years. There has been a rapid growth of specialized programs (approximately 700), and this rapid growth has presented problems to the payers. The expertise in terms of numbers of specialists cannot match the number of facilities opening their doors professing to provide "state-of-the-art" treatment. Marketing took on a new product of rehabilitation for those with brain damage. Although most "for-profit" treatment centers offer quality care, a new breed of entrepreneurs has emerged to seek investors to participate in this venture. These entrepreneurs' primary motivation is financial. Insurance companies became fair game to make money under the guise of providing care for unfortunate victims of head injury and brain damage. Competing for patients seemed to be the rule, rather than improving treatment.

What has started to occur is the uncovering of the wrongs being done in some for-profit treatment settings. The March 16, 1992 edition of the *New York Times*, a major U.S. newspaper, published a front-page article with the following headline: "Centers for Head Injury Accused of Earning Millions for Neglect" (Kerr, 1992). The article cited substantiated information including (a) insurance fraud, (b) overcharging, (c) unethical marketing, (d) bad care, and (e) admitting and keeping patients who cannot benefit simply to gain insurance payments. Some facilities have also instructed medical staff members to file false or misleading progress reports to keep patients in their program. As a result, the U.S. Congress is investigating this entire matter of patient neglect in the rehabilitation setting.

Fortunately, quality ethical facilities and programs do exist. These facilities provide excellent treatment, and are refining their technical skills as more research and knowledge is acquired concerning this young specialty. Unfortunately, those individuals with limited knowledge in treatment for head injuries will be reluctant to pursue this vital area of rehabilitation for individuals in need. Those who have been skeptical will become even more so.

SOLUTIONS SOUGHT

With the continued specialization and refinement in health care and rehabilitation comes a more accurate predictability as to treatment and outcome. Responsibility and accountability is in clearer focus, with the patient and family contributing significantly to the entire treatment process rather than being the product of the process.

Shortened inpatient and residential confinements are occurring with earlier transition and continued treatment taking place in the home and community. An economic advantage to this process is a reduction in costs. Most importantly, however, individuals are returning to the family unit sooner, accelerating the adjustment for both patient and family.

From the standpoint of governmental agencies and the insurance industry, new solutions are sought to reduce the tax burden and cost to the private sector. There is a continuing debate as to whether the United States should adopt a national health-care system. There are problems and inadequacies: Both the present Medicare system, designed primarily for senior citizens, and Medicaid, which is based on financial need, provide only limited benefits.

Insurance companies are reassessing their scope of coverage and are emphasizing closer controls and scrutiny on health-care providers.

Innovative ideas are emerging. One theory to control the escalation in cost was developed by Patrick Rooney, chairman of Golden Rule Insurance Company. In the February 28, 1992 issue of the *Wall Street Journal*, Rooney suggested employers place a sum of money per employee into a "fund" each year specifically for minor medical bills. Insurance would then be used for any major illness or accident exceeding the fund. Monies not spent in a given year would carry over to subsequent years, supplementing the regular yearly contributions. This theory speculates that there will be an overall reduction in insurance costs with this method.

Concerning treatment of head injury, the Department of Health and Human Services (1989) in Washington, DC established an Interagency Head Injury Task Force at the request of Congress to study the issues associated with head injury completely. The task force was asked to recommend solutions to meet the needs of those unfortunate enough to sustain this type of injury. The government is concerned with high cost as well as the recent abuses associated with treatment providers.

The issues addressed by this task force touched on all areas affecting the injured, the families, the treaters, and the payers. The following highlights major areas of challenge:

- Establishment of regional centers of excellence linked with a network of local facilities.
- Additional research in all aspects of the problem to include prevention, basic science, clinical and rehabilitation intervention, and community services.
- Increase of local community programs of emergency care, acute care, rehabilitation, and long-term care.
- Financial and legal reforms to ensure availability and access to needed care.

Other theories and solutions are still being developed and debated. There are no simple answers. We may find that a combination of several options is required. Regardless, the problems and solutions must be jointly shared by the health-care industry, the insurance industry, government, and society. Quick, easy, short-term solutions are not the answer. Our collective responsibility is to ensure a future of appropriate quality care for all in need at a price that is palatable for the taxpayer and consumer. We are at a point where there are many challenges ahead of us.

CHALLENGES

Both treatment providers and payers are faced with challenges of examining type of treatment, benefits, and realistic outcomes. To meet these challenges effectively, a cooperative effort is essential; otherwise there will be a continuation of unsolved and unresolved issues. The focal point must be quality care that is cost-effective, in order to obtain improved or enhanced quality of life for those who are brain damaged. Not only is this humane and moral, but it also makes good business sense. Payers in the private sector should view quality treatment as a financial investment in humanity. Given these challenges, where do we go from here?

FUTURE

With the yearly incidence of brain injury, there has been growing emphasis on treatment. Prevention is being emphasized with increased research and technology in designing safer equipment for the home and workplace, safer transportation, and laws to guard against accident. Continued efforts in this area are essential and constantly evolving.

However, even with these efforts, the long-term needs of individuals with brain damage are still not satisfactorily met. Parents become unable to maintain these individuals in their homes due to aging and death. Spouses frequently choose to dissolve marriages. Children become independent and move away to seek their own professions and begin families. What remains are nursing homes and institutions that for the most part are inappropriate, and many of these unfortunate people become "warehoused" or confined to institutions for life.

Community-based support services, group homes, respite services for families, and avocational activities for those unable to return to competitive employment are approaches that seek to improve the quality of life for the brain damaged. These are areas that require more study and planning. Those individuals with good outcomes may require additional support services years after the injury or illness. We do not yet have a clear understanding of how the aging process will affect people who have suffered head injury and brain damage. This alone may require changes in intervention and support systems as those with brain damage become an aging population with specific needs.

We must become visionaries and plan for the future. Unless this planning occurs, we will continue to drain the economy and ineffectively meet the needs of this population. Planning must take place now before this population becomes a burden to society.

As a society we must achieve a collective interest and a shared responsibility. Neither patient, family, treators, payers, nor community should shift responsibility. Short-term solutions become Band-Aids, only lasting a short time and requiring frequent change.

We now have the attention of all areas of society. We need to seize this opportunity to evaluate and plan for all aspects of these issues: (a) prevention, (b) acute and rehabilitative measures, (c) continued research, and (d) long-term management. The process must be ongoing with reassessment as new information and technology emerge. New methods have to be implemented to meet these evolving issues in order for society to meet and afford the major issues associated with head injury and brain damage.

REFERENCES

Department of Health and Human Services. (1989). *Interagency Head Injury Task Force Report.* Washington, DC: Author.

Kerr, P. (1992, March 16). Centers for head injury accused of earning millions for neglect. *The New York Times,* pp. 1, D4.

National Association of Rehabilitation Facilities & American Hospital Association Section for Rehabilitation Hospitals and Programs. (1988). *Public awareness of medical rehabilitation.* Washington, DC: Author.

Pope, A. M., & Parlor, A. R. (1991). *Disability in America: Toward a national agenda for prevention.* Washington, DC: National Academy Press.

Rejda, G. (1989). *Social insurance and economic security.* Englewood Cliffs, NJ: Prentice-Hall.

Rooney, J. D. (1992, February 28). Give employees medical IRAs and watch costs fall. *The Wall Street Journal,* p. A14.

CHAPTER SEVENTEEN

Social and Economic Consequences of Brain Damage in Denmark: A Case Study

Jill Mehlbye and Anders Larsen

ABSTRACT

We present the results of the consequences of the treatment of brain-injured persons at the Center for Rehabilitation of Brain Injury, Copenhagen University. The evaluation focuses primarily on the economic consequences, but the social consequences are also evaluated. The case study, which covers 3½ years, is based on 20 brain-injured persons who underwent an intensive treatment at the Center in 1987. Our study on the development of the social situation of brain-injured persons confirms the results of similar studies. The evaluation shows that after treatment at the Center, the students' quality of life improved (e.g., more students now live in their own homes). The public costs are reduced due to the training at the Center. The distribution of the gain (reduced expenditures) differs among public authorities. In conclusion, economic indications can be said to support rehabilitative efforts performed at the Center for Rehabilitation of Brain Injury.

"Does Rehabilitation Pay?" was the title of a study carried out by Amternes og Kommunernes Forskningsinstitut (AKF) in 1991. It was based on 20 students who in 1987 underwent intensive rehabilitation and treatment at the Center for Rehabilitation of Brain Damage, Copenhagen University. The main purpose of AKF's study was to evaluate the social and economic consequences of rehabilitation and treatment of brain-injured persons at the Center mentioned previously.

The main questions addressed were:

1. What are the brain-injured students' social and economic situations 1 month, 1 year, and 3 years after treatment and rehabilitation at the Center in relation to their situations immediately prior to rehabilitation?
2. Does the cost of treatment and rehabilitation pay for itself later on in the form of saved expenditure on public help and care of brain-injured persons?
3. If there are savings, in which cost areas and where in the public sector do the biggest savings lie?

The study was instituted by the Center for Rehabilitation of Brain Damage and financed by the Ministry of Social Affairs.

TRADITIONAL TREATMENT AND REHABILITATION IN DENMARK

To put the treatment at the Center in perspective, we sum up the traditional treatment and rehabilitation in Denmark. Usually the acute treatment and rehabilitation directly following the diagnosis of brain damage take place at a hospital. When the brain-injured person is discharged, he or she will, in some cases, have the possibility of continuing rehabilitation with a physiotherapist and ergotherapist on an outpatient basis. Apart from this, the possibilities for continued rehabilitation and treatment depend on what is available for the patient's local county or municipality, and on what national institutions have to offer.

The different sectors offer various schemes at both the county and municipal levels. For example, the social sector can offer a home help, a support person, or a place in a nursing home. The health sector can offer physiotherapy, ergotherapy, and home care. The education sector can offer various training schemes, such as speech training and extensive special training. Thus, the different offers have to be pieced together from the different sectors, and therefore do not stand as a coherent and coordinated offer to the brain-injured persons.

The Center for Rehabilitation of Brain Damage differs from the traditional methods by offering specialized knowledge and expertise on an overall basis—linking different treatment and rehabilitation needs together. The cost of treatment and rehabilitation at the Center is generally funded by the Hospital Act or the Social Assistance Act, depending on whether the referring body is a county hospital or a municipality's social-service administration.

METHODS AND DATA

The 20 students who participated in the Center's intensive rehabilitation and treatment program that lasted 4½ months form the basis of the study. A questionnaire study was completed on the brain-injured persons—the students at the Center and/or their families and of the students' case officers in the home municipalities, social and health services. In addition, information has been gathered from the Center's case records. From 1987 through part of 1991, data were collected on each of the 20 students. Time points for data collection were: (a) 1 month before treatment, (b) 1 month after treatment, (c) 1 year after treatment, and (d) 3 years after treatment (see Fig. 17.1).

The main reason for collecting the data was to obtain as complete a picture as possible of the schemes and services provided for the students by the public sector, including their costs and funding sources. Information was also gathered on the case officers', the students', and their families' perceptions of the students' situation before and after the rehabilitation at the Center. In the case of the families, any changes that had taken place in their work situations as a result of the need for them to support the brain-injured member of their family were recorded.

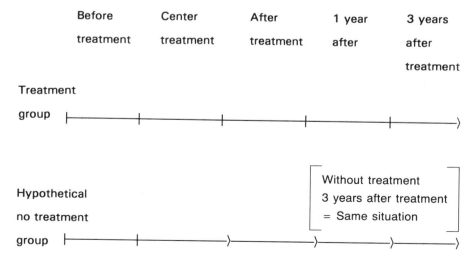

FIG. 17.1. Time points for data collection.

As for the research methods, we are aware that the connection between cause and effect is not quite clear. We cannot know for sure whether factors other than rehabilitation and treatment at the Center have influenced the students' situation. We did not make any attempts to establish a control group. Because of the project's term and budget, we estimated that the advantages of a control group would not outweigh the disadvantages of increased costs and extended term. It would be difficult or impossible to find a group similar to our treatment group who had received no treatment at all.

Instead, we compared the students with themselves, hypothesizing that if they had not received the treatment at the Center their situation would not have changed. On average, the students started at the Center 3 years after suffering their brain damage, so their situation was stabilized in most respects. Using each student as his or her own control is, to some extent, the weak point of our study. On the other hand, this method offers an advantage because matching characteristics of another are not required.

The financial analysis is a so-called prevalence-based, "cost-of-illness" analysis. In this kind of economic analysis, the total amount of costs (caused by illness) is calculated for a period for all the patients studied, regardless of when each patient became ill.[1] A prevalence-based cost-of-illness analysis differs from an incidence-based cost-of-illness analysis in such a way that the latter calculates all costs—caused by the illness—from the time the patient became ill until the recovery or death of the patient.

The cost-of-illness analysis is mainly based on directly measurable costs. The following conditions of the study should be stressed:

- The individual types of therapy cannot be isolated from other therapies, so the different types of therapies outside the Center must be seen as a whole, although at the same time it is assumed that the Center's rehabilitation and follow-up have a substantial effect on the students' future situation.
- If the therapy given at the Center had not been initiated, $3\frac{1}{2}$ years later the students' situation would continue to be as it was before the rehabilitation.

---

[1]Alternatively, this could be called a cost-effectiveness analysis based on the assumption that the outcome (the students' situation) after 3 years is the same in the actual course and in the alternative course (no rehabilitation). Taking the equal outcome for granted, we compare the cost of the actual course and the cost of the alternative cost.

- The basis of the study is relatively confined, and the 20 students should be regarded as an example of a group of brain-injured persons who have participated in intensive rehabilitation and treatment at the Center for Rehabilitation of Brain Damage.

THE STUDENTS' SOCIAL SITUATION DURING THE 3½ YEARS

Most of the students were relatively young, with an average age of 27 years at the start of the treatment. The age distribution goes from 16 to 48 years. More than half were under 30 years of age. The students came to the Center on average 3 years after suffering brain damage. A few started 1 year after, and another few started 8 to 9 years after. The damage consisted of cranial trauma caused by accidents such as traffic accidents and cerebral diseases.

As individuals, the brain-injured persons were quite different from each other. The nature and extent of the damage varied greatly, and the students' educational and occupational backgrounds also differed widely. Some of the most serious consequences of the brain damage mentioned were speech problems and difficulties in expressing thoughts, impairment of memory and concentration, and motoric handicaps. Some had reading and writing problems.

Before rehabilitation and treatment at the Center, the students had received various types of support and rehabilitation of varying intensity. The students' situation when they started at the Center is compared with the situation 1 month after leaving the Center and 3 years later.

When the students started at the Center, half of them were still unable to manage by themselves in their everyday life. Most of them received help from their immediate families, and a few had been granted home help or a support person in their residences. In addition, a number of the students were either in family care or an institution. Thus, only a few of the students had been living alone in their homes. Half were receiving or had just ended treatment and rehabilitation elsewhere, such as speech training, ergotherapy, and physiotherapy. Only a few had jobs, and a small number received occupational training.

Most of the students had been referred to the Center by their respective municipalities' social and public health administrations, whereas only a few had been referred by the county hospitals. Most of them now lived in their own homes. Only two were employed in ordinary jobs, but many more were undergoing rehabilitation or received job training. Slightly more than half of the group had some

TABLE 17.1
The Students' Situation Before Treatment, 1 Month After, and 3
Years After Leaving the Center

Before	1 Month Before	1 Month After	3 Years After
Housing situation			
1. Living alone	3	5	7
2. Living with a partner	4	5	9
3. Living with parents	10	6	1
4. Living at an institution	3	3	1
5. Collective housing	—	1	2
Total	20	20	20
Employment			
1. Employed	2	2	2
2. Job offer	—	—	—
3. Job testing	2	6	4
4. Partial and protected work	—	—	4
5. Education	2	—	1
6. Employment	14	12	9
Total	20	20	20
Public help services			
1. Practical help and support at home	7	5	2
2. Treatment and rehabilitation	10	1	1
3. Education and job training	4	6	10
4. Other (foster care, institution, etc.)	3	3	1
Total[a]	17	14	12
Students without any help from public services	3	6	8
Total	20	20	20

[a]The numbers in this column do not add up to 17 because some of the students enter more than once.

kind of occupation or were receiving education. Only a couple were receiving practical assistance and help from the public authorities, such as home help.

However, most of the students were still living on transfer incomes. Thus, 3 years after their stay at the Center, more than half of the students had been awarded pensions, and most of the others were living on Social Security.

The opinions of the case officers, the students, and their families on the results of the students' stay at the Center were generally positive. All the students and families participating in the questionnaire study were very satisfied with the Center's work, and almost everyone—both students and their families, and the case officers in the municipalities—thought that the students had made progress since rehabilitation and treatment. The students seemed happier and more self-confident, and they did not need as much help and support from their families and public authorities. This result already emerged immediately after the treatment. At the same time, the students' situation generally improved over the following 2 years.

IS THE PUBLIC EXPENDITURE TO INTENSIVE REHABILITATION AND TREATMENT REGAINED?

The financial analysis in the project intends to answer the question of whether the expenses connected with the training given at the Center are later paid for in the form of savings on other public services, such as home help, support person, and family care. In this chapter, we look at the costs and the transfer payments.

The Costs

The public sector's treatment costs and total expenditure before treatment at the Center were used as an alternative course, based on the assumption that the financing would have amounted to the same for the entire period of study (3½ years), had the student not received any training at the Center.

The economic analysis shows that an average saving of approximately DKK 190,000 per student was achieved with regard to the costs of public treatment and care (the costs of the stay at the Center not included).

Some of the services increased costs. In others—the majority—savings were achieved. As mentioned, the saved and increased costs in the period were calculated by comparing the costs in the actual course with the expected costs in the alternative course.

The calculations show that the biggest savings were reached in areas such as (a) speech training at a speech institute, (b) the support person scheme, (c) psychiatric treatment, (d) stay in institution, and

TABLE 17.2
The Costs Before, During, and After the Treatment at the Center

Time Period	Costs Per Month Per Person (DKK)
Before treatment	11,630
During treatment	5,331
Just after treatment	5,843
1 year after treatment	7,802
3 years after treatment	3,675
Reduced costs in the whole period	−190,400

(e) outpatient treatment. In all of these areas, there were savings in relation to the alternative course of events. On the other hand, the costs of rehabilitation and family care rose.

As mentioned earlier, saved costs for support and treatment during the period studied averaged DKK 190,400 per student. (To this savings could be added what each student saved on his or her payment for public services received. This is, on average, about DKK 6,000 per student.) Throughout the study, the price level of 1990 and a discount rate of 3% per annum have been used.

The question then is whether these savings are sufficient to balance the costs of treatment and rehabilitation at the Center, which have been calculated to be DKK 162,000 per student. The costs here defined are staff payments and other costs directly connected to the treatment excluding rent and administration.

In relation to the assumed alternative course of events and after 3½ years, an average saving in public costs of DKK 34,500 was achieved per student, after deduction of the cost of treatment and rehabilitation at the Center. Approximately DKK 28,400 of the saving is attributed to the public sector and DKK 6,100 to the students because, as mentioned earlier, some of the students paid part of the cost of the services they received.

Transfer Payments

If the economic perspective is widened to include so-called transfer incomes, such as sickness and unemployment benefits, we find that these transfer incomes remained at approximately the same level. On average and per person, the increase in public transfer incomes have been very small (i.e., DKK 500 per person).

Three and one-half years after the treatment at the Center, the total expenditure (costs plus transfer income) has furthermore been reduced by an average of DKK 190,000, provided the public payments to the Center are excluded.

TABLE 17.3
Cost Savings After 3½ Years

Costs	Total Saved
Public costs	DKK 190,400
Center costs	DKK −162,000
Public costs	DKK 28,400
Students' costs	DKK 6,100
Total (public and private)	DKK 34,500

TABLE 17.4
Public Expenses Before and After the Treatment

Expense Type	Expenses per Month per Person (DKK)			
	Before Treatment	1 Year After Treatment	3 Years After Treatment	Reduced and Increased Expenses for the Whole Period
Sickness benefit	1,553	0	0	−41,100
Unemployment benefit	532	0	532	−11,700
Social security	861	638	754	−4,800
Others	0	54	4	1,200
Protected work	0	73	229	4,300
State-supported education	0	627	157	11,300
Pension	2,245	2,552	3,459	19,100
Rehabilitation	0	832	1,034	33,100
Paid taxes	−2,700	−2,681	−3,616	−10,900
Total expenses	2,491	2,095	2,553	500
Public costs	11,630	7,802	3,675	−190,400
Total amount of public costs and expenses	14,121	9,897	6,228	−189,900

Regarded from the public sector's view, the total expenditure must also include the municipalities' and counties' expenses connected with the stay at the Center, amounting to about DKK 211,600 per student (treatment costs plus overhead expenses such as rent). Deducting this expenditure from the saved public costs of DKK 190,000 on average per student, we arrive at an extra public expenditure of about DKK 21,000 on average per student.

Costs and Transfer Payments of 5 Years Instead of 3½ Years

Assuming that there are no changes of the situation during the extended period, the calculation of costs and transfer payments during 5 years instead of 3½ years will turn the extras of the public sector of DKK 21,000 into an average public saving of about DKK 69,000 per student after 5 years.

DISTRIBUTION OF THE GAIN ON DIFFERENT PUBLIC AUTHORITIES

The distribution of the reduced costs and transfer payments (during the 5 years) is very important. For instance, if the transfer payments are supposed to be undertaken by the municipality while at the same

TABLE 17.5
The Development in the Total Public Expenditure After 5 Years

Costs	Expenditure After 3½ Years (DKK)	Expenditure After 5 years (DKK)
Saved public costs	−190,400	−280,800
Additional expenses for transfer payments	+500	+500
Total saved public expenses	−189,900	−280,300
Center payments	+211,200	+211,200
Changes of public expenses	−21,300	−69,100

Note. + = additional expenses; − = savings.

time the municipality suffers an economic loss, the economic structure in the Danish public sector has a problem. As shown in Fig. 17.2, this is the case when referring brain-injured persons to the Center.

We find that the counties have gained, whereas the state and the municipalities have had extra costs. This is mostly because the municipalities and the state had been financing the costs of the treatment at the Center and the Social Security support of the students, whereas the counties achieved gains through reduced expenditure on treatment and rehabilitation of the students within the county (e.g., training at a speech institute, psychiatric treatment, and stay in institutions). After 5 years, the counties' gain has increased considerably. The

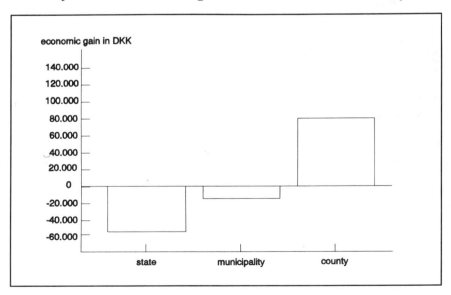

FIG. 17.2. Distribution of additional expenses and savings on public services, average per person.

municipalities are just about to break even, whereas the state's expenses on the whole have remained the same because of the pensions.

The distribution of gain and losses depends to a large extent on who pays for the students' stay at the Center. As long as it is primarily the municipalities and the state (from which the municipalities receive 50% reimbursement) who pay for the stay, the counties will evidently obtain all the economic profits. Provided that the counties pay for the stay at the Center, the municipalities and the state will make the profit, and the county will suffer a loss after 3½ years. However, this loss will be compensated after 5 years, and all three public purses (state, counties, and municipalities) will have achieved a gain. This would be the ideal economic structure.

CHAPTER EIGHTEEN

Federal Planning with Regard to Traumatic Brain Injury in the United States

Leonard Diller

ABSTRACT

Planning in the United States with regard to traumatic brain injury (TBI) has increased at a rapid pace. It has taken place in the context of four larger initiatives during the 1990s. These include the themes of (a) prevention, (b) the decade of the brain, (c) the Americans with Disabilities Act, and (d) rising costs of health care. Within these themes, there has been considerable activity. Federal agencies have taken the initiative to organize existing resources to address these themes even in instances where new funding has been less than optimal. Within this framework, the National Head Injury Foundation has provided a major thrust to articulating the research and service needs of individuals with TBI. Specific legislation to improve the quality of services has been passed.

> *Every 15 seconds, someone suffers head injury in the United States. Every 5 minutes one of those people dies and another becomes permanently disabled. Every year head injury claims the lives of 75,000–100,000 in the United States. Of those who survive approximately 70,000–90,000 suffer lifelong disability, 5,000 develop epilepsy and 2,000 remain in a vegetative state. . . . There are 2,000,000 head injuries a year. . . . 500,000 are severe enough to require admission to a hospital.*
> —Interagency Task Force Report, National Institutes
> of Neurological Disorders and Stroke (1989)

FOUR THEMES DRIVE HEALTH CARE AND SCIENCE IN
THE 1990s

The four themes are (a) prevention, (b) the decade of the brain, (c) the Americans with Disabilities Act, and (d) the rising costs of health care. These themes are fulfilled by different agencies in the government. Their efforts are coordinated by an interagency government task force.

Before describing the themes driving public policy in the United States, it would be useful to look at the process by which policy is translated into action. Someone once said that the philosophy of a program is expressed in its annual budgets. I believe that this is true to some extent at all levels of government, as well as in the actual operations of rehabilitation programs.

How Policy Is Translated into Action

Policy may be traced through two paths in the law: authorization and appropriation. The Congress authorizes the executive branch of the government, which is controlled by the president to carry out a given action, by passing a law. The intent of Congress is stated in the legislation. Congress then appropriates the money to carry out the law. For example, if money to study the brain is given to that branch of the government concerned with basic science, then different kinds of studies would emerge than if it were given to providing services or studying the needs of people who have acquired brain damage. The paths of the legislative and the administrative authorization and appropriation are dynamic, reflecting tensions and pressures within the professional and scientific communities. This suggests two propositions. First, no branch of the government is immune from pressure of one form or another, be it from scientific or professional groups or citizens, including individuals with disabilities. Second, for every dollar that is authorized, there are competing requests for that very same dollar. Passing a law and funding the way it is to be administered is not a simple process.

Prevention

One major player in setting the tone for research is the National Center for Environmental Health and Injury Control, Centers for Disease Control (CDC). Based on an earlier report (Committee on Trauma Research, Commission on Life Science, National Research Council, & Institute of Medicine, 1985) commissioned by The National Academy of Sciences, "Injury in America," the CDC convened a series of seven panels culminating in the "Third National Injury Control Conference," which was held in 1991. The panels were divided into prevention (motor vehicle injury, injuries due to violence, home and leisure injury, occupational injury) and systems of care (trauma care, acute care treatment, rehabilitation of persons with injuries). Each panel followed a format of describing the current state of affairs, including (a) a brief history and a statement of what seems to work, (b) a statement of goals, (c) statements of how goals are to be achieved, and (d) a series of recommendations.

For the rehabilitation section, the goal is to establish by the year 2000 a cost-effective system of rehabilitation care that will permit a person with a disabling injury to achieve optimal health, personal autonomy, and an independent noninstitutional lifestyle. A cost-effective system of rehabilitative care will help achieve an important objective of "Healthy People, 2000," namely the reduction of secondary disabilities as a result of head and spinal injuries. Specific recommendations are presented in Table 18.1. The agenda is broad in concepts as well as in the attempt to include recommendations that draw on branches of the government with diverse interests and funding. Space permits only limited comment on some highlights of the vision. These include funding of basic research such as (a) studying central nervous system (CNS) regeneration, (b) developing injury surveillance systems by the individual states to obtain data pertinent to the epidemiology of injury and mandating the linkage to trauma registries and rehabilitation systems, and (c) improving the quality of research and the information that is disseminated by encouraging the strengthening of peer review process among professionals and access to information by the public. Service delivery should be modeled

TABLE 18.1
Recommendations for Rehabilitation by the
Centers for Disease Control

Domain	Mechanism
Basic research	National Center For Medical Rehabilitation Research
Surveillance	Clinical care database from records of all injured people, including epidemiologic data on etiology, risk factors, treatment, outcomes, and costs
Dissemination	Information dissemination and technology transfer among all participants
Service capacity	Build systems of care from trauma center to community
Service research	Health-system research models: study access, payment, cost–benefit, employment
Training	Trained personnel in research, clinical care, personal services

after the model system programs in spinal cord injury (SCI) and head trauma. Research for all elements of service delivery to include all the services offered by professionals in rehabilitation is to be supported. Long-term studies are to be encouraged. Studies designed to enhance knowledge about living with the long-term consequences of disability are to receive special attention. Of special interest is the study of psychosocial integration and independent living centers. The latter have placed great emphasis on activities such as peer counseling and personal attendant services.

Unfortunately, the government authorization does not have a great deal of money to make a large impact. However, it did permit sufficient funds for critical initiatives so that the effect of funds is magnified. It encourages individual states to set up surveillance systems via state registries, and encourages states through their health departments to meet and develop plans for servicing TBI. In a sense, it draws on existing resources and models derived from experiences with developmentally disabled to address the needs of community integration. Prior to this effort, the only concerned state agency to assist in providing support for TBI was the state vocational rehabilitation agency. This meant that the states were involved in the rehabilitation of TBI only to the extent of supporting vocational efforts. Drawing on models provided by other disability groups, the state could now assist with issues of housing, architecture, and transportation. Although progress in this area varies from state to state, there are at least models being set up, and states are establishing communication with each other. In short, the funds were sufficient to create an atmosphere for planning and dialogue at the state level, where services are actually funded. One current type of program that states are using is the case manager (i.e., someone funded by the state to track an individual so that proper services are delivered from the acute to the chronic phase).

The Decade of the Brain

The National Institutes of Health (NIH) is the branch of Health and Human Services that carries the major mission for the decade of the brain. Within the NIH, there are a number of independent institutes focused on different health-threatening behaviors. The principle institute to carry out the decade of the brain is the National Institute of Neurological Diseases and Communication Disorders (NINDCD). However, other institutes may participate. With extensive lobbying, a new institute on Deafness and Communication Disorders was formed in 1990. Within this institute, much of the research on aphasia is sponsored. In addition, a parallel agency, the National Institute of Mental Health (NIMH), has been the primary federal vehicle for the biological advances in psychiatry over the past two decades. Much of the work on mental illness and health psychology has been sponsored by NIMH. NIH and NIMH are familiar to psychologists and neuropsychologists. Although communication disorders are no longer part of the mission of NINDCD, which changed its name to National Institute on Neurological Disorders and Stroke (NINDS), it is the lead agency in sponsoring research involving a network of clinical centers in SCI and another in head trauma. The support of the clinical centers for head trauma has been particularly influential in tracking recovery during acute care (Levin et al., 1987). It has supplied important data using multiple sites, tracking care from emergency room to operating room. In the past year, NINDS has sponsored a competition to award new programs to establish the feasibility of participating for 3 years in a larger multicenter study that would take place over a 7-year period. Up to this point, the focus has been on biomedical, rather than behavioral, aspects of care. NINDS is also sponsoring a multicenter follow-up study of stroke patients. The most surprising finding thus far is that many stroke patients, even those with disabilities, do not attend rehabilitation programs.

Within the past 2 years, a major development has taken place within NIH in setting up the National Center For Medical Rehabilitation Research (NCMRR) as a center within the National Institute for Child Health and Development. This center was established in the past year to recognize that rehabilitation medicine had developed a sufficient body of practice so as to justify the need for a recognizable entity within NIH. The primary task is to raise the level of research in the field of medical rehabilitation. Although the mandate is to cover a wide range of disabilities besides head trauma and stroke, it is clear from the way disability is conceptualized and the areas of study are categorized that brain damage is an important consideration (Table 18.2).

TABLE 18.2
Terminology in Disability Classification from
National Center for Medical Rehabilitation Research

Impact on person with a disability
Pathophysiology
Impairment
Functional disability limitation
Disability
Impact on others
Family
Community

TABLE 18.3
U.S. Dollars for Medical Rehabilitation Research at
National Institutes of Health

National Institutes of Health	$ (millions)
National Institutes of Child Health and Development	6.4
Center for Medical Rehabilitation Related Research	8.3
National Institute on Aging	12.9
National Institute of Arthritis and Musculoskeletal and Skin Diseases	18.9
National Cancer Institute	14.1
National Institute on Deafness and Other Communication Disorders	19.3
National Institute of Dental Research	7.9
National Institute of Diabetes and Digestive and Kidney Diseases	4.4
National Eye Institute	2.6
National Institute of Neurological Disorders and Stroke	14.4
National Center for Nursing Research	4.0
National Center for Research Resources	8.6
Other Government Agencies	
Centers for Disease Control	1.3
National Institute on Disability and Rehabilitation Research	68.0
Veterans Administration	26.8

As part of its mandate, the NCMRR is coordinating all of the medically related rehabilitation research efforts within NIH. Many of the existing institutes conduct research on populations that involve rehabilitation. For 1992, approximately $138 million, or 1% of the total NIH budget, is directed toward these efforts (Table 18.3).

Americans With Disabilities Act

This act, which was passed in 1990, requires the removal of all barriers, particularly architectural, and all obstacles for people with disabilities. It plays a strong role in helping to guide the research agenda in rehabilitation.

Research in rehabilitation up to this point has been largely sponsored by the Department of Education instead of by Health and Human Services, because the rehabilitation movement originated from a background in vocational rehabilitation, which has its roots in education rather than in health. The major research activity is directed by the National Institute of Disability and Rehabilitation Research (NIDRR), which is a subbranch of the Department of Education, rather than Health and Human Services. It operates under a different set of ground rules than NIH. For example, because education is the right of all citizens, the utilization and dissemination of any research sponsored by this department is an important consideration in evaluating research proposals. Although scientific merit is a significant consideration in peer review, applicability of findings for service delivery carries a heavier weight than it does in NIH. Under the new guidelines, research review panels include persons with disabilities. Thus, a proposal involving brain injury or stroke must have a disabled person or a family member participate in the discussions. As the movement has evolved in the United States, the disabled see themselves less as patients and more as a minority group fighting to overcome barriers in the environment.

Throughout its history, there have been a number of tensions with regard to priorities in funding. These include the question of which disabilities are to be given priorities and whether rehabilitation services and their research arms should be directed to the less severely disabled, who will yield a higher probability of returning to work, or to the more severely disabled, who have less prospect for return to gainful employment. The tensions in the evolution of services occurred when an earlier emphasis on the mildly disabled caused statistics on return to work to look very impressive. Many people with severe disabilities took matters into their own hands and wrote to their congressmen. There was a change in attitude that is reflected in the amendments to the Rehabilitation Act passed in 1973. Since then, there have been a number of laws that have profoundly affected the status of the disabled.

1973—Disabled civil rights—serving severely disabled

1978—Creation of Independent Living Centers as alternative to employment for severely disabled; creation of NIDRR as an independent agency

1986—Mandating supported employment for severely disabled

1990—Americans with Disability Act—a major civil rights law in which employment could not be denied on the basis of disability. Provision had to be made for reasonable adaptation of the environment to meet the needs of people with disabilities.

1992—All discrimination to cease for government-funded programs as well as private employment.

In the course of these legislative changes, a number of factors have emerged within NIDRR. There is a decreased emphasis on medical components of rehabilitation. There is less emphasis on research in the areas of pathology and impairment, and more weight is given to research on disability and handicap. As the committee of the American Congress of Rehabilitation concerned with long-term planning has noted, there had been very little study of living with a disability over the long term. There is heightened emphasis on research on technologies to assist people with disabilities.

As a principal research agency in the field of rehabilitation research, NIDRR sponsored a conference on the state of the art in TBI rehabilitation that took place in 1987 (Bach-Y-Rita, 1989). That meeting sketched some of the current issues to be resolved from a research perspective. It reviewed topics ranging all the way from agreeing on the definitions of severity of brain damage, from pathophysiology, assessments, and interventions, to outcomes. NIDRR currently sponsors three major research initiatives in the field of TBI, aside from individual grants that are awarded for unsolicited proposals. These include: (a) research and training centers in head trauma and stroke, (b) model systems for service delivery (Thomas, 1988), and (c) regional head-trauma programs. They each have different mandates.

Each research and training center (RTC) is supposed to have a series of interrelated research projects that together offer a sufficient mass that could not be obtained by individual studies. In addition, each is supposed to have a series of training projects primarily to disseminate the findings to appropriate audiences. For 1993–1998 in the area of brain trauma, one research training center will involve studies of interventions, another will involve studies of employment, and a third will involve community integration. There will also be one concerned with stroke. Each RTC is to be funded annually for at least $500,000. They are open to competition every 5 years. There are five model-systems programs in TBI, and 14 in the field of SCI. The key idea in model-systems programs is that each patient who is admitted to a trauma program is followed through neurosurgery, acute and subacute rehabilitation, and an outpatient basis. The treatments may vary a great deal from patient to patient and from program to program. The programs share common protocols for assessing patients at given points in time. They must also have prevention and dissemination projects. In addition, the programs might collaborate with each other in research projects of limited scope. The point is to gather sufficient cases to permit meaningful data analysis. These programs are funded annually at $300,000 each.

The newest approach involves the development of regional programs that are designed to provide targeted research to enhance service programs (e.g., studies of alcohol abuse in a given population), as well as to provide information networks so that a person living in a given geographical area might have access to the benefits of a program outside the area. These programs in effect subcontract research or disseminate funds to other programs to participate. All of these programs work very closely with different service providers (e.g., medical centers, state-operated vocational employment services, and other institutions in the community).

With regard to service programs, the state employment services that are funded by individual states and the federal government have given a high priority to vocational rehabilitation of individuals with brain trauma. In many states, the funds from state vocational rehabilitation agencies are used to pay for the rehabilitation of individuals with TBI if it has a vocational goal.

As a sign of the current atmosphere, at a meeting sponsored by NIDRR for all research projects funded in rehabilitation, all project directors were asked to identify meaningful outcomes for their research. This is part of a larger trend for the government to show results for investment of research dollars.

At an address to a more recent meeting of all project directors of RTCs, the director of the agency (Graves, 1992) urged Participatory Action Research (PARS). The goal of PARS is to involve greater participation by the disabled in the actual formulation of the research. The model is taken from industrial psychology and sociology in attempting to win acceptance of change in an organization by having the recipients or those affected by the change participate in the design of a study that is aimed to bring about change. This move fits well with the changes in legislation regarding the disabled, many of whom view rehabilitation research as not very meaningful in terms of affecting the lives of those people who are supposed to benefit. If the consumer of research is involved in its production, the chances are enhanced for greater utilization.

Years ago, Tamara Dembo, a pioneer of rehabilitation psychology, argued that, unlike clinical psychology, which studied the psychopathology of everyday life, rehabilitation psychology has as its mission the development of a psychology of everyday life. To be meaningful, rehabilitation psychology must incorporate the person with the disability as a central player, not just as a subject for study or a patient for treatment. A distinction was made between the insider and the outsider. The insider is closer to the situation and is much more aware of the details than the outsider. The insider has a frame of reference that must be understood in order to be involved in problem solving. Rehabilitation professionals have been able to work productively with individuals and family members through the National Head Injury Foundation (NHIF) to help achieve much of the legislative gains and the changes in public policy. They have been effective in part because they have learned to appreciate the position of the insider who must live with consequences of TBI.

Rising Health Costs

It is no secret that brain-injury rehabilitation is expensive, and that rising health-care costs are matters of concern at both public and private levels. Who pays, how much does it cost, and is it worth it are questions for everybody in rehabilitation, including patient and family, providers of services, researchers, and third parties who are concerned with finances. The matter receives heightened attention because rehabilitation may be conducted as a profit-making venture. Three points might be noted. First, systems of managed care are becoming popular: Once a severe injury or condition occurs, a case manager is assigned to work with the patient and family to help guide them through reasonable paths in the treatment process (i.e., to see that proper services are obtained and that funds are not spent for useless treatments). The case manager is emerging as an important member of the team. It is too early to tell whether this will result in better care or more effective use of money. In California, for-profit health maintenance organizations (HMOs) now manage 35% of health-care services. It is estimated that this figure will reach 80% over the next few years. This trend may well determine the kinds of settings where rehabilitation takes place.

Second, at a political level, there is a well-known attempt by the state of Oregon to give priorities for funding selected medical conditions. Other states are examining this proposition very carefully. This has a certain popular appeal in terms of fairness. But the weight of opinion favors acute medical procedures and tends to ignore needs of people with disabilities, which might be chronic, costly, and yield unspectacular results. It may work against the needs of individuals with TBI.

Third, the Agency for Health Care Policy and Research (AHCPR), which has a strong voice in shepherding many of the federally funded clinical quality initiatives, has organized study groups to develop a research agenda and identify key issues in quality assurance and quality improvement. The study groups review the professional and scientific literature to examine the evidence for clinical practice. They may look at the procedures in assessment and treatment and the contexts of clinical decisions in terms of tables of evidence generated by the literature. They use the results to set guidelines for care. The power of the approach is great. The initial panel on management of acute pain published a guide with 100,000 copies, which were distributed within the first 6 months of publication (Clinical Practice Guideline, 1992). The approach is too new to judge its effectiveness. Thus far, 12 expert panels have been organized to examine content areas. Among the areas that are of relevance is a panel that is considering stroke rehabilitation. This panel examines (a) documented evidence for the benefits of interventions, (b) the validity of the instruments for assessments, and (c) the outcome measures as the basis for providing parameters for care.

With more than 1,500 head-trauma programs in the United States, if the approach is viable there will be considerable pressure to use it to look at rehabilitation in brain trauma.

Epilogue

Rehabilitation of TBI has received a great deal of support from managed care systems that are profit seeking; this has led to a number of abuses that have resulted in congressional hearings and unfavorable publicity. As a result, Congress recently passed laws to correct this: (a) the Brain Injury Rehabilitation Quality Act of 1992, which protects the rights of each brain-injured patient in rehabilitation with a national set of standards and oversight; and (b) a bill to develop a national definition for TBI. This bill, "the TBI Act," mandates all states to add TBI to their data-reporting structures. It identifies the need for federal, state, and local resources to develop services for a defined condition.

CONCLUSIONS

Rehabilitation of people with TBI has received increasing attention and support. Structures have been put into place with regard to service delivery and research. An important immediate challenge is to implement the initiatives that have been undertaken in the coordination of efforts at the federal agency level. The steps must capitalize on (a) initiatives of an emphasis on prevention, (b) results from the research on the decade of the brain, (c) heightened awareness of the disabled as a minority group coming to the attention of the public, and (d) how to do this in a cost-conscious atmosphere.

ACKNOWLEDGMENT

This chapter was supported, in part, by the U.S. Department of Education National Institute on Disability and Rehabilitation Research, Research and Training Center on Head Trauma and Stroke, grant no. H133B80028.

REFERENCES

Bach-Y-Rita, P. (1989). *Traumatic brain injury.* New York: Demos.

Clinical Practice Guideline. (1992). *Acute pain management: Operative or medical procedures and trauma* (AHCPR Pub. No. 92-0032). Rockville, MD: Agency for Health Care Policy and Research, U.S. Department of Health and Human Services.

Committee on Trauma Research, Commission on Life Science, National Research Council, & Institute of Medicine (1985). *Injury in America: A continuing public health problem.* Washington, DC: National Academy Press.

Graves, W. H. (1992, May). *Participatory action research: A new paradigm for disability and rehabilitation research.* Annual conference of National Association of Research and Training Centers, Washington, DC.

Levin, H. S., Mattis, S., Ruff, R. M., Eisenberg, H. M., Marshall, L. M., Tabbador, K., High, W. M., & Frankowski, R. F. (1987). Neurobehavioral outcome following minor head injury: A three center study. *Journal of Neurosurgery, 66,* 234–243.

Thomas, J. P. (1988). The evolution of model systems of care in traumatic brain injury. *Journal of Head Trauma Rehabilitation, 3,* 1–5.

CHAPTER NINETEEN

A European Chart for Evaluation of Patients with Traumatic Brain Injury

Jean-Luc Truelle
D. Neil Brooks
C. Potagas
Pierre-Alain Joseph

ABSTRACT

In 1988, 40 European, Scandinavian, and North American experts (physicians, psychologists, social workers, lawyers, family association representatives, etc.) met in Brussels to derive guidelines for a minimum assessment of head-injured people. This workshop led to a research contract between the European Brain Injury Society (EBIS) and the European Economic Community (EEC) Directorate for Science to develop a European Evaluation Chart. A preliminary chart was constructed. After reliability studies were achieved, a more definitive version was completed, and this has been used to examine 495 patients within the various countries of Europe. Validation studies have shown excellent agreement between severity of injury and many different aspects of outcome and between disability, social, vocational, and family handicap. Further developments of the chart continue to make it shorter and more "user friendly."

BACKGROUND

Head injury causes severe and prolonged disability (Brooks, 1991), yet the deficits may be invisible or minor to the naive examiner (Brooks, 1984). Such patients are evaluated by many different specialists, but all too often the specialist has little knowledge or experience of traumatic brain injury (TBI), therefore evaluation may be skimpy, inappropriate, and inaccurate. As a direct consequence, the patient's real needs are not identified, and therefore those needs simply cannot be met. In view of this, a chart was developed with two general purposes: clinical and scientific (Truelle, 1988; Truelle & Brooks, 1991; Truelle, Joseph, Brooks, & McKinlay, 1990). The clinical purposes were as follows:

1. to develop a common terminology for assessing impairments, disabilities, and handicaps after TBI;
2. to derive a profile of assets, disabilities, and handicaps of the injured patient at different stages after injury;
3. to guide the various specialists concerned with the initial management, and with rehabilitation and community reentry of people with TBI; and
4. to enable the preparation of detailed clinical and medicolegal reports.

The scientific purposes were as follows:

1. to supply data to improve knowledge of the consequences of TBI within Europe and elsewhere;
2. to define the specific needs of patients with TBI; and
3. to assist in establishing profiles and quality-assurance standards for judging the value and effectiveness of specific TBI programs.

To achieve these aims, it is clear that the chart has to be simple, specific, and reliable. These criteria are discussed in brief detail next.

Simplicity, Specificity, and Reliability

It was intended that the chart should contain only directly relevant information. Indeed, there has already been one ruthless "pruning," when items with low reliability, high frequencies of missing data, or low frequencies of appearance were removed. Second, the chart must be simple enough to be able to be readily used by the many different professionals who have to manage the patient with TBI, and this usage should be without detailed preliminary training. Furthermore, the chart should be able to be completed in as short a time as possible (it is currently around 1 to 2 hours), and this is already being shortened.

The specificity criterion is met by ensuring that the chart covers aspects that relate specifically to TBI rather than to disability in general. Furthermore, it draws on knowledge that the brain-injured person may be an unreliable informant, particularly when reporting cognitive and behavioral disability. Therefore, the chart has to be completed by examining both the head-injured patient and a further informant (if at all possible, the relative who early after the injury had responsibility for the patient) (Brooks, 1984).

The third criterion of reliability was met early on by carrying out reliability studies in Germany, Portugal, and Scotland. In each case, five patients were evaluated by two examiners, and discrepancies between the results were identified. The discrepant items were then removed.

Structure of the Chart

The chart is divided into two main sections as follows: (a) initial information; and (b) follow-up, dealing with Impairments, Disabilities, and Handicaps (a World Health Organization [WHO] classification). Within each of these two areas, there are detailed subdivisions as follows.

Initial Information. Normally this information should be completed during the period when the patient is first in hospital, but many patients are evaluated much later than this. Then the information in this section may need to be completed by perusal of the patient's early clinical records.

This part of the examination begins with a preliminary interview with the patient and accompanying person (seen separately). It is designed to allow them to tell their own story, so that the examiner can begin to construct a history. The examiner is then guided by the chart to identify important details of the pretraumatic situation, such as work level, occupational history, and any previous problems in a variety of areas (medical, psychological/psychiatric, social, family, occupational, etc.). Also, this part of the chart includes a brief examination of the patient's pretraumatic personality, activities, and achievements (at work, in leisure, trade union, other activities), because these can be a very important basis for rehabilitation. The type of accident is noted (road traffic, assault, etc.), as well as whether others (whether known to the patient or not) were injured or killed in the accident.

A detailed examination of severity of injury is made, beginning with a scoring on the Glasgow Coma Score (GCS; worst score on the first day). By accepting that in patients seen late after injury, access to such information may be very difficult; and in those who were sedated, the score cannot be interpreted. Bearing this in mind, the examiner is also instructed to score the patient on the duration of posttraumatic amnesia (PTA), both in terms of actual days of PTA and broad categories of PTA. A detailed assessment is made of the nature, locations, distributions, and so on, of brain damage and damage to the skull. The chart is intended to be generic in that any professional should be able to complete it. However, this part of the chart does require some specialist knowledge, and it may be that this (and only this) part of the chart will need the assistance of a physician skilled in the evaluation of head-injured patients.

Follow-up. Following the examination of the initial state, the next part of the chart is the follow-up, which can be carried out at various stages after acute management. This part of the chart is organized under the World Health Organization (WHO) classification of Impairments, Disabilities, and Handicaps. Within each of these areas, the chart identifies the most likely sequelae of TBI. In various places in the chart, the examiner is instructed to identify management and treatment strategies.

Impairments and Disabilities

This part of the chart begins with an explicit assessment of the patient's current medical state, including current complications in a variety of relevant areas (neurological, respiratory, gastrointestinal, urinary, and dermatological). The examiner is then prompted to identify any current treatment that the patient has, including medication and clinical management, and the examiner is asked to identify a case manager. Many patients do not have a case manager, therefore items such as this fulfill a didactic as well as a clinical role.

Following the assessment of the current medical situation, the chart proceeds to assess impairments and disabilities. These are organized under the broad headings of Physical State, Intellectual State, and Affective and Behavioral State.

Physical State. Here the examiner's assessment is based on the patient's presentation during the examination (does the patient report, or are there signs of, motor disturbances, sensory disturbances, or specific syndromes such as Parkinsonism, etc.). The views of the relative are then sought out, and the examiner is cautioned to base his or her assessment on the presentation of the patient during the examination and on the information supplied by the accompanying person. If these do not correspond, the examiner is instructed to base his or her assessment on the responses and behavior of the patient, and is urged to use clinical judgment.

Intellectual State. This is subdivided into a number of areas including (a) arousal and vigilance, (b) slowness, (c) attention and concentration, (d) language and oral communication, (e) memory, (f) perception and construction, and (g) logical reasoning. Within each of these areas, the examiner is instructed to ask a small number of key questions. He or she is also given a brief cognitive screen to carry out, which requires the patient to perform the following: (a) read a short passage, (b) write a sentence, (c) perform simple calculation, (d) perform simple reasoning test, and (e) perform two simple learning and memory tests. The specific tests include word fluency (naming animals in 60 seconds), learning 10 words over three trials, "serial 7s," and a simple visual memory test.

Affective and Behavioral State (see Appendix 1). Affective and behavioral state is assessed by having the examiner identify some of the most common changes (Prigatano, 1987; Truelle & Robert-Pariset, 1990) in these areas. Also, the examiner is instructed to have the patient and informant separately rate their levels of stress or subjective burden (Brooks & McKinley, 1983). The areas include behavioral disturbance (irritability, aggression, inappropriate or embarrassing behavior, impaired social behavior), mood, emotion, and feeling (depression, rapid mood swings, anxiety, fear, suspiciousness, etc.). For each of these areas, the patient is examined separately, and then the informant is asked about the presence of changes in any of the appropriate areas.

Disability and Handicap (see Appendix 2). The next section is entitled Disability and Handicap. It is designed to identify the main disabilities and their handicapping consequences, ranging from the most simple disturbances of activities of daily living, to high-level disabilities concerning community reintegration (planning a week, dealing with one's own finances, etc.).

This section begins with simple activities of daily life, starting with the most primitive (swallowing, chewing, grasping, etc.) and moving up to the most complex (mobility in the home and outside the home, shopping, writing a letter, own financial management, etc.). The chart then moves to the area of the family, relatives, and the living situation, recognizing that all too often the family is left alone to cope with the disabled patient after he or she leaves the rehabilitation unit. Therefore, the examiner is instructed to identify whether there have been any significant changes in family roles (Lezak, 1986), whether the current accommodation is appropriate, and whether changes would need to be made. The examiner is also instructed to identify whether there have been additional problems in the family (behavior problems in children, etc.), and whether there is a need for respite admissions for the patient to reduce the burden on the family. This part of the chart also examines the current statutory and voluntary resources, looking particularly at whether anyone has been appointed to coordinate further input, and whether the patient is benefiting from continuing rehabilitation or attendance at day centers. Educational and vocational aspects are addressed by identifying whether the patient's learning or work skills have been assessed, and whether there is a program under way dealing with community reentry (social skills, vocational skills, etc.). Finally, this section deals with litigation and financial aspects, looking at the current financial situation of the family, whether they are receiving social allowances, and whether there is a claim for compensation.

VALIDATION STUDY

Following the institution of the initial database of 412 patients (in January 1993, 495 patients), a detailed validation study was carried out during the period of July 1990–April 1991. This involved data on patients from eight European countries (France, United Kingdom, Spain, Italy, Denmark, Belgium, Germany, The Netherlands), together with Canada. Of the 412 cases, most were male (75%), and as might be expected most were rather young, with a mean age of 26 and 62% between the ages of 16 and 30. Most (63%) were single, and most (83%) had suffered the injury in a traffic accident. Severity of injury was assessed in the validation study using duration of PTA (there were large numbers of cases with missing data on the GCS), with 13% having a PTA under 8 days, 21% between 8 and 28 days, and the remainder having PTAs longer than this, showing that this was a very severely injured group. In terms of the Glasgow Outcome Scale (GOS; Jennett, Snoek, Bond, & Brooks, 1981), 26% had good recovery, 35% had moderate disability, 34% had severe disability, and 3% recorded being in a persistent vegetative state. The latter cases were excluded from further analysis.

In terms of simple aspects of physical outcome, 11% of patients were reported as having epilepsy, 29% as having a right or left hemiparesis, and 32% as having at least some disturbance of visual or auditory function.

As far as the intellectual situation was concerned, the most common disturbance was mental slowness. Sixty-four percent reported having mental slowness problems, and at least 50% reported having (a) mental fatigue, (b) difficulty in following a conversation, (c) disturbances of attention and memory, and (d) poor word fluency.

Behavioral disturbances were addressed in a number of ways in the validation study. The most fruitful was to carry out a principal components analysis to identify clusters of items. This produced a number of different groups, including items indicating (a) anger (aggressiveness, bad temper, hostility, etc.), (b) excessive behavior (agitation, talkativeness), (c) avolitional state (withdrawn, etc.), or (d) affective change (depression, anxiety). Of these four areas, the more salient problems were affective, followed very closely by anger and avolitional changes. As an additional check on validity, the relationship between these aspects of disability and handicap, and severity of injury, were examined. Factor scores were created for the four areas, and one-way analysis of variance (ANOVA) was carried out to assess the difference in mean levels of each of the factors as a function of three levels of PTA (1 week or less, 8–28 days, over 28 days). In each case, the F ratio was highly significant, and Scheffe tests showed that the significant difference arose largely from the disproportionate deficits in the most severely injured patients.

Finally, the relationship between measures of disability and the global assessment of outcome (GOS) were examined. The results showed very clearly that, with increasing levels of disability, the patients were increasingly likely to be in the more severe outcome categories. This can be illustrated by the relationship between advanced aspects of activities of daily living and the GOS. These aspects (community reentry) were assessed by combining different items to form one scale, which was scaled to have a minimum score of 0 and a maximum score of 10. When the GOS was divided into six levels of conscious survival (upper and lower levels of good recovery, upper and lower levels of moderate disability, and upper and lower levels of severe disability), there was a stepwise relationship. The mean score in Activity Daily Living (ADL) of the most severely injured patients was 1.2, and the scores of the remaining groups in order of decreasing disability on the GOS were 1.8, 1.0, 3.9, 5.4, and 9.8.

DISCUSSION

By its very nature, an evaluation chart such as the one described here imposes restrictions on an examiner, and some examiners may wish to use their own form. Of course there is nothing to stop any examiner from using his or her own scheme in addition to the one proposed in the chart. However, there are many potential advantages to using the chart, most particularly that it is reliable and valid, and is designed to be completed by any professional who works with head injury. There is only one area dealing with medical matters that will need perusal of the case sheet and the assistance of a physician, but it must be a physician skilled in the assessment of TBI.

Although the chart has demonstrated satisfactory reliability and validity, it is still under further development. The current database (495 patients) has been derived from the version of the chart reported in this chapter, but already a further version is being developed that will have a number of changes. It will be shorter: Items with high numbers of missing values or low frequency of endorsement are removed. A user's manual is being developed to supply specific operational definitions for the presence and severity of particular problems, and the layout is to be changed to make it as easy as possible to administer.

Work on the current chart has identified a number of areas that need further development. The chart is readily used by specialists in TBI, but few nonspecialists use it currently, although one aim of the initial research contract was to develop a procedure that could be used by nonspecialists. The latter have not used it because it is simply too long for their needs. Therefore, the intention now is to develop a further "mini" chart in which the main problems contributing to outcome are outlined—a chart that the nonspecialist can complete in a very short time (chart having perhaps only 20 items). Furthermore, it is obvious that the chart is not totally appropriate for children. It does not allow a detailed examination of the family and educational situation, and therefore we are keen to develop a chart aimed specifically at the head-injured child. A further area of development concerns emotional and behavioral symptomatology. Certainly the chart contains a substantial amount of information here, but it is not in any particular taxonomic scheme. Therefore, we plan to develop a chart based on the *DSM-III-R* to allow formal diagnoses of mental disorder to be made. Clearly this will require specialist examination by a clinical psychologist or psychiatrist. These developments form the basis of further research proposals that are being submitted to the European Community.

ACKNOWLEDGMENTS

The work of achieving the final document is supported by a grant from the Directorate of Scientific Affairs of the Commission of the European Communities, and coordinated by the European Brain Injury Society (EBIS). The following experts were most particularly involved in the initial development: Andrews (UK), Attal (F), de Barsy (B), Berrol (US), Betts (IRE), Bori (SP), Boucand (F), Bricolo (I), Brooks (UK), Bryden (UK), Castro-Caldas (P), Chadan (F), Chevrillon (F), Chiron (F), Danze (F), Dartiques (F), Dessertine (F), Drouin (CAN), Eames (UK), Eyssette (F), Fugelmeyer (SW), Gerhard (GER), Grondard (F), Guerreiro (P), Hall (UK), Hamonet (F), Held (F), Janzik (GER), Jennett (UK), Joseph (F), de Labarthe (F), Laloua (F), Lay (B), Leclercq (B), McKinlay (UK), McLellen (UK), Mathe (F), Mazaux (F), Mondain-Monval (F), Morris (UK), Nadeau (F), Potagas (GR), Remy-Neris (F), Richer (F), Schmieder (GER), Talbott (UK), Thomsen (DK), Truelle (F), Vanier (CAN), and Van Zomeren (HOL).

(Excerpts of the evaluation chart)

APPENDIX 1
AFFECTIVE AND BEHAVIORAL STATE

This section should be completed at 3 months or later after injury. The questions are designed to identify some of the most common emotional/ behavioral changes, and levels of stress in the patient, and family.

Problems are only scored as present if they have appeared since the injury. Start with a general discussion of positive behaviors and work toward identifying negative behaviors.

Base your assessment both on your direct examination and on the informant's opinion on the patient's behavior during the 3 months up to the examination (excluding the patient's opinion here).

Exceptions are indicated for specific items. Otherwise, code as follows:

0 = None
1 = Mild/Moderate : reported by the informant
2 = Severe : observed by the examiner

RECORD 5

129	Loss of emotional self-control Is he/she verbally aggressive or showing anger over trivial annoyances or without reason failing to control his temper when something upsets him?		_	01
130	Mental excitement; talkativeness Does he/she talk rapidly and excessively without making much sense?		_	02
131	Lack of personal hygiene Is he/she dirty, ill-groomed, careless of dress or personal cleanliness?		_	03

132   Avolitional, aspontaneous
        Does he/she lack initiative or motivation?
        For example, does he/she stand or sit for
        long periods without doing anything? |__| 04

133   Emotional withdrawal
        Does he/she show diminished emotion?
        Is he/she isolate him/herself?
        Is he/she retiring within him/herself, becoming
        withdrawn, avoiding relations with others? |__| 05
            Score if any of these is present.

134   Depression
        Does he/she express sadness, gloominess,
        pessimistic ideas, feelings of hopelessness
        or total incapacity? |__| 06

135   Anxiety
        Does he/she show anxiety or overconcern? |__| 07

APPENDIX 2
HANDICAP

ATTENTION! This section should be completed when planning discharge from hospital/rehabilitation center or at a later date. The form is designed to help the interviewer identify the services that will be needed in the community. It also suggests ideas for using existing resources in flexible and imaginative ways. The assessment should be based on both data from the examination and the informant's opinion considering the 3 last months. If these do not correspond, the interviewer must exercise clinical judgment in answering the questions and selecting a course of action.

Exceptions are indicated for specific items. Otherwise, code as follows:

    0 = Normal/independent (as before the accident)
    1 = Independent but less possibilities (e.g. slowness or
        need for technical help)
    2 = Partly independent (needs human help or stimulation)
    3 = Severe dependence (most of the time)

2.5.1   *ACTIVITIES OF DAILY LIFE*   RECORD 6
        Elementary activities of daily life
137   Eating, drinking |__| 01
138   Sphincter control |__| 02
139   Toileting |__| 03
140   Dressing |__| 04

141	Transfer (getting up, going to bed, going from the bed to the arm chair)	|__| 05
142	Mobility in the home	|__| 06
143	Mobility outside the home	|__| 07
	Complex activities of daily life	
144	Going out shopping	|__| 08
145	Using public transportation	|__| 09
146	Driving a car	|__| 10
147	Writing a letter	|__| 11
148	Own financial management and administrative tasks	|__| 12
149	Keeping the house	|__| 13

Copyright Truelle & Brooks (1991).

REFERENCES

Brooks, D. N. (1984). *Closed head injury: Psychological, social and family consequences.* New York: Oxford University Press.

Brooks, D. N. (1991). Editorial. The effectiveness of post-acute rehabilitation. *Brain Injury, 5*(2), 103–109.

Brooks, D. N., & McKinlay, W. W. (1983). Personality and behavioural change after severe blunt head injury: A relative's view. *Journal of Neurology, Neurosurgery and Psychiatry, 46*, 336–344.

Lezak, M. D. (1986). Psychological implications of traumatic brain damage for the patient's family. *Rehabilitation Psychology, 31*, 241–250.

Prigatano, G. P. (1987). Psychiatric aspects of head injury: Problem areas and suggested guidelines of research. In H. S. Levin (Ed.), *Neurobehavioral recovery from head injury* (pp. 215–231). New York: Oxford University Press.

Truelle, J-L. (1988). L'Evaluation des Traumatises Craniens [The Evaluation of Head Injured]. In Proceedings of the 3rd European Conference on Traumatic Brain Injury. *Readaptation, 355*, 7–17.

Truelle, J-L., & Brooks, D. N. (1991). Traumatic brain injured people: A European evaluation chart. In J. Pelissier, M. Baral, & J. M. Mazau (Eds.), *Traumatisme cranien grave et Medecine de reeducation* (Vol. 19, pp. 287–295). Paris: Masson Publishers.

Truelle, J-L., Joseph, P. A., Brooks, D. N., & McKinlay, W. W. (1990). European initiative to develop services for the rehabilitation of brain injured patients. *Brain Injury, 4*(3), 305–306.

Truelle, J-L., & Robert-Pariset, A. (1990). A Questionnaire assessment of neurobehavioral problems: European head injury evaluation chart. In R. Wood (Ed.), *Neurobehavioral sequelae of traumatic brain injury* (pp. 69–88). Hillsdale, NJ: Lawrence Erlbaum Associates.

CHAPTER TWENTY

Visions for Rehabilitation

Anne-Lise Christensen

ABSTRACT

Visions and plans for neuropsychological rehabilitation were developed initially on the basis of experiences in neurology and neurosurgery and in psychiatry. However, the most important experiences stem from work in an intensive outpatient program affiliated with the Psychology Department at the University of Copenhagen. Areas of concern for further development in neuropsychological rehabilitation are: (a) the concept of brain injury and its sequelae, (b) the methods selected for treatment, (c) professional areas necessary to provide the most effective treatment, (d) the initiation and duration of treatment, (e) the plan for effective rehabilitation, and (f) the outcome hoped or expected given the optimal conditions for treatment.

Until the last 20–25 years, brain injury and its sequelae have been in the hands of the medical profession. Damages to the brain have been treated neuromedically and neurosurgically with increasing success, increasing the survival rate after brain injury. The prospects for survivors have been discouraging largely due to early neurophysiology, where, in particular, Nobel Prize winner Cajal (1928) stated that dead brain cells do not regenerate. The subsequent negative conclusion that rehabilitation of an injured brain is impossible has had a very lasting, pernicious influence. Goldstein's (1973) important contributions to the early understanding of the mental sequelae was also influenced by this notion. It was his view that the most effective help the brain-injured individual could get was a restriction of the surroundings to match the diminished potentialities resulting from the decline from the abstract to the concrete attitude.

However, the growing research in the neurosciences has provided a new outlook on brain injury, where the importance is stressed of "the contextual situation" in which the injury takes place. The notion of context presented by Stein (1988) and the complexity of interrelated variables have changed the concept of brain injury from a static event into a dynamic process, where plasticity of the brain has become a key concept.

The development in neurosciences has yielded results and ideas that are, to a great extent, in correspondence with those stemming from the work of A. R. Luria. His principles of functional systems, which are social in origin, mediated in structure, and changeable through development, opened new ways to consider the cerebral organization of the higher psychological processes. Lashley's principles of mass action and equipotentiality were no longer satisfactory as models of brain organization. It was stated that symptoms must be analyzed and "qualified"—there is no one-to-one relationship with specific points in the brain. Luria's development of a neuropsychological instrument to qualify the symptoms brought brain-injury rehabilitation into the hands of neuropsychologists. The qualification of symptoms had further implications for the understanding of the sequelae of brain injury, and created possibilities for a more comprehensive planning of the rehabilitation.

From this short description of background data, it can be concluded that treatment of brain injury in its first stages is a task for the medical profession, and subsequently a task for neuropsychologists. The brain is an organ in the body, but it is also the seat of the higher cortical processes and the human mind. The injured brain as an organ needs medical care, but sequelae of the injury require neuropsychological rehabilitation. Given the newest insight provided by the neurosciences, and by the neuropsychological concept of *functional systems,* the prospects for recovery from brain injury need no longer be as gloomy as they formerly have been.

The methods selected for treatment need to rest on a thorough qualification of the symptoms, both psychological and physical. Luria's Neuropsychological Investigation (Christensen, 1975) proved to serve the purpose regarding the psychological symptoms. At the Center for Rehabilitation of Brain Injury in Copenhagen, it is the analysis of symptoms into syndromes that has made it possible to build the structure of the Center's cognitive training program. The investigation enables differentiation between preserved and disturbed functions through the clusters that the functional systems form. The compensatory mechanisms that the patients have developed in their attempt to overcome their disturbances can be illuminated and discussed with the patients against the background of this investigation. The inquiries, feedback, and explanations from this method are important tools in making a patient aware of his or her situation and as a consequence motivated for training. The exploration of conditions under which a task can be solved by the patient creates a special mutual acceptance between patient and therapist that can make it possible for a patient to abandon an evasive attitude and work with problems in a new way. Knowledge regarding preserved functions and primary versus second-ary disturbances is incorporated into the individual cognitive tasks, but it can also be applied in the physical and social training.

The physical training can be more effective if the physiotherapist is properly informed about the patient's pattern of neuropsychological functioning. A thorough description of the practice of physiotherapists in the Center's program is given in chapter 10.

Another aspect of the cognitive training method of an additional character that has been found of great importance is the introduction of educational principles. In some ways, the Center's location at a university has made this approach natural, but it has become clear that much of the work in cognitive training can be improved by a more comprehensive use of educational methods. A consequence is to consider the patient as a student taking a course. Ben-Yishay and Diller (1981) were the first to practice this: The patients in their program are called *trainees*.

Luria's Neuropsychological Investigation does not directly focus on emotional and social functioning. Questions in these areas are asked during the preliminary conversation with the patient. The syndrome analysis can provide some information within these areas, which can be included in the planning of the program. These areas are of great importance. This is most clearly evidenced in American neuropsy-chological training in the programs of Ben-Yishay and Diller (1981) and with special refinement in the Prigatano et al. (1986) program. However, it seems that further emphasis on the understanding of the emotional reactions attached to the cognitive syndromes might improve rehabilitation. Numerous brain-injured patients have de-scribed their very early experiences as damaging to their confidence in therapy and future recovery. Lack of abilities that were part of the individual's self-image is most often projected to the surroundings, such as in the case of an impressive aphasic patient who believed that he or she had been transferred to another country. The experiences of catastrophic anxiety described by Goldstein (1973) are another reaction. If after brain injury the first contact with relatives and therapists rested on more understanding and knowledge, it seems that much fear could be avoided. Thus, before deciding on specific methods within the training areas (i.e., the cognitive, physical, emotional, and social), more basic and individualized knowledge is needed to formulate an overall plan.

It is now evident that training programs need to be tailored to the individual. However, the individual also needs training to regain his or her social skills, and for this purpose group training in various kinds of groups seems to be the most appropriate. This approach has inherent possibilities to widen the world of the brain-injured person when employed by knowledgeable, well-trained, and experienced therapists. The goal must be to promote awareness and to shake egocentricity, concreteness, and the field dependence so well described by Goldstein. If these traits are not understood in their origin and nature, they can make life difficult for the relatives of the brain-injured person, and often can lead to the most unfortunate belief that life after injury will never be the same.

Group situations can lead to gaining an increasingly realistic view of the actual situation after brain injury. In the world outside the rehabilitation program, the brain-injured person may experience con-fused reactions (e.g., relatives and friends can respond to unsuitable or uncharacteristic behavior without apparently noticing or even sometimes with approval or amusement, and most often to concealing their own embarrassment or from fear of hurting the brain-injured person's feelings).

Individual or group training are the basic formats for the neuro-psychological rehabilitation. The areas are (a) cognitive, (b) physical, (c) emotional, and (d) social re-adaptation. The content has to be arranged pedagogically in such a way that preserved functions can form the building blocks in the reorganization of abilities. New information has to be looked for regarding the right time for the right procedure. It has been advocated that training directed toward the defect may be the right procedure in the very early stages to mobilize the residuals.

Professionals areas mentioned so far need to be incorporated, and more can be added. Medical staff are first on the scene to deal with the acute event, but to secure the most effective course of recovery, the psychologist, physiotherapist, and occupational therapist are thereafter necessary. Because the psychological sequelae are those that are the longest lasting, the rehabilitative task needs to be carried on by the neuropsychologist as soon as the acute care has been completed. Other professionals who may join the interdisciplinary team are (a) speech therapists, (b) special education teachers, (c) recreational therapists, and (d) vocational therapists. The multifaceted situation that real life demands is a well-coordinated team. The vision in this area is that the one who best knows the brain injured and his or her relatives should be the responsible party, delegating work to the others, but all the time keeping a close and respectful therapeutic alliance with the patient.

Initiation and duration of treatment are most important. At the first conference in Copenhagen 5 years ago, the issue was much debated whether neuropsychological rehabilitation should be initiated as soon as possible, promoting brain work and preventing immediate and accidental compensatory mechanisms that might prove destructive. The view of early rehabilitation has gained support, and seems today close to worldwide acceptance. The question of duration of treatment is still debated. Visions in this respect could be treatment provided within a time frame, with a follow-up of contact that could provide emotional stability and advice including supervision of social reorganization. The main advantage would be that the brain-injured person would not need to change allies in his or her rehabilitative efforts. An attempt according to this model has been adapted at our Center, and we believe it has strongly added to the generally good outcome that has been obtained. The fear that neuropsychologists might be overwhelmed by the brain-injured person's needs has been dissipated. The system, with its inherent security, seems to strengthen the wish of brain-injured persons to manage on their own terms.

The course of rehabilitation and how it may most efficiently be planned has been touched on already. Advanced knowledge within the various stages of the course of recovery is a must, and therefore there is a need for highly skilled, well-trained providers of treatment. Furthermore, a frame is needed within which plans can be made on individual terms binding the stages together and passing on information. A very important part of the course is the start of neuropsychological rehabilitation that needs to be performed in such a way that the alliance between the brain-injured person and the therapist is established. This is a necessity for the creation of motivation and awareness, these being essential for a successful outcome. Through the whole rehabilitation period, collaboration with the relatives on a realistic basis is critical because it will possibly correlate highly with the overall outcome.

It is my vision that brain injury in the years to come will be treated more comprehensively and more effectively. It is also my vision that the sequelae will be managed in such a way that re-adaptation to the intellectual, emotional, and social challenges of life can be obtained in many cases. The realistic view of life as a dynamic process, where changes—even dramatic ones—can occur and be overcome, should also hold true for brain injury.

This chapter has been written without hard facts or numbers. It has advocated the inclusion of humanistic principles into a formerly mainly medical area. I end with a quotation from Luria's last book (Luria, Cole, & Cole, 1979):

> Classical scholars looked at events in terms of their parts. Step by step they singled out important units and elements until they could formulate abstract general laws that were seen as the governing agents in their respective fields. As a result, living reality with its richness of detail was reduced to dry and abstract schemes. The living whole was lost which prompted Göethe to pen his well-known saying: "Grau, lieber Freund, ist jede Theorie, und grün des Lebens goldener Baum (Grey, dear friend, is every theory, evergreen is life's tree)." (p. 174)

The second type of scholar of sciences was just the opposite. These men of sciences did not follow reductionism, which was the leading philosophy of the "classics." Romantics in sciences wanted neither to split living reality into elementary components nor to compress the whole wealth of life's concrete events into dry schemes or overly abstract concepts devoid of real impressions. They thought that preserving the whole wealth of living reality was of utmost importance, and they tried to ascend to a science that would not lose this richness of living reality.

REFERENCES

Ben-Yishay, J., & Diller, L. (1981, May). *Working approaches to remediation of cognitive deficits in brain damage.* Supplement to 9th annual workshop for rehabilitation professionals, New York University, Institute of Rehabilitation Medicine, New York City, NY.

Cajal, R. Y. (1928). *Degeneration and regeneration of the central nervous system.* London: Oxford University Press.

Christensen, A.-L. (1975). *Luria's Neuropsychological Investigation. Textbook, manual and test materials* (4th ed.). Copenhagen: Munksgaard.

Goldstein, K. (1973). Biophysical theories: Effect of brain damage on personality. In T. Millon (Ed.), *Theories of psychopathology and personality* (2nd ed., pp. 54–62). Philadelphia: Saunders.

Luria, A. R., Cole, M., & Cole, S. (1979). *The making of mind.* Cambridge, MA: Harvard University Press.

Prigatano, G. P., Fordyce, D. J., Zeiner, H. K., Roueche, J. R., Pepping, M., & Wood, B. C. (1986). *Neuropsychological rehabilitation after brain injury.* Baltimore: Johns Hopkins University Press.

Stein, D. G. (1988). Contextual factors in recovery from brain damage. In A.-L. Christensen & B. P. Uzzell (Eds.), *Neuropsychological rehabilitation: Current knowledge and future directions* (pp. 1–18). Boston: Kluwer.

CHAPTER TWENTY-ONE

Visions for International Support Organizations

George A. Zitnay

ABSTRACT

This chapter provides a historical overview of the development of American and international disability advocacy groups, as well as discussing the National Head Injury Foundation (NHIF). It presents a model for a new International Brain Injury Association, and discusses its purposes and functions. In addition, new brain-injury research ideas are presented.

Before I can talk to the future of international support organizations for people with disability, it is necessary to recount a short history of this major movement.

In the United States, one of the first voluntary support organizations was the Association for Retarded Children (ARC). Founded over 41 years ago by parents of children with mental retardation because of their frustration in getting needed services, this voluntary, not-for-profit organization, composed of affiliate chapters across the United States, has grown into one of the most effective advocacy and lobbying organizations working on behalf of persons with mental handicaps. Through the efforts of the ARC, legislation providing for construction of community facilities was enacted by the U.S. Congress in 1963. The most sweeping legislative accomplishment was the passage of the Education for All Handicapped Children's Act in 1975, which provided for free public education of all children under 21 years of age with disabilities. The Developmental Disabilities Assistance and Bill of Rights Act of 1975 established legal rights for all persons with mental handicaps and created a federally supported protection and advocacy system. Most recently, the Americans with Disability Act, enacted into law in 1990, established the right of all people with disability to have access to public buildings and forbids discrimination in housing and employment. How did this voluntary organization, founded by parents, have such success? Simply put, they have used public awareness, especially the media, to get their message out to the public. It has worked (West, 1991).

One of the first international support organizations, the International League of Societies for the Mentally Handicapped, was founded in 1969. It brings together parent-sponsored associations from all over the world. More than 100 member societies participate with the League. These societies all have in common the desire to get "help" for their children with disabilities. All of these voluntary support associations work to get (a) educational services, (b) vocational services, (c) medical services, (d) residential services, (e) guardianship services, and so on.

To secure them, they have learned that parents or concerned friends must (a) band together with other parents; (b) keep the pressure on public officials and legislators; and (c) enlist the aid of professionals in the field, the support of civic organizations, and the support of the corporate and business world if they are to succeed. It is this basic similarity of their needs and concerns that has provided the strong impetus for parent organizations; it has made them the most visible and potent consumer groups in the field of human services throughout the world, including the former Soviet Union states. The International League of Societies for the Mentally Handicapped is an action-oriented organization that serves as an exchange of information and a clearinghouse for model service and legislation. This service orientation distinguishes the League from "professional" organizations. The most notable of its accomplishments was the *Declaration of Rights of Mentally Retarded Persons*, adopted by the United Nations (UN) in the latter part of 1976 (Dybwad, 1990).

I want to talk briefly about one other movement that has impacted all voluntary associations around the world. This movement, which was started in Denmark in the late 1960s by Niels Bank-Mikkelsen and Karl Grunvald in Sweden, has had a profound impact on how services should be delivered and on how people with disability are involved in designing and managing the services. This is the normalization principle that has been accepted worldwide as a guideline to the provision of services for people with disability. Simply stated, normalization aims to provide people with disabilities with patterns and conditions of everyday life that are as close as possible to the norms and patterns of the society or culture of which they are a part. In the field of brain injury, this principle is emerging as a major factor in determining the role of persons with brain injury, in their rehabilitation, and in their living arrangements and vocational choices.

I turn now to the development of the National Head Injury Foundation (NHIF) in the United States. As is well known, NHIF was founded on April 20, 1980, when 13 people (e.g., doctors, psychologists, and parents of children with head injury) gathered at the home of Marilyn Price Spivak. Mrs. Spivak, the founder of NHIF, started the organization out of the same frustration and concern for the lack of services for people with head injuries, as did the parents of persons with mental retardation some 41 years earlier. However, much had changed in terms of social acceptance and public policy. NHIF was established for the same purposes as well: (a) to make the public aware of head injury, (b) to provide a clearinghouse for information, (c) to develop support groups for families, and (d) to establish rehabilitation services and programs (Kreutzer & Wehman, 1990).

Today, 12 years later, NHIF has grown to an association of over 25,000 members, chapters or affiliated groups in every state, and a multimillion dollar budget. A Provider of Rehabilitation Services Council, a Professional Council, a Survivors Council, and a Family Council support the activities of NHIF and represent the various constituencies of the association.

The primary mission of NHIF continues to be to improve the quality of life for persons with head injury and their families, and to promote prevention. However, NHIF has become more sophisticated with time. With the move to Washington, DC, it has developed a strong public policy program, an effective lobbying effort using professionals, and a strong public awareness and public education program. This has resulted in increased federal funding, passage of safety and prevention legislation, and the creation of community-based, regional brain injury centers.

In addition, NHIF has worked to involve people with head injury in all aspects of the association, including membership on the board of directors and on all standing committees. NHIF has convened international groups, has brought international experts to speak at the NHIF National Symposium, and has hosted international guests. In addition, NHIF has participated in conferences throughout Europe. NHIF has worked with Dr. Robert Voogt in sponsoring his International Brain Injury Symposium held in New Orleans, which has brought together experts in brain injury from throughout the world to exchange information on services and research.

To strengthen the work of NHIF, the association is working in close association and collaboration with other professional organizations such as the Neurotrauma Society, the Academy of Rehabilitation Medicine, the Congress of Rehabilitation Medicine, the Neurosurgeon Association, the National Coalition for Research in Neurological Disorders, and the National Institutes of Health. NHIF has served as a model for the development of similar support associations throughout the world.

As a voluntary support organization that conducts professional seminars, symposia, and other forms of education, NHIF has learned first and foremost that it must: (a) keep the pressure on public officials and legislative bodies; (b) enlist the support of professionals and providers of service; and (c) use the media, especially television, for public awareness and acceptance of head injury as an important cause that needs to be supported by the public.

What about the future? What is the vision? As the world becomes more and more a "global village," I see the need for the creation of a strong international support organization composed of all voluntary support organizations for persons with brain injury and their families. The major function of this new International Brain Injury Association would be to:

- serve as a clearinghouse for information;
- serve as an international exchange of information and people;
- serve to stimulate world support through media and multinational corporations;
- serve to create an international "Be Head Smart" prevention campaign;
- lobby for safe cars, gun control, helmet use, seat belt use, etc.;
- promote international laws on safety through the UN;
- conduct family support and empowerment conferences;
- advocate for rights of all people with TBI;
- educate the public about TBI as the number one killer of young people through multicultural educational programs;
- publish an international family support journal;
- work with the governing bodies of member nations to develop community services and to support research;
- use the "Decade of the Brain" to move an international agenda on TBI forward;

- convene a world congress with delegate representatives to develop an international Bill of Rights for persons with TBI, and for international understanding and acceptance work with the UN to adopt this declaration of rights; and

- develop a forecast of how brain injury in the year 2000 might look if research and services are developed and supported.

With an International Brain Injury Association working with the World Health Organization (WHO), the UN, the scientific community, and national governments, the following list of scientific achievements and medical breakthroughs may be possible by the year 2000. This is not an exhaustive list, but it can serve as a stimulus for research, governmental action, and a vision for the future.

1. Direct sensory prostheses will increase sensory input and stimulus ranges, and will enhance memory performance of persons with brain injury.
2. Neuron regeneration in the brain and direct repairs for some types of damage to the brain may provide a cure for some individuals with brain injury.
3. Drugs will be used to raise intelligence artificially.
4. Drugs such as the second or third generation of Freedox will prevent continuing brain damage after initial trauma.
5. Computer-assisted instruction specifically designed for persons with brain injury will be available in the home. Instruction will be provided for both academic and vocational areas.
6. Extensive reliance on technical advances may result in the isolation of persons with brain injury. That is, devices that allow them to stay at home could actually work against their integration.
7. Interactive televisions in the home will allow individuals to receive on-the-job training, physical therapy, instructions, and medical and legal consultation.
8. Miniature communication devices will enable persons with brain injury to remain in constant contact with a specific person or location. The devices will include emergency numbers and signals to aid in personal navigation.
9. Computers will have become so "simplified" in terms of their operation that persons with cognitive impairment will be able to carry out complex intellectual tasks without having the usual necessary background knowledge.

10. "Virtual Reality," the new enhanced interactive computer program, may make all tasks possible for people with brain injury.
11. Traumatic brain injury becomes the largest disability group due to increased automotive accidents, violence, and assaults.

Why is an international support organization needed?

To achieve this impressive list of goals on a global basis, we must come together, unite, and raise the level of public awareness about TBI. This can best be done by creating an international support association that provides the leadership required to get the job done. Is an international support organization needed? In response to this question, I offer the following.

First, the most important reason is the increasing number of persons sustaining a traumatic head injury in the United States as well as around the world. For example, in the United States, a head injury occurs every 15 seconds, resulting in 2 million a year. In the Bronx, New York area, the incident rate is 407 per 100,000. The annual costs exceed $25 billion. Second, the proliferation of motor vehicle use around the world is leading to increased numbers of accidents, resulting in higher incidence rates of head injury. Third, with violence against persons on the increase, there is a concomitant increase in head injury. Fourth, there are no international public policies or support services. Fifth, there is the need for multicultural public education programs. Sixth, there is a need for multicultural prevention programs. Seventh, through collaboration and by banding together, there is strength.

In conclusion, let me say that I applaud the effort started in Copenhagen.[1]

REFERENCES

Dybwad, R. F. (1990). *Perspectives on a parent movement*. Brookline, MA: Brookline Books.
Kreutzer, J. S., & Wehman, P. (1990). *Integration following traumatic brain injury*. Baltimore: Paul H. Brooks.
West, J. (1991). *Americans with Disability Act—From policy to practice*. New York: Milbank Memorial Fund.

---

[1]The International Brain Injury Association (IBIA) was established in 1993.

CHAPTER TWENTY-TWO

Panel Discussion

Moderator:
Barbara P. Uzzell

Panel Members:
Leonard Diller, Aase Engberg, Ritva Laaksonen,
José Leòn-Carrion, Claudio Perino, George P. Prigatano,
Jean-Luc Truelle, Tom W. Teasdale, Barbara Wilson

Discussants from the Audience:
Anne-Lise Christensen, Nathan Cope,
Hallgrim Kløve, Donald Stein

B. P. Uzzell

Many questions need to be addressed in the field of rehabilitation. But none is as urgent as the one I posed to members of the panel and audience. This question is pervasive, and answers to it also provide answers to other questions.

Throughout history, there have been, and will continue to be, individuals who sustain brain injuries. In the past two decades, more of these individuals than ever are surviving. Many of them are young people whose life expectancy may be a further 50 or 60 years. What can be done for them? Neuropsychological rehabilitation is a human, personal activity both for individuals needing services and therapists providing them. It is costly both in terms of requiring therapists to be well educated and experienced, and in the operation of centers in many different areas of the world. Some individuals do not believe it produces satisfactory results. Others laud its benefits. It has developed a core of knowledge over the years, as is evident by the chapters in this book.

The question I want to pose is: Is rehabilitation worthwhile and appropriate for all brain-injured persons? The latter part of the question has ethical and economic overtones, which most individuals associated with neuropsychological rehabilitation have to consider at one time or another. Let me begin the discussion of this question, which penetrates every aspect of rehabilitation.

Claudio Perino

My first answer is yes, but this may be an emotional response that needs to be divided into subsets. From a clinical point of view, rehabilitation may or may not be effective, depending on different variables that can be controlled. Rehabilitation may also be unethical in some cases where general neurorehabilitation techniques to some extent may be harmful.

Regarding economics in health care, it is very different in Europe, in comparison with what happens in the United States. The medical health systems are profoundly different. Socialized medicine is common in Europe. The economic burdens of rehabilitation are mainly on public finances, and in some cases on private or personal resources of the client. Generally speaking, insurance companies do not yet pay for rehabilitation. There is no competition in treating patients. No widespread organization makes a profit from rehabilitation in Europe.

However, there are critical questions for the patient and family in rehabilitation. First, how much awareness can we promote without taking away any hope? Second, is the conflict brought about by the participation of the family in the rehabilitation process? What is best for the injured person may not be the best for the spouse or the family, or vice versa. Should the patient and the family each have an advocate, or should the interests be taken care of by the same person?

Aase Engberg

I am here on behalf of Hovedcirklen, the Danish Head Injury Foundation, which is an association and support group for people with severe head injuries. I am also a family member and a medical doctor.

Rehabilitation is worthwhile. When such an overwhelming event has taken place, the family has to be able to say that every serious and qualified effort has been made to do everything to eliminate the deficits. When we look around Denmark today, physical rehabilitation is good or fairly good. When it comes to psychological deficits, this is not the case. Today, most brain-inured people do not receive a qualified assessment or treatment for their mental deficits. The task of tomorrow will be to treat these patients who today are housed in nursing homes.

José Leòn-Carrion

At our Human Cognitive Neuropsychology Laboratory of the University of Seville, we are currently setting up a rehabilitation system for traumatic brain injured (TBI) patients. Almost all of our patients present cognitive deficits and personality problems during the first year after hospital discharge.

Family structures are fairly stable in Spain. Divorce and separation rates are not very high, and marriages have been traditionally "for the rest of one's life." Family relations are very close, and offspring usually live at their parents' homes until they get married.

In our experience, the greater the socioeconomic and cultural status (SECS), the better the prognosis for the patient. In low SECS, family members have different ideas about life and death, medicine, and illness than at high SECS. Although low SECS assumes that health staff are responsible for the patient's recovery, high SECS never assume this and always try all the possible means of recovery. Even when one sees a better prognosis in the low-SECS patient, the high-SECS patient with a worse prognosis usually recovers better than the former.

Barbara Wilson

The World Health Organization (WHO) definition of *rehabilitation* is: "Rehabilitation implies the restoration of patients to the highest level of physical, psychological and social adaptation attainable. It includes all measures aimed at reducing the impact of disabling and handicapping conditions and is enabling disabled people to achieve optimum social integration" (1987, p. 1). That is the very broad definition, but if that is what we are working toward, it is unethical not to do rehabilitation. A professor of rehabilitation in Southampton says that rehabilitation is not something given to disabled people, but that they are part of the process. It is an interactive, two-way process, and there really should be a disabled person here answering the question with us. You should never say a patient is untestable or untreatable, and similarly you should not say a patient is not worthy of rehabilitation.

Jean-Luc Truelle

Several issues are raised by the overriding question of whether rehabilitation is worthwhile. The first issue is finding the appropriate neuropsychological assessments and methods for developing a scale especially adapted to measure the quality of life of both patient and family. A second issue addresses the formulation of a neuropsychological program to manage behavior and cognitive sequelae. The principal professionals in our program include a psychiatrist, a neuropsychologist, and a case manager. The case manager system has been successfully used in France due to the attention to community reentry after discharge from rehabilitation centers.

Tom W. Teasdale

In evaluating whether rehabilitation is worthwhile, one can attend to leisure activities of brain-injured patients. Based on self-report from interviews with patients, we have found leisure activities to fall into three categories: (a) no reported leisure activities, indicating a poor outcome; (b) performance of socially isolated hobbies during leisure time, indicating a moderately successful outcome; and (c) social interaction during leisure time, indicating the most desirable outcome.

George P. Prigatano

In evaluating the efficacy of rehabilitation, awareness needs to be considered. However, the question is whether awareness is psychologically motivated or a part of the neurologic insult to the brain. If it is psychologically motivated, then you have to ask the question: Do patients want to know? If they do not want to know, what are the good reasons? Are you being unethical if you force or try to force them to face something that they are not yet ready to emotionally face? It would be unethical to push awareness under those kind of circumstances. It raises the question: How much of a commitment are you willing to make to the patient? If you are simply going to force awareness and walk away from the patient, it is highly unethical behavior. But if you believe that the awareness problem has a neurological component to it, such as aphasia, would it be unethical to help the aphasic patient as much as possible with word retrieval, or repetition of words? Clearly not. Brain functioning of some patients contains lack of insight as to what is going on, and this is the central issue in helping them. It is not unethical to help a patient understand what is wrong. But you always have to ask the question: What is the goal? Awareness for what reason? The goal is a better adaptation to life.

The awareness issue is also, in my mind, highly connected to the acceptance issue. Neurologically, we make a distinction between these two words and give definitions that separate them. But in my clinical experience, as patients truly become aware they gain hope and acceptance. They then see a complex picture clear, and that is the essence of a positive approach to their therapy. Other things include: what cost issues are important, and who will do the therapy? Although some therapies cannot be done by nonprofessionally trained people, this is a highly delicate area, just as you would not want a medical student to perform neurosurgery on you. When it comes to helping you face what is wrong after brain injury, you need a highly trained person. You cannot reduce cost over this issue. It is very important to have people who are adequately trained to do the work. Perhaps this is one of the most powerful ethical issues.

Leonard Diller

I was thinking about Dr. Prigatano's distinction between psychological and neurological unawareness in relation to this question: If the person who is unaware on a neurological basis, would that person be legally competent?

George P. Prigatano

The question that Dr. Diller asked, if I understood it correctly, is: "Is the person who is not aware for neurological reasons legally competent?" It is the extent of the unawareness. They do not see aggression as inappropriate behavior. Therefore, they are perfectly justified in attacking. This is a legal, not a totally medical/scientific, issue. Awareness is truly the highest of all the cerebral functions. When it is altered, there is limited or no understanding. Rehabilitation efforts would progress easier if understood. Awareness is the most difficult problem because it goes to the heart of consciousness.

Aase Engberg

It is extremely important to have highly educated, well-trained specialists treating the brain-injured. Insight into problems of brain injury and proper methods for treatment from these specialists provide good outcome and enhance societal awareness. Without appropriate education and training of specialists, there will be a shortage, making rehabilitation outcomes dismal.

Nathan Cope

A prevalent issue in rehabilitation that raises ethical concern is the demand for the execution of the medical model for treatment versus no treatment in a random-assignment study. If failing to treat some individuals is unethical, then what alternatives do we have available to convince public policymakers that rehabilitation is worthwhile?

George P. Prigatano

The medical model study of treatment versus no treatment needs to be done. Without performing such studies, we will never earn the respect of medical specialists and never get funding for patient treatments. Because we do not feel that we have the "powerful treatment," the consequences of withholding it may not be jeopardizing patients' care.

Ritva Laaksonen

Careful consideration has to be given in designing a treatment versus no-treatment, randomized study. Many factors have to be considered: (a) ages and selections of the patients, (b) frequency of therapy, (c) location of therapy either in a center or at home, (d) training and experience of the therapist, and (e) selection of tests to measure outcomes. If the study is not carefully designed and executed, the field of rehabilitation will suffer from the consequences for many years.

Aase Engberg

The family's point of view has to be considered in execution of the treatment versus no-treatment, randomized study. No family would agree to have its relative be a member of the no-treatment group. The study that needs to be done at this time is one that compares different treatments to determine the most effective one.

Leonard Diller

Another alternative to the treatment versus no-treatment, randomized study is to have a multicenter effort where experiences from similar cases from different centers are shared. Studying the successes from different kinds of treatments would be more useful. It should be understood that, unlike other aspects of medical care, rehabilitation continuously has to prove to skeptics that it works.

Anne-Lise Christensen

My colleague, Jarl Risberg, has measured cerebral blood flow in an identical group of young TBI patients from our center. Each of these patients had a different pattern of cerebral blood flow. From this we conclude that a program must be adapted for each brain-injured person.

Hallgrim Kløve

Another point worth mentioning, when designing a study to show that rehabilitation is worthwhile, is that control of all aspects postinjury is impossible. Clinical and animal experimental evidence has shown the dependence of outcome on early management.

Tom W. Teasdale

Regardless of the scientific method chosen, critics will find flaws. For instance, if a single blind study is performed because patients know they are brain damaged, critics might say the study should have been double blinded, although this of course is impossible. If you show a 4-month program to be effective, critics will ask whether the same effect could be achieved while reducing the program to 2 months.

George P. Prigatano

Even if there are multiple problems and no one study solves all problems, studies need to be done. Otherwise, policies will be made by those outside the field.

Ritva Laaksonen

Different programs need to exist for different problems with regard to time, length of treatment, and method.

Donald Stein

Turning to another field provides an example of the question that has been raised. Regulations regarding animal research are imposed not by peers, but by people who have nothing to do with the field, because the scientific community did not regulate its own affairs. Neurorehabilitation decisions in the United States may be taken out of the hands of rehabilitation people by the American Academy of Neurology, which has the endorsement of the medical establishment.

Claudio Perino

Studying the brain is not the same as studying other bodily organs. Brain lesions cannot be matched exactly in humans, and it would be impossible to get two comparative groups for a study. The scientific community will have to acknowledge that the medical model cannot be applied. Multiple, baseline, single-case design is an alternative that is not well accepted by many who fund research.

Barbara P. Uzzell

This ethical problem may not be easily solved, and it also is present for medical professionals.

Barbara Wilson

Models have been presented where groups of patients are selected for specific neuropsychological rehabilitation programs, such as those in Phoenix, Arizona, and Copenhagen, Denmark. In Great Britain, there is an alternative model where everyone referred receives treatment. The task for the therapist is to solve the patient's problems. If problems are not solved, then the therapist has not shown imagination and creativity in addressing the problems.

Donald Stein

Before reacting to the rehabilitation methodological questions of ethical importance, one has to investigate acute-care management of patients immediately following injury. At present, a mismanagement is taking place in various areas, physiologically and pharmacologically, that is confounding outcome evaluations. The burden of outcome responsibilities should not rest with rehabilitation specialists alone. For example, the administration of large continuous doses of benzodiazoephines has neurotoxic and psychotoxic implications. Additionally, decisions for keeping severely impaired patients chemically restrained are made for economic and social reasons, not for medical ones.

Jean-Luc Truelle

With success of treatment may come additional problems, including the consequences for separation of family members. If the treatment has made the patient autonomous, allowing a wife to divorce her husband saying, "He can live alone, and I can survive myself," is this an ethical intervention?

Ritva Laaksonen

One case was a man in a wheelchair who had a large infarct in the region of the left, middle cerebral artery. Treatment was given for 4 weeks without any effect and then discontinued. The wife became angry at the discontinuation. She would have sued if there had been a law requiring treatment. What is ethical in this case? Is it to treat the patient or to follow family demands or professional judgment?

Barbara P. Uzzell

Is there any connection between the question of whether rehabilitation is worthwhile and for everyone and its cost-effectiveness?

George P. Prigatano

The issue of cost containment cannot be dealt with as long as effectiveness of therapies are not proved. The question of who can be treated cannot be solved without scientific evidence as to what treatments are effective with certain individuals.

Barbara P. Uzzell

A need exists for an international task force to develop guidelines for neuropsychological rehabilitation. The panel and audience agree that neuropsychological rehabilitation is worthwhile and should be given to those who need it, as stated in the WHO definition for rehabilitation and following ethical considerations. Furthermore, it is cost-effective for individuals and society when alternatives without it are considered.

Other factors in rehabilitation noted during the discussion include an increasing need to assist patients in becoming more aware of their circumstances without taking away hope so they can deal realistically with their individual situations and recover. To do this requires trained specialists with a high level of knowledge and experience. It also requires an interactive, two-way process between patients and specialists.

REFERENCE

World Health Organization (1987). *Optimum care of disabled people.* Report of a WHO meeting, Turku, Finland.

Postscript

Barbara P. Uzzell
Anne-Lise Christensen

A single approach for rehabilitating brain-damaged individuals has not met with success in the past, as evidenced by individuals who have been nonproductive to themselves and to societies in which they live. The complexity of the brain and any injury to it requires an integrated, multidisciplinary approach for rehabilitation and a highly qualified staff.

During the past 5 years, knowledge about brain injuries has increased, making it possible to plan and execute more effective treatments. Lack of reality awareness of the brain injured has caused an increase in group methods and psychotherapy, which have been incorporated into neuropsychological rehabilitation when required by the premorbid personality and neuropsychological characteristics of an individual. Research in neuropharmacology is underway to discover how the brain and external agents administered at an optimum time course may promote recovery and improve functioning. Understanding the pathophysiology from current and future imaging techniques is critical to this process. The severity of the injury, acute-care treatment, age at time injury, and the presence of multiple injuries are factors affecting neuropsychological rehabilitation. Computers are being utilized successfully in treatments and as orthotic devices, but we need to know more about these treatments and devices.

Brain-damaged individuals do not live in a vacuum, but in families and societies throughout the world. Many factors impinging on brain-damaged individuals need to be addressed in treatment. Rather

317

than be isolated, brain-damaged individuals need to be strong participants in the societies in which they live. This makes family-coach models as well as community-based, cognitive, and physical treatments attractive. Such techniques require clear operational definitions and careful selection of patients who will benefit from neuropsychological treatments, plus the recognition of those who will not benefit, in order to achieve return-to-lifestyle objectives and contain escalating costs. Although job coach and supportive employment may be extremely costly, they are beneficial in the long run. Certainly we can anticipate more work in this area in the future.

As the field of neuropsychological rehabilitation has progressed, more brain-damaged individuals have been able to fulfill more of their goals and aspirations, making it cost-effective. Progress in rehabilitation has been shown by increased work return and decreased government and private payer costs in Denmark, the United States, and elsewhere. Subjective evaluations of the quality of life of brain-injured survivors are correlated with vocational status. The groundwork has been laid for international communication and support during the past 5 years, and will be more visible in years to come. Government studies funded in the United States and elsewhere are directed toward (a) finding the right treatment for the right patient, (b) delivering cost-effective quality service, and (c) controlling the rising cost of health care. Governments and private funds would have borne these costs were it not for the effectiveness of neuropsychological rehabilitation.

As we enter the 1990s, we certainly know more about neuropsychological rehabilitation than we did during the 1980s. Certainly, the same treatments cannot be applied to all brain-injured individuals. Treatments are now more adaptable to the individual than ever before, through consideration of a host of factors.

Neuropsychological rehabilitation is dynamic in its nature, and will continue to improve so that today's treatments will not be those of tomorrow. The past 5 years have borne witness to the ever-evolving neuropsychological rehabilitation that has offered hope for an improved lifestyle for brain-injured persons.

Author Index

Subject Index